Laser and Light Source Treatments for the Skin

Laser and Light Source Treatments for the Skin

Editors

Mathew M Avram MD JD
Director, MGH Dermatology
Laser and Cosmetic Center
Massachusetts General Hospital
Assistant Professor of Dermatology
Faculty Director
for Procedural Dermatology
Harvard Medical School
Boston, Massachusetts, USA

Paul M Friedman MD
Director, Dermatology and Laser Surgery Center
Clinical Assistant Professor of Dermatology
University of Texas Houston Medical School
Houston, Texas, USA
Clinical Assistant Professor of Dermatology
Weill Cornell Medical College, The Methodist Hospital
New York, NY, USA

Series Editor

Marc R Avram MD
Clinical Professor of Dermatology
Department of Dermatology
Weill Cornell Medical College, New York
Presbyterian Hospital, New York, NY, USA

JAYPEE

JAYPEE BROTHERS MEDICAL PUBLISHERS (P) LTD

New Delhi • London • Philadelphia • Panama

Jaypee Brothers Medical Publishers (P) Ltd

Headquarters

Jaypee Brothers Medical Publishers (P) Ltd
4838/24, Ansari Road, Daryaganj
New Delhi 110 002, India
Phone: +91-11-43574357
Fax: +91-11-43574314
Email: jaypee@jaypeebrothers.com

Overseas Offices

J.P. Medical Ltd
83, Victoria Street, London
SW1H 0HW (UK)
Phone: +44-2031708910
Fax: +02-03-0086180
Email: info@jpmedpub.com

Jaypee-Highlights.
Medical Publishers Inc
City of Knowledge, Bld. 237
Clayton, Panama City, Panama
Phone: +1 507-301-0496
Fax: +1 507-301-0499
Email: cservice@jphmedical.com

Jaypee Medical Inc.
The Bourse
111 South Independence Mall East
Suite 835, Philadelphia, PA 19106, USA
Phone: +1 267-519-9789
Email: jpmed.us@gmail.com

Jaypee Brothers
Medical Publishers (P) Ltd
17/1-B Babar Road, Block-B
Shaymali, Mohammadpur
Dhaka-1207, Bangladesh
Mobile: +08801912003485
Email: jaypeedhaka@gmail.com

Jaypee Brothers
Medical Publishers (P) Ltd
Shorakhute, Kathmandu
Nepal
Phone: +00977-9841528578
Email: jaypee.nepal@gmail.com

Website: www.jaypeebrothers.com
Website: www.jaypeedigital.com

Inquiries for bulk sales may be solicited at: jaypee@jaypeebrothers.com

Laser and Light Source Treatments for the Skin

First Edition: 2014

ISBN: 978-93-5090-995-9

Printed at : Ajanta Offset & Packagings Ltd., New Delhi

Dedicated to

My entire family

My parents
Morrell and Maria Avram
who gave me love and
support throughout my life

My beautiful wife
Alison, and

My children
Rachel, Alexander and Noah
who inspire me everyday, and

My brothers and sister
Marc, Eric, David and Rella
I owe everything to each and
every one of you

—Mathew M Avram

My wife and soulmate
Joanna
for her love, devotion and steadfast encouragement
My life has been enriched in so many ways since meeting you

My son
Geoffrey Ray
for teaching me the truly important things in life

My parents
Irving and Diane
for teaching me the value of hard work and
for their enduring affection, and

My siblings
Robin Friedman-Musicante MD *and Edward Friedman* MD
for their inspiration and support

—Paul M Friedman

My wife
Robin, and

My two children
Robert and Jacob
for their love and support
They are an inspiration to me everyday, and

My parents
for a lifetime of love and support

—Marc R Avram

Contributors

Tina S Alster MD
Dermatology and Pediatrics
Georgetown University
Medical Center, Washington
Institute of Dermatologic
Laser Surgery
Washington DC, USA

Mathew M Avram MD JD
Director
MGH Dermatology Laser and
Cosmetic Center
Massachusetts General Hospital
Assistant Professor of Dermatology
Faculty Director for Procedural
Dermatology
Harvard Medical School
Boston, Massachusetts, USA

Marc R Avram MD
Clinical Professor of Dermatology
Department of Dermatology
Weill Cornell Medical College
New York, Presbyterian Hospital
New York, NY, USA

Eric F Bernstein MD MSE
Laser Surgery and Cosmetic
Dermatology Centers, Marlton
New Jersey, USA; University of
Pennsylvania, USA

Henry HL Chan MD Specialist in Dermatology MBBS (London) MD (London) PhD (HK) FRCP (London, Edinburgh, Glasgow) FHKCP FHKAM (Medicine)
Honorary Clinical Professor
Division of Dermatology
Department of Medicine
University of Hong Kong
Honorary Consultant
Dermatologist
Queen Mary Hospital, HKSAR
Visiting Scientist, Wellman Center
for Photomedicine, Massachusetts
General Hospital
Harvard Medical School
Boston, Massachusetts, USA

Paul M Friedman MD
Director, Dermatology and
Laser Surgery Center
Clinical Assistant Professor of
Dermatology
University of Texas Houston
Medical School
Houston, Texas, USA
Clinical Assistant Professor of
Dermatology
Weill Cornell Medical College
The Methodist Hospital
New York, NY, USA

Elizabeth R Geddes MD MS
Dermatology Resident PGY-4
University of Texas at Houston
and MD Anderson Cancer Center
Houston, Texas, USA

Mitchel P Goldman MD
Cosmetic Laser Associates of
La Jolla, Inc., La Jolla and
University of California
San Diego, California, USA

Omar A Ibrahimi MD PhD
Director
Connecticut Skin Institute
Stamford, Connecticut, USA

Tobin C Island PhD
Chief Operating Officer
TRIA Beauty, Inc
Dublin, California, USA

H Ray Jalian MD
Clinical Instructor
Division of Dermatology
UCLA Clinical Fellow
Wellman Center for Photomedicine
Boston, Massachusetts, USA

Suzanne L Kilmer MD
Laser and Skin Surgery Center of
Northern California
Sacramento, California, USA

Jennifer L MacGregor MD
Clinical Professor of Dermatology
Georgetown University Hospital
Associate
Washington Institute of
Dermatologic Laser Surgery
Washington DC, USA

Ane BM Niwa Massaki MD
Aniwa Dermatology, Private
Practice
Votuporanga-SP, Brazil
Former Fellow at Goldman,
Butterwick, Fitzpatrick,
Groff and Fabi Cosmetic Laser
Dermatology
San Diego, California, USA

Andrew A Nelson MD
Nelson Dermatology
Saint Petersburg, Florida, USA
Assistant Clinical Professor
Department of Dermatology
Tufts University School of Medicine
Boston, Massachusetts, USA

Arisa Ortiz MD
Procedural Fellow
Division of Dermatology
UC San Diego
Clinical Fellow
Dermatology Cosmetic and Laser Center
Massachusetts General Hospital
Harvard Medical School
Wellman Center for Photomedicine
San Diego, California, USA

Jennifer D Peterson MD FAAD
Board Certified Dermatologist
Dermatology and Laser Surgery Center, Fellowship-Trained Cosmetic Surgeon
Houston, Texas, USA

Parisa Ravanfar MD MBA MS
Department of Dermatology
Dartmouth-Hitchcock Medical Center
Houston, Texas, USA

Sara Risner-Rumohr MD
Houston Dermatology Associates
Houston Methodist Hospital
Houston, Texas, USA

E Victor Ross MD CDR MC USN
Dermatology Department, Naval Medical Center San Diego and Division of Dermatology
University of California
San Diego, California, USA

Iris Rubin MD
Director
Dermatologic and Vascular Laser Surgery Service
Children's National Medical Center, Washington DC, USA

Nazanin Saedi MD
Assistant Professor
Department of Dermatology and Cutaneous Biology
Thomas Jefferson University
Philadelphia, Pennsylvania, USA

Fernanda H Sakamoto MD PhD
Wellman Center for Photomedicine
Massachusetts General Hospital
Harvard Medical School
Boston, Massachusetts, USA

Joshua D Shofner MD
Department of Dermatology
Massachusetts General Hospital
Harvard Medical School
Boston, Massachusetts, USA

Kelly Stankiewicz MD FAAD
The Dermatology Institute
DuPage Medical Group
Naperville, Illinois, USA

Foreword

Laser and Light Source Treatments for the Skin represents the inaugural topic in a series dedicated to cosmetic dermatology. Twenty-first century dermatology utilizes lasers for both esthetic and medical applications. No longer is there a separation between esthetic and medical training in dermatology. Lasers are a central treatment modality to treat a wide variety of skin diseases ranging from vascular malformations to acne.

Paul M Friedman MD and Mathew M Avram MD JD have assembled an outstanding group of contributors who have created a state-of-the-art comprehensive review of lasers in the treatment of skin diseases. This textbook will be an invaluable resource for both the novice and experienced laser surgeon.

I want to thank Paul and Mathew for their unrelenting dedication to create the finest textbook in print covering the topic of lasers in dermatology.

Marc R Avram MD
Clinical Professor of Dermatology
Department of Dermatology
Weill Cornell Medical Colege, New York
Presbyterian Hospital, New York, NY, USA

Preface

Laser and Light Source Treatments for the Skin provides a comprehensive, clinically relevant survey of cutaneous laser surgery written by the top authorities within this field. Importantly, this text focuses not only on lasers but also light sources and other energy-based devices such as radiofrequency, intense pulsed light, ultrasound and cryolipolysis.

Topics range from vascular lesions to laser hair removal to noninvasive fat removal. New techniques and clinical pearls are emphasized throughout the text. Chapters have numerous charts, tables and clinical photographs to assist the reader in understanding these new techniques in a user-friendly manner. The text begins with an overview of the basic science principles behind these laser and energy-based technologies. From there, it is organized by clinical topics and includes chapters detailing treatments for: acne, acne scars, vascular lesions, pigment, tattoos, laser hair removal, rhytides, noninvasive fat removal, tissue tightening, ethnic skin, and a myriad of other topics. We feel that these chapters will benefit both the neophyte as well as the experienced laser surgeon because there is an emphasis on basic principles at the same time as there are many cutting-edge treatments that are detailed. Extensive verbiage is eschewed in favor of straightforward explanation. In all cases, the safe and effective use of these treatments is detailed by experienced laser surgeons in order to avoid patient injury.

This book provides an excellent, comprehensive, practical overview of the field of laser, light source and other energy-based treatments within the field of dermatology.

Mathew M Avram
Paul M Friedman

Acknowledgments

We are grateful to our esteemed colleagues and friends who generously shared their wealth of experience and expertise as reflected in the high quality of the chapters they contributed. We sincerely appreciate their invaluable assistance and the editorial team at M/s Jaypee Brothers Medical Publishers, New Delhi, India. We would like to extend our special thanks to Ms Chetna Malhotra Vohra (Senior Manager—Business Development) and Ms Saima Rashid (Development Editor) for their tremendous assistance and cooperation. In addition, the efforts and support of our families and office staff were invaluable in making this project so successful. We are grateful to all of you.

Contents

HAPTER

1

Introduction to Lasers: Light–Tissue Interaction and Laser Safety

Joshua D Shofner

INTRODUCTION TO LASERS

Light–Tissue Interaction

The use of lasers and light sources in dermatology has expanded rapidly in the past twenty years. As our understanding of the field has grown, lasers have progressively become more effective and selective in their ability to treat unique dermatologic targets. Lasers are now used worldwide in many clinical settings, and better understanding of laser physics and laser-skin interactions has led to the continued development of novel devices. The term "laser" or "LASER" is itself an acronym, which stands for Light Amplification of Stimulated Emission of Radiation.[1] This acronym describes the fundamental process by which laser light is generated.

The first device to incorporate the concept of optical amplification of emitted electromagnetic radiation was the MASER (Microwave Amplification by Stimulated Emission of Radiation), developed in the early 1950s by Charles Hard Townes. This device used microwave amplification in an energized stream of ammonia particles.[2] The MASER and the physical underpinnings behind it ultimately led to the Nobel Prize in Physics in 1964 for Charles Townes. Owing to the excitement generated over the MASER, multiple research groups undertook the search to develop the first device capable of light amplification. The first laser was developed in 1960 by Theodore Maiman, in which he noted laser emission of red light in a flashtube-pumped ruby laser.[3] Medical applications soon followed, and their regular use for skin conditions was pioneered by Leon Goldman.[1] He utilized continuous wave ruby lasers in the early treatment of tattoos, nevi and skin cancer.[4-6] The use of early lasers, however, was complicated by an unacceptably high risk of scarring and disfigurement. It was not until the theory of selective photothermolysis was proposed in 1982 that the current understanding of lasers began to take shape. This theory, proposed by Anderson and Parrish, states that precise targeting of tissue can be achieved using a specific wavelength of light that is selectively absorbed by the target of interest, resulting in minimal damage to surrounding tissue.[7] What began as the search for a nonscarring approach to pediatric port-wine stains now forms the mechanism behind an effective treatment modality for a number of different dermatologic conditions.[8]

Any discussion of laser fundamentals must first begin with a background in the physical properties of light. Visible light is a form of electromagnetic radiation with wavelengths from 400 nanometers (nm) to 750 nm.[9] While early lasers were developed in the visible light spectrum, newer devices span a wide range of wavelengths of electromagnetic radiation, from the ultraviolet to the infrared. The fundamental particle that defines the properties of light and lasers is the photon. A photon is the emitted form of light energy, and it exists in tiny "packets" of energy, known as quanta. Photons are governed by the rules of quantum mechanics and exhibit wave-particle duality possessing properties of both waves and particles. Particles of light propagate in a sinusoidal wave, whereby the frequency and wavelength of the photon are inversely related. Despite wave-like propagation, light maintains the ability to be emitted or absorbed as a discrete particulate element, the photon. Thus, light can act as a wave and a particle simultaneously. Photons travel, fittingly, at the speed of light (3×10^8 meters/second).

Laser light is created through a complex chain of events. That chain of events centers on the energy gained and subsequently emitted from an electron when it is stimulated by a photon. When light energy (photon) collides with an electron, the energy possessed by the photon is transferred to the electron, increasing its energy by a single quanta to an excited state. In the excited state, the electron is quasi-stable and eventually relaxes to its more stable ground state, and in doing so, emits a photon of random phase. This process of relaxation of quasi-stable excited electrons back to their ground state in the absence of an external stimulus is known as spontaneous emission, and is the mechanism behind fluorescence. If, however, emitted photons relax to the ground state in a cavity containing incident light, the emitted photons are in identical phase to each other and the original incident light. Owing to their particulate properties, photons have the unique ability to stimulate an excited atom to emit a photon of the same energy and wavelength as itself, thus creating a multiplicity of photons with identical energies, wavelength, and the ability to travel in phase together. As more energy is pumped into a laser, a larger and larger quantity of emitted photons is produced, until over half of the electrons are in an excited state. This is known as population inversion and allows for the amplification of light and the delivery of high energies of focused laser light. This is the physical underpinning of a laser.

The construction of a laser begins with a highly reflective optical cavity containing a gain medium, typically a gas, solid, or liquid. The medium is a substance that can be stimulated via an energy source, allowing amplification of light energy by stimulated emission of radiation. In the simplest form, imagine two mirrors containing the gain medium and an energy source between them. The medium is then excited by an energy source, which creates a multitude of emitted photons with identical wavelength, coherence and collimation. Those emitted photons then reflect off the wall of the optical cavity and pass back through the medium. They can travel back-and-forth inside the optical cavity, each time passing through the excited medium, thus exponentially amplifying the original signal and creating a highly intense beam of focused laser light.

Laser light possesses several unique properties that differentiate it from other sources of light energy—monochromicity, coherence and collimation.[10] Monochromicity refers to laser output consisting of a single wavelength of light. Coherence refers to the identical sinusoidal movement of light waves in space, traveling completely in phase in both time and space. Collimation refers to the nondivergent parallel nature of the light beam, allowing it to travel long distances without significant loss of energy. Laser light must possess all of these characteristics to be deemed a laser.

The mechanistic underpinning of laser–skin interactions is derived mainly from the theory of selective photothermolysis, first introduced by Anderson and Parrish in 1982.[7] It states that selective heating of a target of interest can be achieved with appropriate choice of both the wavelength and pulse duration. The wavelength of the laser must correspond with the absorption spectra of the target, and the pulse duration must be chosen so that it is shorter than the thermal relaxation time (the time required for the target to lose 50% of heat) of the target. By picking a wavelength of light that is selectively taken up by the target of interest and by choosing a pulse duration that allows for heating of the target (and not the surrounding tissue), one can selectively destroy dermatologic lesions with a very low risk of damage to surrounding tissue.

Laser–skin interactions form the foundation of understanding therapeutic uses of lasers. When laser light reaches skin, one of the following four things happens: the light is either reflected, scattered, transmitted, or absorbed. To some extent, each of these variables can be manipulated to maximize the therapeutic effect of the laser and to minimize collateral damage to surrounding tissue. A beam of light striking the skin typically loses 4–7% of its energy due to reflection. This is due to the difference between the refractive indices of air and skin.[11] The remaining energy then enters into the skin, where it is either scattered, transmitted, or absorbed. Determining which of these actions occur is dependent upon what the photon interacts with. Transmission occurs when light energy passes through a medium unaltered, neither changing its energy or direction. Scattering occurs when the light interacts with particles containing differing concentrations of water and proteins, thus possessing different refractive indices, allowing the light beam to be scattered in numerous directions. Scattering has no effect on the target tissue. Absorption, the desired effect, only occurs when light is absorbed by a target chromophore, converting light energy to heat.

When absorption occurs, the energy of the photon is then transmitted to the target in the form of heat. Heat induces denaturation of essential structures within cells, namely proteins and nucleic acids. As these vital components denature, the cell eventually will undergo necrosis. The goal of laser therapy is to selectively induce necrosis of the target of interest and only minimally damage surrounding tissues. A target's thermal relaxation time is directly proportionate to the diameter of the target of interest. Larger structures such as hair follicles have longer thermal relaxation times than smaller structures such as tattoo particles. Thus, larger diameter targets require longer pulse durations. Different lasers are capable of producing either intense, short pulses of light or longer millisecond pulses of light. The ability of the laser to selectively target the target chromophore is dependent upon the choice of fluence, wavelength of light and the pulse duration.

Different chromophores in the skin, such as melanin, water and hemoglobin, preferentially absorb certain wavelengths of light.[12] Ablative lasers typically target water as the primary chromophore and vaporize tissue by the rapidly heating water in the target tissue. Nonablative lasers can target either water or other chromophores such as melanin or hemoglobin. Based on the unique absorption spectra of the most common chromophores in skin, lasers can be designed to emit specific wavelengths of light, allowing for selective heating of the target of interest. Other parameters, including pulse duration, fluence and spot size, can be manipulated to specifically target lesions of interest. The pulse duration is defined as the length of time that the laser energy is being delivered to the target of interest, and fluence is the energy delivered by the laser. If the pulse duration is too long, the energy absorbed by the target will be transferred to the surrounding tissues as heat and can potentially lead to nonspecific thermal damage and scarring. If the pulse duration is too short, insufficient heat is generated to destroy the target. Fluence is the amount of energy delivered per unit area (defined as joules/cm^2) and is the intensity of the laser beam. Higher fluences correspond with greater thermal damage rendered upon the target. The ability to change the spot size, or diameter of the laser pulse delivered to the skin, allows for changes in the energy delivered and depth of penetration. Smaller spot sizes allow for greater fluences to be used while larger spot sizes allow for greater depth of penetration of the laser energy due to decreased scattering. An appropriate pulse duration and fluence will be sufficiently high to induce thermal damage to the target and target alone. Manipulation of the fluence, wavelength spot size and pulse duration allows for the selective destruction of pigmented lesions, hair, vascular lesions, and the skin itself.

Other techniques are also employed to minimize damage to the surrounding tissues during laser treatments. Epidermal melanin is a strong chromophore that can absorb a significant portion of laser energy when the pulse is emitted. Damage to the epidermis can be minimized through the judicious use of cooling before and during emission of the laser light. Cooling can be accomplished with gas, liquid or solid phase components. Spray cooling involves the use of a directed coolant at the skin just prior to emission of the laser. Solid contact cooling typically involves the use of solid medium, such as a sapphire crystal, which is placed onto the skin and held in contact during the laser treatment. Often, cold gels or forced cold air will be applied to the skin prior to laser treatment to additionally reduce the risk of epidermal damage.

There are numerous ways in which lasers emit their energy. Lasers can be operated in either a continuous or pulsed mode. Continuous mode lasers produce a constant beam of energy, whereas pulsed mode lasers are operated with discrete pulses of energy, typically in terms of a pulse duration allowing for the generation of very high energy pulses of light delivered in different pulse intervals. Quality-switched (Q-switched) lasers are able to generate extremely high energy pulses over a very short, typically nanosecond, pulse duration. The generation of such short pulses allowed for the destruction of miniscule targets, such as tattoo pigments and even melanocytes. Newer technology has incorporated the use of fractional technology, in which the laser output is produced in a pixilated grid-like fashion, creating thousands of microscopic channels of microthermal energy instead of a broad beam typically millimeters across.[13] By heating these tiny columns of tissue, one can induce dermal remodeling and production of collagen I and III. Fractional lasers have been successfully used for the treatment of scars and photoaging. Compared to older ablative lasers, this new concept in skin restoration has led to faster healing times and a decreased risk of adverse events.

Laser Safety

Lasers represent not only a tremendously precise and effective surgical tool but also a dangerous instrument in the hands of untrained users. The high intensity and focused nature of laser light presents a work hazard to both the skin and eyes of users.[14] Incident laser light that is misdirected and fired at a nonintended target can cause unintended consequences. Since laser light is collimated and coherent, it can travel long distances without loss of intensity, and thus can strike a person standing across the room, causing pain and even scarring of the skin depending upon the laser being operated.[15] Laser safety standards are now legal requirements for operation of a laser. Practice regulations are adopted from the American National Standards Institute.

The most dangerous side-effect of laser operation is damage to the eye itself. In the visible and near-infrared spectra (370–1000 nm), laser light penetrates the cornea and is strongly absorbed by the pigmented cells of the choroid and retina. The light beam, already intensely focused, is even more greatly focused by the natural convexity of the lens itself, whose job is to focus light onto the retina. This can lead to retinal burn and blindness. At wavelengths greater than 1000 nm, laser light is prefentially absorbed by water, thus poses a greater risk to the cornea, which can lead to corneal burns and cataract formation. If operating a nanosecond-domain Q-switched laser, misdirected laser light can penetrate the eye faster than the blink reflex occurs.

As a result, all laser systems necessitate the use of appropriate eye protection for both users and patients. All people in the room at the time of laser operation must wear safety goggles. Laser goggles will clearly state on them the wavelengths that they are protecting and the optical density the lens provides. Optical density (OD) is based on a logarithmic calculation that describes the percentage of laser light that is transmitted through the lens of the laser goggles. Current recommendations require an OD of at least 4 at the wavelength of the laser being used. The color of the goggles is not a sufficient determinant of whether it is appropriate for the laser being used.

Another consideration when dealing with lasers is the fire hazard they may pose. Fire risk is greatest with CO_2 and Erbium lasers. The most common cause of fire is failure to put the laser into "standby" mode. When operating a laser that poses significant fire risk, operators should use wet drapes around all treatment zones. If an endotracheal tube is placed and treatment is being delivered in the perioral region, the FiO_2 should be as low as can be tolerated by the patient. Endotracheal tube fires have been reported with the use of ablative lasers.

Lasers remain tremendously complicated treatment devices. Careful consideration must be made before treating any patient. Complications can occur, and will be discussed in greater detail in another chapter. A thorough understanding of the mechanisms of laser action and laser–skin interactions is paramount when using these devices, both to ensure proper usage but also to ensure your and your patient's safety.

REFERENCES

1. Goldman L, et al. Effect of the laser beam on the skin. Preliminary report. J Invest Dermatol. 1963;40:121-2.
2. Townes CH. The present status of microwave spectroscopy. Ann N Y Acad Sci. 1952;55(5):745-50.
3. Fine S, et al. Biological effects of high peak power radiation. Life Sci. 1964;3: 209-22.
4. Goldman L, et al. Radiation from a Q-switched ruby laser. Effect of Repeated Impacts of Power Output of 10 Megawatts on a Tattoo of Man. J Invest Dermatol. 1965;44:69-71.
5. Goldman L, Igelman JM, Richfield DF. Impact of the laser on nevi and melanomas. Arch Dermatol. 1964;90:71-5.
6. Goldman L, Wilson RG. Treatment of basal cell epithelioma by laser radiation. JAMA. 1964;189:773-5.
7. Anderson RR, Parrish JA. Selective photothermolysis: precise microsurgery by selective absorption of pulsed radiation. Science. 1983;220(4596):524-7.
8. Morelli JG, et al. Tunable dye laser (577 nm) treatment of port wine stains. Lasers Surg Med. 1986;6(1):94-9.
9. Fitzpatrick RE, Goldman MP. Cosmetic laser surgery. St Louis, Mo: Mosby. 2000;xi:239.
10. Carroll L, Humphreys TR. LASER-tissue interactions. Clin Dermatol. 2006; 24(1):2-7.
11. Anderson RR, Parrish JA. The optics of human skin. J Invest Dermatol. 1981; 77(1):13-9.
12. Rapini RP, Jorizzo JL, Bolognia J. Dermatology. St Louis,Mo, London: Mosby. 2003;2:2500.
13. Manstein D, et al. Fractional photothermolysis: a new concept for cutaneous remodeling using microscopic patterns of thermal injury. Lasers Surg Med. 2004; 34(5):426-38.
14. Powell CH, Goldman L. Recommendations of the Laser Safety Conference. Arch Environ Health. 1969;18(3):448-52.
15. Goldman L. Progress in laser safety in biomedical installations. Arch Environ Health. 1970;20(2):193-6.

HAPTER

2

Laser and Light Treatment for Cutaneous Vascular Lesions

Iris Rubin

INTRODUCTION

Laser surgery for vascular lesions was revolutionized with the introduction of the theory of selective photothermolysis by Anderson and Parrish in the 1980s.[1] Pulsed lasers allow for treatment of the target of interest, while minimizing damage to surrounding tissue and structures. There are three requirements for selective photothermolysis: (1) a wavelength of light with preferential absorption of the chromophore of interest; (2) a pulse duration appropriately matched to the size of the vessel target. The ideal pulse duration is equal to or somewhat shorter than the thermal relaxation time of the target vessel. The thermal relaxation time in seconds is approximately equal to the square of the vessel diameter in millimeters; and (3) adequate fluence to achieve photothermolysis. If the fluence is too high, nonspecific thermal damage can occur.

Oxyhemoglobin has traditionally been the target chromophore for vascular lasers. More recently, other hemoglobin species have been identified as useful targets for photothermolysis, including deoxyhemoglobin and methemoglobin.

Vascular lasers have evolved to incorporate epidermal cooling, allowing for safer treatment of cutaneous vascular lesions by reducing the risk of pigmentary changes and scarring. Epidermal cooling also increases treatment efficacy by allowing the use of relatively higher fluences. Newer generation pulsed-dye lasers also have the advantage of higher energies that provide adequate fluence for larger spot sizes. Larger spot sizes can be beneficial by increasing the depth of penetration due to less scattering of light.

Pulsed-dye lasers (PDL) are the most commonly implemented lasers for vascular lesions. Pulsed-dye lasers were originally developed at 577 nm to target an oxyhemoglobin peak. It was later found that 585 nm was more useful for treatment of port-wine stains. The next generation PDL at 595 nm improved depth of penetration due to the longer wavelength. Other lasers and light sources to treat vascular lesions include potassium titanyl phosphate (KTP 532 nm), intense pulsed light source, and near-infrared long-pulsed lasers, specifically alexandrite (755 nm), diode (800–810 nm), and neodymium: yttrium aluminum garnet (Nd:Yag 1064 nm) (Table 2.1). The near-infrared lasers are implemented for vascular lesions to achieve a greater depth of penetration associated with the longer wavelengths. While absolute absorption of hemoglobin species is lower at these wavelengths, selective photothermolysis can still be achieved.

Table 2.1: Devices implemented to treat vascular lesions
• Vascular lasers – Pulsed-dye laser (585 nm, 595 nm) – KTP laser (532 nm)
• Near-infrared lasers – Alexandrite (755 nm) – Diode (800–810 nm) – Nd:Yag (1064 nm)
• Intense pulsed light devices (500–1200 nm)
• Dual wavelength laser (595 nm/1064 nm)

Parameters will be discussed in various sections, and it is important to note that parameters vary by device and by the individual patient. Color of a lesion, location on the body, a patient's age, response to prior treatment, skin type, and laser endpoint all guide the appropriate parameters for an individual patient. A cookbook approach can cause complications. It is essential to follow the appropriate endpoint for the device being implemented. In addition, caution is advised in patients with darker skin types as there is increased risk for pigmentary complications. Longer pulse durations, lower fluences and test pulses are advised in darker skin types.

PORT-WINE STAINS

Port-wine stains are slow-flow vascular malformations that are composed of ectatic capillaries and postcapillary venules in the superficial vascular plexus. Port-wine stain vessels are characterized by diminished vascular tone and decreased density of nerves. In most cases, port-wine stains are congenital, though in rare cases they may be acquired. The prevalence of port-wine stains is 0.3–0.5% of newborns. The majority appear on the head and neck and can be quite disfiguring. Port-wine stains persist throughout life, and many thicken with time. There may be associated soft tissue overgrowth. Vascular blebs can form and may bleed, especially with shaving. Port-wine stains in the V1 distribution prompt evaluation for Sturge-Weber syndrome which can have ocular and neurologic involvement, and referral to ophthalmology and neurology is appropriate. Port-wine stains on the lower extremity can be associated with venous malformations and bone/soft tissue hypertrophy in Klippel-Trenaunay-Weber syndrome. Associated lymphatic malformations may also be seen in Klippel-Trenaunay-Weber syndrome.

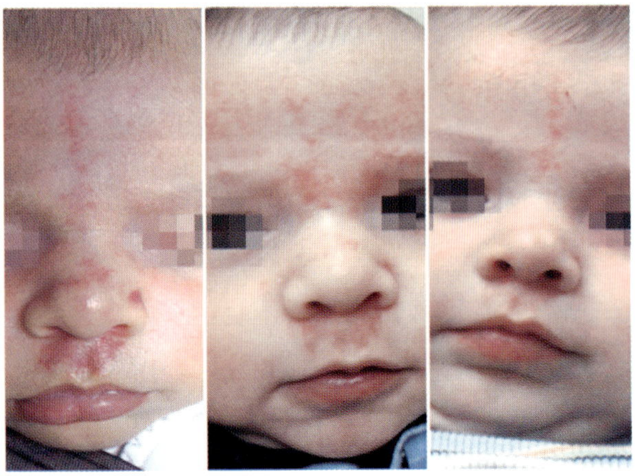

Fig. 2.1: Port-wine stain treated with pulsed-dye laser in infancy, starting at 6 weeks of age. Right photo after four treatments

The goal of treatment for port-wine stains is to improve the vascular color (Fig. 2.1) and to minimize potential psychosocial distress associated with the port-wine stain. It has been theorized that early treatment of port-wine stains may also prevent hypertrophy as well as development of vascular blebs. The pulsed-dye laser, which is strongly absorbed by oxyhemoglobin, is the most commonly used laser for port-wine stain treatment. The theory of selective photothermolysis guides treatment parameters. Port-wine stain vessels vary in size from approximately 10 microns to 150 microns, and older patients tend to have larger vessels. In practice, the ideal pulse duration is typically between 0.45 milliseconds and 6 milliseconds. The pulse duration may be varied between treatments depending on clinical response. Longer pulse durations are advisable for darker skin types.

While the pulsed-dye laser is effective, it is limited by the depth of penetration. The alexandrite laser at 755 nm is advantageous due to the greater depth of penetration and may be used to target deeper vessels. In practice, the alexandrite laser may be implemented for port-wine stains refractory to treatment with the pulsed-dye laser, or for initial treatment of hypertrophic, violaceous port-wine stains. The endpoint for the alexandrite laser has been described by Izikson et al.[2] as a subtle gray-blue color that evolves to purpura over several minutes. The range of fluences with the alexandrite laser is quite broad and the risk of scarring is increased compared to the pulsed-dye laser.

Other lasers that have been used to treat port-wine stains include the Nd:Yag laser at 1064 nm, again the longer wavelength allows for a greater depth of penetration. There is, however, a very narrow therapeutic window with the Nd:Yag laser and the risk of ulceration, and scarring is not insignificant. Yang et al.[3] have demonstrated that fixed fluence dosing is risky. The Nd:Yag laser has greater absorption for oxyhemoglobin compared to deoxyhemoglobin, making it relatively more artery selective, which may explain the tendency for ulceration. The combined 595 nm/1064 nm laser has also been implemented to achieve a greater depth of penetration, and has a narrow therapeutic window as well. Intense pulsed light treatment with appropriate vascular filters has also been reported to be effective for treatment of port-wine stains, though is not considered to be the first-line treatment.

While the majority of port-wine stains can be improved with a series of laser treatments, most do not clear completely. Early laser treatment can improve outcomes. A retrospective study by Chapas et al.[4] of 49 infants who started treatment before or at the age of 6 months demonstrated an impressive average clearance of 88.6% after 1 year.

While port-wine stains may redarken after laser therapy, the laser treated areas remain lighter than before treatment.[5] Other treatment modalities that are being investigated include photodynamic therapy and anti-angiogenesis medications. Port-wine stains are composed of postcapillary venules and a vein-selective laser that targets deoxyhemoglobin is in the early stages of development to optimize port-wine stain treatment.[6]

Parameters

Treatments are done at 4–6 week intervals, and it is not uncommon for 6–10 treatments or more to be performed. While most port-wine stains improve, the minority clear completely. Parameters vary by device. Lower fluences and longer pulse durations are advisable for darker skin types.

While it is always imperative to follow clinical endpoints when treating a port-wine stain, the range of fluences may include: Pulsed-dye laser at 595 nm, 7–10 mm spot, 0.45–6 msec, 5–9.5 J/cm^2, appropriate cooling. Perform test spots on the darkest portion of the port-wine stain, and assess for the clinical endpoint. Utilize lower fluences with shorter pulse durations and larger spot sizes. The endpoint is immediate purpura (Fig. 2.2). A confluent gray color signifies that the fluence is too high.

Since larger spot sizes can penetrate deeper, it is advisable to implement the largest spot size that provides adequate fluence and confines treatment to the area of interest. It is helpful to mark the borders of the port-wine stain with a marking pen prior to treatment as laser pulses can induce erythema blurring the border. In addition, topical anesthetics can cause erythema outside of port-wine stain border. Port-wine stains may also blanch under general anesthesia. Table 2.2 presents port-wine stain treatment hints.

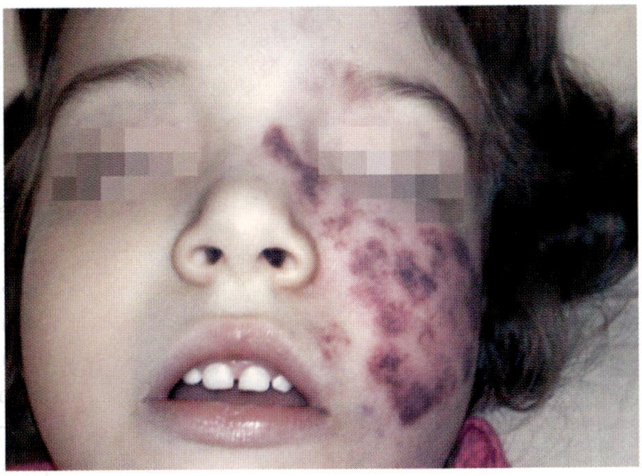

Fig. 2.2: Expected purpura post pulsed-dye laser for port-wine stain. Purpura typically lasts up to 7–14 days

Table 2.2: Port-wine stain treatment hints
• Outline the port-wine stain prior to treatment
• Follow your endpoint
• Appropriate cooling is essential
• Use the largest spot possible that confines treatment to area of interest
• Use appropriate eye protection
• Metal intraocular shields must be inserted when treating within the orbital rim. Never use plastic eyeshields
• Apply surgilube to hair bearing areas to minimize singing
• Pulsed-dye laser can cause PERMANENT hair removal of eyelashes. Pulsed-dye laser can cause PERMANENT hair removal on the scalp in infants with dark hair.
• Minimize NSAIDs pre- and post treatment. Platelet function is important for effective photothermolysis
• If a patient is anemic, treatment will not be as effective since there is less target chromophore
• Do not treat when tan. Sun protection must be emphasized pre- and post treatment
• General anesthesia tips: – Oxygen and hair can be flammable. Minimize oxygen in the field when performing laser treatment. Wet hair or apply surgilube to hair.

INFANTILE HEMANGIOMA

Infantile hemangiomas (IH) are benign endothelial cell proliferations that represent the most common tumor of infancy, occurring in 4–10% of infants. Infantile hemangiomas typically present within the first few weeks of life. An early macular stain that is hypopigmented, red, or telangiectatic may be present at birth. There is a proliferative period usually until 3–12 months of age. Involution then occurs more slowly over years. Approximately 50% of IH have regressed by age 5 and 90% have regressed by age 9. After regression, there is often residual fibrofatty tissue and/or telangiectasias.

Observation is appropriate management for many IH. Indications for treatment include functional difficulties, bleeding, ulceration and cosmetic disfigurement. Functional difficulties can occur when important anatomical structures are involved or obstructed. Potential complications include, but are not limited to, airway compromise, symptomatic liver involvement and visual axis obstruction. PHACE (posterior fossa malformation, hemangioma, arterial anomalies, coarctation of the aorta, eye abnormalities, sternal or supraumbilical raphe) syndrome must also be considered in patients that present with large facial IH.

Treatment options for IH include topical medications, specifically topical steroids and the beta-blocker timolol, intralesional corticosteroid injection, systemic medications, propranolol and corticosteroids most commonly as first-line treatment, surgery, and laser. There is no standard treatment protocol for IH, and treatment is determined on a case-by-case basis.

Pulsed-dye laser can be implemented by itself or in conjunction with other treatments. Studies have shown that pulsed-dye laser can expedite healing of ulcerated IH,[7] and the associated discomfort (Figs 2.3A and B). It is expected that most ulcerated IH will heal with a scar due to the underlying ulceration. Laser treatment is also beneficial for involuted IH. Pulsed-dye laser can be implemented to treat residual erythema or telangiectasias, and fractionated ablative or nonablative lasers can improve residual textural and fibrofatty changes.[8]

The role of laser in the proliferating and involuting phases of IH has been more controversial. A recent retrospective case review by Rizzo et al.[9] of 90 patients with childhood hemangiomas and a median age of 3 months showed positive results. Eighty-one percent had near-complete or complete clearance in color, and 64% in thickness. The mean number of treatments was 6.7 for superficial hemangiomas and 8 for mixed hemangiomas. Hyperpigmentation was seen in 4% and hypopigmentation in 14%. Relatively high fluences were implemented. There has yet to be a randomized controlled trial supporting the early use of laser treatment for uncomplicated IH.

There has been debate about whether to use high or low fluences for laser treatment of IH. An

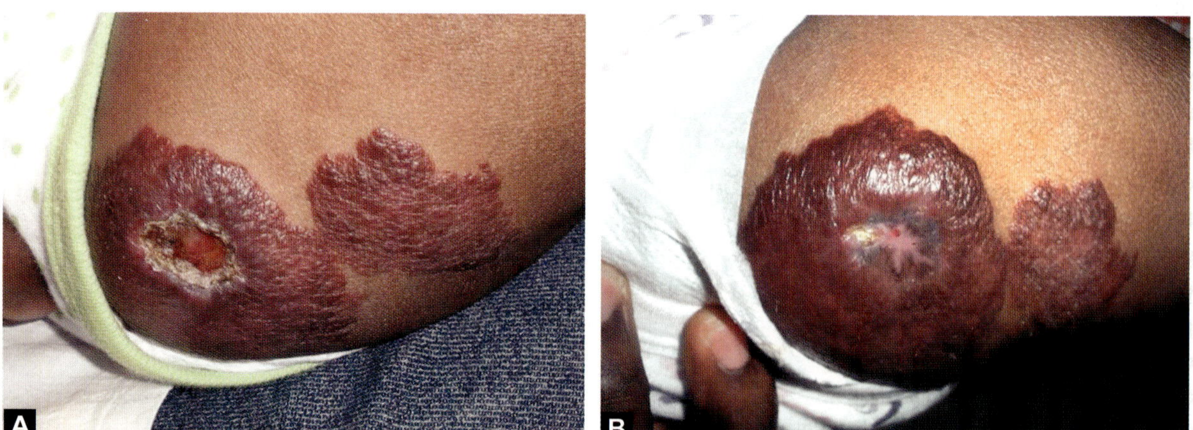

Figs 2.3A and B: Ulcerated infantile hemangioma treated with pulsed-dye laser. The ulceration had been present for 2 months and was refractory to local wound care. Treatment was initiated at a low fluence and a long pulse duration, with a single pulse. Healing occurred within 1 week. Caution is advised when treating darker skin types due to the increased risk of hypo- and hyperpigmentation. In this case a pigmentary change was expected from scarring due to the ulceration, and the risk of further hypo-hyperpigmentation was discussed with the parents

editorial by Dr Rox Anderson in Lasers in Surgery and Medicine in 2006 advocated a low fluence approach, citing that the goal of treatment is to "trigger an active process of regression," rather than to heat and destroy vessels as with a port-wine stain.[10]

Potential risks of pulsed-dye laser treatment for IH include hypopigmentation, hyperpigmentation, ulceration and scarring. Multiple treatments are generally required and may be done at 2–6 weeks intervals, with proliferating hemangiomas treated at shorter intervals. Given the depth of penetration of PDL, one would expect PDL to be more effective for superficial IH.

TELANGIECTASIAS

Facial telangiectasias are highly prevalent and are one of the most common vascular lesions to present for treatment. Telangiectasias consist of small dilated vessels in the superficial dermis approximately 0.1–1 mm in diameter. The most common causes of facial telangiectasias are dermatoheliosis and rosacea. Other causes include trauma, a host of genodermatoses including hereditary hemorrhagic telangiectasia, radiation dermatitis, liver disease, and connective tissue diseases including lupus, scleroderma, and CREST syndrome.

There are a variety of laser and light sources that may be implemented for the treatment of telangiectasias. Treatment must be tailored, taking into account vessel caliber and skin type. A series of 2–4 treatments with pulsed-dye laser or intense pulsed light is typically very effective. In the past, purpuric settings were often implemented to treat telangiectasias. With modern pulsed-dye lasers that offer higher energies and longer pulse durations (0.45–40 msec), it is often possible to clear telangiectasias with minimal or no purpura. A new generation pulsed-dye laser has 8 subpulses per pulse, limiting high energy peaks that may cause purpura. Pulse durations of 0.45–3 msec are likely to cause purpura, and pulse durations 6 msec or longer are less likely to cause purpura. When treating at subpurpuric parameters, the desired endpoint is a transient blue coagulum (Fig. 2.4), vessel clearance, and/or erythema. Techniques that have been implemented for subpurpuric treatment include longer pulse durations and multiple, typically 2, passes.

Rosacea patients frequently have telangiectasias, and may also have background erythema, flushing, and/or acneiform papules. Laser and light-based treatment for rosacea is aimed at improving telangiectasias, as well as facial erythema. Flushing may also improve in some patients, though has a tendency to recur. Rosacea patients can be counseled that their skin will be expected to improve significantly, though laser is not a cure for rosacea and maintenance treatments will be required. It is best to advise patients that physiologic flushing will likely continue after treatment.

Parameters to consider for facial erythema associated with rosacea are pulsed-dye laser at 595 nm, 10 mm spot, 6 msec, 6–7.5 J/cm^2, appropriate cooling, 1–2 passes. Note that patients with more erythema have more target chromophore and require lower fluences. It is helpful to apply ice post treatment to minimize potential swelling. Telangiectasias can be treated before or after background erythema. Parameters to consider when treating telangiectasias with the pulsed-dye laser at 595 nm are 7 mm spot, 3–10 msec, 7–10 J/cm^2, appropriate cooling. Some devices also have a 3 × 10 mm elliptical spot that can be useful for telangiectasias. Higher fluences and longer pulse durations may be implemented with the 3 × 10 mm spot.

The intense pulsed light (IPL) source with appropriate vascular filters may also be used for treatment of background erythema and for telangiectasis. Poikiloderma of Civatte has both telangiectasias and pigmentation and most commonly occurs on the neck. Poikiloderma tends to respond well to IPL treatment. Nonablative fractional treatments are also effective, especially for pigment.

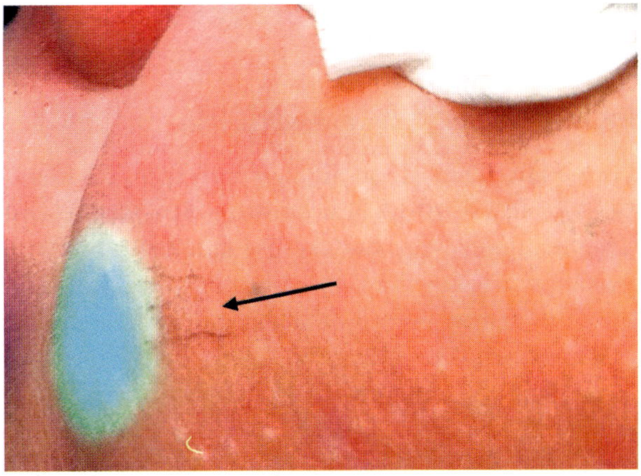

Fig. 2.4: Transient blue coagulum after pulsed-dye laser to treat telangiectasias on the cheek associated with rosacea. This blue color disappears within a few seconds

Individual vessels may be traced with the KTP laser, with the advantage of no purpura. There is relatively stronger absorption of hemoglobin at 532 nm and caution must be taken in patients with darker skin types. The Nd:Yag laser has deeper penetration due to their longer wavelength and has been implemented to treat larger caliber telangiectasias, though caution is advised as the risk of scarring is increased. It is essential not to overlap pulses with the Nd:Yag as this can increase the risk of scarring.

While complications are rare when treating telangiectasias, potential complications include hyperpigmentation, hypopigmentation, a polka-dot effect and scarring. The risk of hyperpigmentation and hypopigmentation are increased in darker skin types. The leg also has a higher risk of hyperpigmentation. Avoiding treating patients that are tan can help minimize the risk of pigment change. Scarring is more likely with deeper penetrating lasers. The risk of scarring is also increased with high fluences, pulse stacking and devices that do not incorporate cooling. Of note the IPL and near-infrared lasers can cause hair removal and it is advised not to use these lasers in locations where this outcome may be undesirable, such as on the cheeks and neck of males.

CHERRY ANGIOMAS

Cherry angiomas are the most common vascular growths of the skin. Cherry angiomas are benign proliferations that tend to be highly responsive to laser treatment. The pulsed-dye laser is commonly used to treat angiomas. The endpoint is purpura. The KTP laser or intense pulsed light treatment may also be utilized.

Parameters that may be Appropriate

Pulsed-dye laser at 595 nm, 5–7 mm spot, 1.5 msec, 8–10 J/cm^2, appropriate cooling. For larger and thicker angiomas, an initial pulse may be placed with diascopy (a glass slide) to compress the lesion and treat the deeper component. After time for cooling, a second pulse may be placed to treat the more superficial component. The endpoint is purpura.

SPIDER ANGIOMAS

Spider angiomas are benign proliferations of capillaries in the dermis with a central arteriole. Clinically, they appear as vascular papule with radiating vessels. These lesions also tend to be highly responsive to laser treatment.

Parameters that may be Appropriate

Pulsed-dye laser at 595 nm, 5–7 mm spot, 1.5 msec, 8–10 J/cm^2, appropriate cooling. Diascopy with a glass slide is performed and the first pulse is aimed at the central feeding arteriole. Additional pulses without diascopy are then placed to treat surrounding radiating vessels. The endpoint is purpura.

VENOUS LAKES

Venous lakes are acquired vascular malformations that consist of ectatic venules in the superficial dermis. Venous lakes appear clinically as compressible violaceous papules, and are most commonly located on the lip. Treatment may be initiated for cosmetic purposes or may be prompted by bleeding.

Laser treatment options include with pulsed-dye laser for more superficial lesions. Pulsed-dye laser, however, is ineffective for deeper lesions. For deeper lesions, the diode laser achieves deeper penetration and is more effective.[11] Alternatively, the alexandrite or Nd:Yag laser may be used for deeper lesions.

Pulsed-dye laser parameters are similar to the cherry angioma parameters above.

VENOUS MALFORMATIONS

Venous malformations present clinically as compressible blue-violaceous papules or nodules that increase in size with measures that increase venous pressure, such as the dependent position. Vessel walls may exhibit calcifications and phleboliths that are considered pathognomonic. Venous malformations are present at birth. Venous malformations may be clinically apparent in infancy, or not until years later. Laser treatment can be indicated. The goal is to decrease the size of lesion. For localized lesions complete clearance may be possible, though venous malformations have a tendency for recanalization. Diode lasers can be effective given their preferential targeting of deoxyhemoglobin in addition to oxyhemoglobin, and their ability to target more deeply than pulsed-dye lasers. Laser treatment may also be performed for larger venous malformations with the goal of debulking prior to surgery.

SPIDER VEINS

In general, the gold standard for the treatment of spider veins in the absence of deep varicosities is sclerotherapy. Spider veins may be defined as telangiectasias, small red vessels 0.03–0.3 mm in diameter, and venulectasias, red or blue vessels 0.4–2 mm in diameter. Lasers such as the long-pulsed alexandrite and Nd:Yag laser may be implemented for the treatment of spider veins, though there is a risk of side effects such as pigmentary alterations. Scarring is also a risk, in particular with the Nd:Yag laser which has a narrow therapeutic window. The newer generation pulsed-dye laser with longer pulse durations composed of 8 subpulses may improve spider veins with several treatment sessions, though hyperpigmentation can occur.[12]

Lasers do have a role to play in the treatment of spider veins in specific clinical settings. For example, in patients afraid of needles, laser treatment may be useful. Other indications include fine red telangiectasias that are too small to be cannulated by a sclerotherapy needle or telangiectatic matting that may be seen as a complication from sclerotherapy. If lasers are used, the pulsed-dye lasers are suggested for fine red telangiectatic vessels or telangiectatic matting. Larger and/or more violaceous spider veins may respond better to the long-pulsed alexandrite or Nd:Yag laser. Relatively higher fluences must be used with the Nd:Yag laser due to decreased absolute absorption of hemoglobin. Careful technique with appropriate skin cooling and no pulse stacking is essential.

If deep venous disease is present, it is advisable to treat the deep venous disease first.

ANGIOKERATOMAS

Angiokeratomas are characterized by ectatic superficial dermal vessels and overlying hyperkeratosis. Subtypes include solitary or multiple angiokeratomas which often occur on the lower extremities; angiokeratoma of Fordyce affecting the genital region; angiokeratoma of Mibelli, an autosomal dominant condition typically affecting the dorsal surface of the hands and feet; and angiokeratoma circumscriptum. Angiokeratomas may also be seen in association with Fabry's disease, an X-linked recessive disorder characterized by a deficiency of alpha-galactosidase A.

Treatment with vascular specific lasers such as the pulsed-dye laser may be initiated to treat the vascular component, though a residual keratotic component may persist. Ablative lasers such as the CO_2 or Erbium laser may be implemented, though there is a risk of scarring.

CONCLUSION

In summary, lasers and intense pulse light can be very effective in treating a range of cutaneous vascular lesions. The pulsed-dye laser was developed to target oxyhemoglobin and demonstrates a high safety profile and good efficacy; however its main limitation is depth of penetration. Near-infrared lasers have more recently been implemented as well to achieve a greater depth of penetration. It is essential to follow the appropriate endpoint of the device being implemented. Future directions include research on developing a vein-selective laser that targets deoxyhemoglobin. Photodynamic therapy and anti-angiogenesis inhibitors are also being studied for port-wine stains.

REFERENCES

1. Anderson RR, Parrish JA. Selective photothermolysis: precise microsurgery by selective absorption of pulsed radiation. Science. 1983;220:524-7.
2. Izikson L, Nelson JS, Anderson RR. Treatment of hypertrophic and resistant port wine stains with a 755nm laser: a case series of 20 patients. Lasers Surg Med. 2009;41:427-32.
3. Yang MU, Yaroslavsky AN, Farinelli WA, et al. Long pulsed neodymium:yttrium-aluminum-garnet laser treatment for port-wine stains. J Am Acad Dermatol. 2005;52:480-90.
4. Chapas AM, Eickhorst K, Geronemus RG. Efficacy of early treatment of facial port wine stains in newborns: a review of 49 cases. Lasers Surg Med. 2007;39:563-8.
5. Huikeshoven M, Koster PHL, de Borgie CA, et al. Redarkening of port-wine stains 10 years after pulsed-dye laser treatment. N Engl J Med. 2007; 356:1235-40.
6. Rubin IK, Farinelli WA, Doukas A, et al. Optimal wavelengths for vein-selective photothermolysis. Lasers Surg Med. 2012;44:152-7.
7. David LR, Malek M, Argenta LC. Efficacy of pulse dye laser therapy for the treatment of ulcerated hemangiomas: a review of 78 patients. British Journal of Plastic Surgery. 2003;56:317-27.

8. Laubach HJ, Anderson RR, Luger T, et al. Fractional photothermolysis for involuted infantile hemangioma. Arch Dermatol. 2009;145(7):748-50.
9. Rizzo C, Brightman L, Chapas AM, et al. Outcomes of childhood hemangiomas treated with the pulsed-dye laser with dynamic cooling: a retrospective chart analysis. Dermatol Surg. 2009;35:1947-54.
10. Anderson RR. Infant hemangiomas: a controversy worth solving. Lasers Surg Med. 2006;38:92-3.
11. Wall TL, Grassi AM, Avram MM. Clearance of multiple venous lakes with an 800-nm diode laser: a novel approach. Dermatol Surg. 2007;33:100-3.
12. Bernstein EF. The new-generation, high energy, 595nm, long pulse-duration, pulsed-dye laser effectively removes spider veins of the lower extremity. Lasers Surg Med. 2007;39:218-24.

ADDITIONAL READING

1. Kunishige JH, Goldberg LH, Friedman PM. Laser therapy for leg veins. Clin Dermatol. 2007;25:454-61.
2. McCoppin HH, Goldberg DJ. Laser treatment of facial telangiectasias: an update. Dermatol Surg. 2010;36:1221-30.

CHAPTER 3

Pigmented Lesions: General Considerations and Epidermal Lesions

Nazanin Saedi

PIGMENTED LESIONS: GENERAL CONSIDERATIONS

Melanin is the target chromophore in most epidermal and dermal pigmented lesions, and it has a broad absorption spectrum extending from the ultraviolet range through the visible and infrared spectrum. Across the wide range of absorbing wavelengths, many lasers and light devices with sufficient energy levels can target melanin. It is necessary to use wavelengths that avoid absorption by other skin chromophores and penetrate to the desired depth in order to be most effective and avoid adverse effects.

Targeting cutaneous pigmentation with lasers and light devices is dependent on several parameters, including absorption characteristics, the distribution in tissue, and the location in the skin (epidermis, dermis, or both). Separating pigmented lesions into discrete lesions or diffuse pigmentation can help guide the optimal treatment. This approach is described in this chapter.

Discrete Pigmented Lesions

For treating discrete pigmented lesions, Q-switched (QS) lasers can be very effective. The Q-switched lasers release high-powered pulses within the nanosecond range (one billionth of a second, 10^{-9} s), which leads to a combination of photoacoustic, photothermal and photochemical effects. Q-switched laser systems are preferable as they have the ability to destroy melanosomes with limited spread to surrounding structures on the basis of selective photothermolysis.[1] In addition to the thermal damage from selective photothermolysis, photoacoustic effects produced by QS lasers can lead to pigment destruction. The irradiated fragments are then eliminated transepidermally and through the lymphatics.[2]

The QS KTP, ruby, alexandrite, and Nd:YAG lasers can effectively treat epidermal melanocytic lesions due to the high affinity of these wavelengths for melanin. The desired endpoint is immediate whitening, which is achieved by employing an appropriate spot size for the target lesion and by using the lowest fluence possible. Higher fluences can result in unnecessary thermal spread, hemorrhage and epidermal damage with little change in efficacy.[3]

Melanin has good absorption at 532 nm, which increases the risk of dyspigmentation with KTP compared to longer wavelength lasers, especially in patients with darker skin types. The QS KTP laser is effective in the treatment of epidermal pigmented lesions. These include lentigines and ephelides, café au lait macules, Becker's nevus, postinflammatory hyperpigmentation, melasma, and tattoos. One controlled multicenter trial showed greater than 75% pigment removal achieved in 60% of lentigines treated at fluences of 4–5 J/cm^2.[3] Responses were more variable in other lesion types such as café au lait macules, which showed fair to moderate improvement. Mild erythema was noted, and several patients had transient hypo- or hyperpigmentation, although all dyspigmentation resolved spontaneously within 3 months. The treatment was found to be safe with no evidence of scarring or other textural change.

Lentigines can be treated with the QS alexandrite laser in most skin types. The QS alexandrite laser has a wavelength of 755 nm, which falls in the selective window for targeting melanin. The longer wavelength allows for deeper penetration, resulting in clinical efficacy and removal of the epidermal and dermal pigmented lesions. In Fitzpatrick Skin Types III and IV, the severity of postinflammatory hyperpigmentation using a QS alexandrite laser can be lower with a 4-mm spot and lower fluence than with a 3-mm spot size with higher fluence.[4] The technique involves making a single pass over the target area with minimal overlap. The clinical endpoint for this treatment is immediate whitening. As with other pigment targets, dark-skinned patients can be treated safely with QS 1064 nm Nd:YAG laser.

Anderson et al. demonstrated the efficacy of the QS Nd:YAG laser for the treatment of cutaneous pigmentation.[5] Most QS Nd:YAG laser systems have pulse durations ranging from 10 ns to 20 ns, spot sizes of 1.5–4 mm, and repetition rates of 1–10 Hz. Treatment parameters to consider for pigmented lesions include fluences from 3 J/cm^2 to 6 J/cm^2 with a 4–8 mm spot size.

Other discrete epidermal pigmented lesions, such as café au lait macules (CALMS), can be treated with the QS ruby,[6] QS Nd:YAG,[7] and the QS alexandrite laser.[9]

Q-switched lasers are effective for treating discrete pigmented lesions and selecting the appropriate wavelength depends on the patient's skin type along with the location of the pigment.

New on the Horizon: Picosecond Laser

The thermal relaxation time of tattoo pigment particles and melanosomes is less than 10 ns, suggesting that energy delivery in the picosecond range (one trillionth of a second, 10^{-12} s) should be effective.[8,9] Picosecond (PS) laser treatments can cause significant photomechanical effects and lead to mechanical breakup of melanosomes. By using a picosecond pulse duration and lowering treatment fluences, the risk of side effects should decrease while keeping the peak tensile stress induced substantially higher than that typically produced with QS laser. This is an ideal combination of higher efficacy and less adverse reactions. Recently, the FDA (Food and Drug Administration) has cleared the first picosecond laser (Picosure, Cynosure, Westford, MA) for the treatment of tattoos and benign pigmented lesions. In the coming years, there may be a shift to using the picosecond lasers for the treatment of benign pigmented lesions, and it might allow for fewer treatments to clear the lesions.

Diffuse Pigmentation

When approaching diffuse pigmentation, a global approach that involves treating the uninvolved skin can be taken. Diffuse pigmentation often blends in with the background skin, and there is a subtle difference between the affected and unaffected skin. Options can include the use of nonablative fractional resurfacing or intense pulsed light (IPL).

Nonablative Fractional Resurfacing

Nonablative fractional resurfacing (NAFR) delivers narrow beams of high-energy light at a variety of wavelengths targeting tissue water. This results in small cylindrical columns of thermal damage, the so-called "microthermal zones" (MTZs), distributed across the treatment area in a pixilated pattern. The columns of thermal damage are surrounded by normal skin.[10] The surrounding "skip areas" act as a nutritional and structural reservoir to provide the framework necessary for rapid healing.

The prototype device was a 1550-nm erbium-doped nonablative fractional device, and it was originally thought to be promising for the treatment of diffuse hyperpigmentation, such as melasma. In the initial reports on the efficacy of NAFR in treating melasma, ten female patients (Fitzpatrick Skin Types III–V) were treated at 1–2 week intervals with the Fraxel Re:Store (Solta Medical, Inc, Hayward, CA).[11] Following four to six sessions, physician evaluation confirmed that 60% of patients achieved 75–100% clearance. In another study, ten patients with melasma (Fitzpatrick Skin Types III–IV) were treated with a NAFR device (Fraxel Re:Store, Solta Medical, Inc), and the histology was examined.[12] Patients received a total of four treatments at 2-week intervals, and biopsies were obtained from all subjects both before and 3 months following treatment. Histologically, post-treatment specimens demonstrated a relative decrease in melanocyte quantity compared to pretreatment samples on light microscopy. Furthermore, post-treatment electron microscopy revealed fewer melanocytes and less melanin in the surrounding keratinocytes than in the pretreatment specimens. Not surprisingly, clinical improvements in melasma were less extensive in patients with progressively darker skin types. While these initial studies showed promise for the treatment of melasma with NAFR, more recent reports have suggested limitations in its efficacy due to the high recurrence rates after treatment, especially in those patients with darker skin types.[13]

A newer addition to nonablative fractional resurfacing, the 1927-nm thulium fiber laser (Fraxel DUAL, Solta Medical, Hayward, CA), does show efficacy in treating superficial processes such as lentigines, melasma and photodamage. This wavelength possesses a higher absorption coefficient for water than the 1550-nm, conferring greater ability to target epidermal processes. The 1927-nm fractional laser creates relatively superficial zones of thermal coagulation underneath intact stratum corneum. This superficial injury and the preservation of stratum corneum help to minimize the potential risk for scarring or infection. The maximum depth of penetration is approximately 206 microns at 20 mJ per pulse.[14] In addition to applications for dermatoheliosis and dyschromia, this device is quite effective at removing widespread facial actinic keratoses.[15]

Polder and Bruce studied the efficacy of the 1927-nm fractional thulium fiber laser for the treatment of melasma in fourteen patients.[14] The patients received three to four laser treatments (at 4-week intervals) at energies of 10–20 mJ and densities of 20–45% surface area coverage. A statistically significant 51% reduction in Melasma Area Severity Index (MASI) score was seen 1 month after the last treatment. There was still greater than a 30% reduction in the MASI at the 3- and 6-month post-treatment visits. There were no reports of scarring or post-inflammatory hyper- or hypopigmentation.

Masski et al. conducted a retrospective study of twenty women (Fitzpatrick Skin Type II–IV) with the clinical diagnosis of melasma treated with the 1927-nm fractionated thulium laser with energies of 10–20 mJ and high densities of 60–70% surface area coverage.[16] There was a significant reduction in the MASI that was maintained up to 10 months after the treatment. The patient self-assessments revealed that 12 of the 20 subjects had more than 50% clearance of their melasma. There was recurrence in 7 out of 15 patients who were successfully followed-up (mean 10.2 months). Two patients developed postinflammatory hyperpigmentation that subsided with topical bleaching after 3 months. In this study, high-density treatment with the fractional 1927-nm thulium laser appears to be effective for melasma with long-term remission. Given the recurring nature of melasma, there is a need for larger studies with long-term follow-up.

Intense Pulsed Light

The use of intense pulsed light (IPL) has grown significantly in recent years. Intense pulsed light systems emit filtered polychromatic light with wavelengths ranging from visible to near-infrared range (500–1200 nm), which falls into the absorption spectrum for melanin. The filtering and pulsing systems prevent unwanted wavelengths from damaging the skin and make this device more specific. Some devices have handpiece cooling, which is a useful feature that can be employed to provide epidermal protection, while at the same time allowing greater fluences to reach deeper targets. The IPL systems can be used to treat a number of conditions, including rosacea, port-wine stains, hemangiomas, poikiloderma of Civatte and lentigines, as well as provide overall photorejuvenation. Intense pulsed light becomes effective when treating diffuse pigmentation that is not in sharp contrast with the patient's natural skin. There are several reports demonstrating the effectiveness of IPL devices in the treatment of pigmented lesions.

Li et al. studied the efficacy and safety of an IPL device (Lumenis One, Lumenis, Inc, Santa Clara, CA; 560-/590-nm filters, pulse duration: 3–4 msec, pulse delay: 25–40 msec) in the treatment of melasma in Chinese patients.[17] The patients received IPL treatments at 3-week intervals, and 69 out of 89 patients (77.5%) showed 51–100% improvement according to the overall evaluation by dermatologists. Patient self-assessments indicated that 63 of 89 patients (70.8%) considered 50% or more improvement. The MASI decreased substantially.

Bjerring and Christiansen evaluated the effectiveness of an IPL device (Ellipse Flex, Danish Dermatologic Development; 400–720 nm; spot size: 10–48 mm; pulse duration: 2–7 msec, delay: 25 msec; fluence: 10–20 J/cm^2) in the treatment of solar lentigines (18 patients) and benign melanocytic nevi (8 patients).[18] Two months after one single treatment, 96% of patients had pigment reduction and an average clearance of 74.2% for solar lentigines and 66.3% for melanocytic nevi.

CONCLUSION

There are several laser and light devices that can be successfully used for treating epidermal pigment. Q-switched lasers are effective in treating discrete epidermal pigmented lesions, and the picosecond laser has an exciting new application for the treatment of pigmented lesions. For diffuse pigmentation, NAFR can be effective for treating the pigmentation while also leading to textural improvement. Intense pulsed light will treat the pigmentation but also offer the benefit of photorejuvenation. There may be benefit in combining these treatments to maximize the outcomes in a single treatment session. With advances in technology, we continue to strive to optimize treatment options for targeting pigment.

REFERENCES

1. Murphy GF, et al. Organelle-specific injury to melanin-containing cells in human skin by pulsed laser irradiation. Lab Invest. 1983;49(6):680-5.
2. Anderson RR, Parrish JA. The optics of human skin. J Invest Dermatol. 1981;77:13-9.
3. Kilmer SL, Wheeland RG, Goldberg DJ, et al. Treatment of epidermal pigmented lesions with frequency doubled Q-switched Nd:YAG laser: a controlled, single-impact dose-response multi-center trial. Arch Dermatol. 1994;130(12):1515-9.
4. Wang CC, Chen CK. Effect of spot size and fluence on Q-switched alexandrite laser treatment for pigmentation in Asians: a randomized, double-blinded, split-face comparative trial. J Dermatolog Treat 2011; Jul 14 (Epub ahead of print).
5. Anderson RR, et al. Selective photothermolysis of cutaneous pigmentation by Q-switched Nd-Yag laser-pulses at 1064, 532, and 355 nm. J Invest Dermatol. 1989;93(1):28-32.
6. Shimbashi T, Kamide R, Hashimoto T. Long-term follow-up in treatment of solar lentigo and café-au-lait macules with Q-switched ruby laser. Aesthetic Plast Surg. 1997;21(6):445-8.
7. Levy JL, Mordon S, Pizzi-Anselme M. Treatment of individual café au lait macules with the Q-switched Nd:YAG laser: a clinicopathologic correlation. J Cutan Laser Ther. 1999;1(4):217-23.
8. Ross V, Naseef G, Lin G, et al. Comparison of responses of tattoos to picosecond and nanosecond Q-switched neodymium: YAG lasers. Arch Dermatol. 1998;134(2):167-71.
9. Herd RM, Alora MB, Smoller B, et al. A clinical and histologic prospective controlled comparative study of the Q-switched alexandrite (752 nm) laser for removing tattoo pigment. J Am Acad Dermatol. 1999; 40(4):603-6.
10. Manstein D, Herron GS, Sink RK, et al. Fractional photothermolysis: a new concept for cutaneous remodeling using microscopic patterns of thermal injury. Lasers Surg Med. 2004;34:426-38.
11. Rokhsar CK, Fitzpatrick RE. The treatment of melasma with fractional photothermolysis: a pilot study. Dermatol Surg. 2005;31:1645-50.
12. Goldberg DJ, Berlin AL, Phelps R. Histologic and ultrastructural analysis of melasma after fractional resurfacing. Lasers Surg Med. 2008;40:134-8.
13. Tierney EP, Kouba DJ, Hanke W. Review of fractional photothermolysis: treatment indications and efficacy. Dermatol Surg. 2009;35:1445-61.
14. Polder KD, Bruce S. Treatment of melasma using novel 1,927-nm fractional thulium fiber laser: a pilot study. Dermatol Surg. 2012;38(2):199-206.
15. Weiss E, Bauer JA, Anolik R, et al. 1927-nm fractional resurfacing of facial actinic keratoses: a promising new therapeutic option. J Am Acad Derm. 2013; 68(1):98-102.
16. Masski N, Eimpunth S, Fabi SG, et al. Treatment of melasma with the 1,927-nm fractional thulium fiber laser: a retrospective analysis of 20 cases with long-term follow-up. Lasers Surg Med. 2012; Dec 19. (Epub ahead of print).
17. Li YH, Chen JZ, Wei HC, et al. Efficacy and safety of intense pulsed light in treatment of melasma in Chinese patients. Dermatol Surg. 2008;34(5):693-700.
18. Bjerring P, Christiansen K. Intense pulsed light source for treatment of small melanocytic nevi and solar lentigines. J Cutan Laser Ther. 2000;2(4):177-81.

CHAPTER

4

Tattoos, Melasma and Dermal Pigment

Kelly Stankiewicz

INTRODUCTION

Removal of endogenous and exogenous pigment requires the selective destruction of cellular and subcellular targets. Knowledge of this process rapidly advanced after the introduction of the theory of selective photothermolysis in 1983. This theory predicted that lasers with extremely short pulse durations, like Q-switched (QS) lasers with pulse durations in the nanosecond domain, were needed for the destruction of very small targets, like cells, melanosomes and pigment particles, without collateral damage. This advanced the treatment for many pigmented lesions and tattoos tremendously, giving an important option outside of destruction and scar formation.

The principles for the removal of tattoos and dermal pigment are quite similar, from selection of wavelength and pulse duration, to clinical endpoints and complications.

TATTOO REMOVAL

The art of body tattooing is ancient. It has transcended time periods and civilizations to become a prominent fixture in today's society. The most astounding confirmation of ancient tattooing was the discovery of a five thousand years old bronze age mummy found frozen in the Alps with thirty-nine well-preserved tattoos. Tattooing tools and instruments have been found that date back even further than that—from 38,000 to 10,000 BC.[1] Today, one quarter of the US population between the ages of 18 and 50 has a tattoo, with this number trending upward.[2] For some, permanent tattooing comes with regret. One fifth of tattoo owners are dissatisfied and have considered removal. So, with the increase in placement of tattoos comes the inevitable increase in removal. The most common reasons for tattoo removal are compelling and include the following: embarrassment, feelings of shame or that the tattoo represents a stigma, inability to hide the tattoo with clothing when needed, negative impressions of the tattoo in the workplace or a desire to find a new career or job.[3]

Tattoo removal began as a nonselective and destructive procedure, which aimed to replace the tattoo with scar. Techniques like excision, dermabrasion, salabrasion and CO_2 laser resurfacing were the only options for those who wanted to rid their body of tattoo art. The first treatment of a tattoo with a Q-switched (QS) laser was in the late 1960s, before the physics of laser–skin interactions were truly understood.[4] It was not until after the introduction of the theory of selective photothermolysis in 1983 that the selective removal of tattoos with laser progressed. The theory predicted that lasers with extremely short pulse durations were needed for the selective destruction of tattoo particles without collateral damage. Q-switched lasers with pulse durations in the nanosecond domain were found to successfully treat tattoos without scarring. The widespread use of QS lasers for tattoo removal began in the early 1990s. More than 20 years later, the same techniques are used, but increasing interest in improving tattoo removal has sparked recent advancements.

Laser Principles

Tattoos are exogenous pigment particles found intracellularly within fibroblasts and macrophages distributed perivascularly in the dermis (Fig. 4.1).[5] The particle size ranges from 2 nm to 400 nm with smaller particles grouped into larger membrane-bound granules measuring 0.5–4.0 μm.[5] Selective destruction and elimination of tattoo particles largely depends on two parameters: (1) laser wavelength, which should match the maximum absorption of the tattoo particle, and (2) pulse duration, which is optimized based on the target size. Absorption of laser energy by tattoo particles destroys pigment-containing cells and fragments the tattoo particles. This is accomplished through photomechanical effects, including cavitation, which is the evaporation of water leading to steam bubbles, and shock or acoustic waves, which result from thermal expansion caused by sudden heating. After the laser pulse, the tattoo particles are found extracellularly or within damaged cells, and many of the particles have an altered appearance.[5] Shortly after treatment, an inflammatory infiltrate is seen and the pigment particles are repackaged within phagocytes. The exact mechanism of tattoo lightening is unknown. It is proposed that a combination of phagocytosis and transport of pigment-laden cells, transepidermal elimination, and alteration of the tattoo particle into smaller and less dense fragments, account for tattoo lightening.

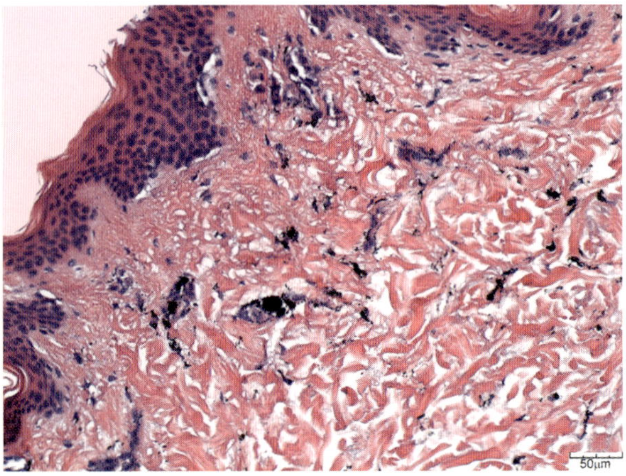

Fig. 4.1: Histologic image of a tattoo showing pigment particles within fibroblasts and macrophages distributed perivascularly within the dermis

Photo Courtesy: H Ray Jalian

Wavelength Selection

Commercially available QS lasers for tattoo removal are the ruby laser (694 nm), alexandrite laser (755 nm), and the Nd:YAG laser (532 nm, 1064 nm). The appropriate wavelength is chosen based on the predicted maximum absorption of tattoo particle, which is dictated by tattoo color. When determining the wavelength of maximum absorption, it is helpful to think of the color wheel, which places complementary colors across from one another. A color absorbs maximally at the wavelength of its complimentary color (Fig. 4.2). For instance, red tattoos absorb green light (450–560 nm) maximally, making the frequency double Nd:YAG (532 nm) the laser of choice. Black ink absorbs all wavelengths of light, making it the easiest color to remove. Orange and yellow absorb at the shortest wavelengths of visible light (400–480 nm) which do not correspond to a commercially available laser, making these tattoo colors the most difficult to remove (Table 4.1).

When selecting wavelength, it is also important to consider skin phototype. Melanin is a chromophore absorbed by all available tattoo lasers. Absorption decreases with increased wavelength (Fig. 4.3) Darker skin types should be treated with longer wavelengths, like the 1064 nm Nd:YAG laser, which has the lowest melanin absorption.

Pulse Duration Selection

According to the theory of selective photothermolysis, a target can be selectively destroyed without collateral

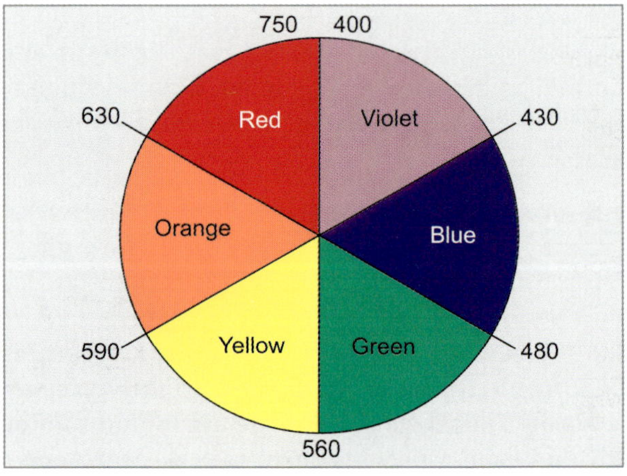

Fig. 4.2: The color wheel. A color absorbs maximally at the wavelength of its complimentary color. The selected wavelength should match the wavelength of complimentary color as closely as possible. Some colors are more difficult to remove because there is no commercially available laser matching the wavelength of maximum absorption

Table 4.1: Ink color and wavelength selection

Ink Color	*Ink Composition*	*Measured Max. Absorption*[53]	*Laser Selection*	*Treatment Notes*
Red	• Mercury sulfide (cinnabar) • Cadmium selenide (cadmium red) • Sienna (red ochre, ferric hydrate and ferric sulfate) • Azo dyes • Hematite (ferric oxide)	500–570 nm	532 nm	Most likely to cause adverse inflammatory reactions
Orange	• Azo dyes • Cadmium seleno-sulfide	420–540 nm	532 nm	
Yellow	• Cadmium sulfide • Ochre • Curcumin yellow • Azo dyes • Limonite • Anthraquinone	470–485 nm	532 nm	
Green	• Chromium oxide (casalis green) • Hydrated chromium sesquioxide (guignet green) • Malachite green • Lead chromate • Ferro-ferric cyanide • Curcumin green • Phthalocyanine dyes (copper salts with yellow coal tar dyes)	570–800 nm	694 nm 755 nm	
Blue	• Cobalt aluminate (azure blue) • Phthalocyanine • Ferric ferocyanide • Indigoid	590–770 nm	630 nm 694 nm 755 nm	
Violet	• Manganese violet • Indigoid	500–570 nm	532 nm 630 nm	
Black	• Amateur: carbon (soot) or India ink • Professional: iron oxide, carbon or logwood extract	600–800 nm	694 nm 755 nm 1064 nm	
Brown	• Ochre	410–550 nm	532 nm 694 nm 755 nm 1064 nm	Immediate ink darkening
White	• Titanium dioxide • Zinc oxide	790 nm	532 nm 755 nm	Immediate ink darkening
Flesh	• Iron oxides	None	532 nm	Immediate ink darkening

damage when the pulse duration of the laser is less than or equal to the thermal relaxation time of the target. The thermal relaxation time is approximately equal to the squared diameter of the target. Given that tattoo particle size ranges from 2 nm to 400 nm, with 40 nm being the most commonly found size,

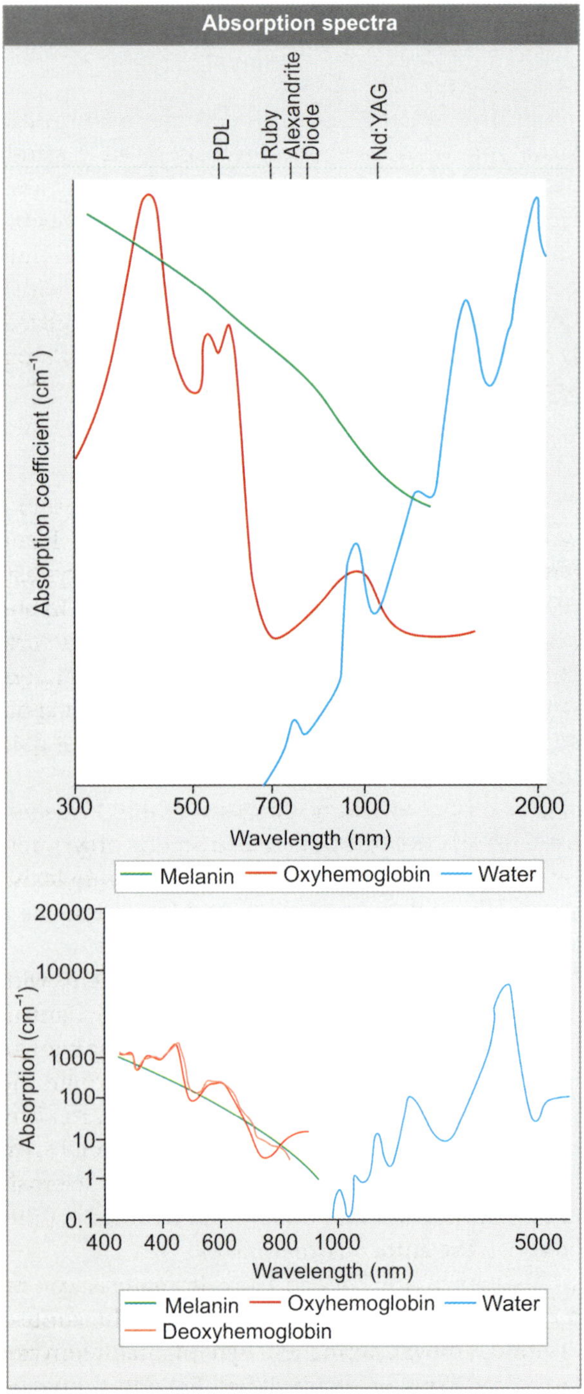

Fig. 4.3: Melanin absorption curve

and granules range from 0.5 μm to 4.0 μm, the ideal pulse duration for destruction of tattoo pigments is in the nanosecond and picosecond domains. Today, the gold standard for tattoo removal is once monthly treatments with QS lasers, which have pulse durations in the nanosecond domain, at wavelengths appropriate for the color of the tattoo and the patient's skin phototype. Picosecond pulse durations may actually be more ideally matched for tattoo removal, especially given the 40 nm particle size most commonly found in professional tattoos. Recent studies have indeed shown greater lightening with picosecond pulse durations when compared to nanosecond pulse durations.[6]

Alternative Treatments

In addition to QS lasers, tattoo removal can be achieved with fractional resurfacing lasers. Fractional lasers destroy a small microcolumn of skin taking the laser ink held within it. When destroying 25% of skin, you can also vaporize 25% of tattoo ink. The concomitant use of QS lasers and fractional lasers in a sequential fashion has been shown to increase patient tolerance for tattoo removal and it may have the potential for enhanced tattoo lightening.[7] Additionally, removal of tattoo by fractional resurfacing is a colorblind process and may be used for cases of resistant ink. Lastly, fractional lasers are a safer option than QS lasers for the removal of allergic tattoos. In one case series, multiple treatments with fractional laser significantly lightened allergic tattoos.[8]

Clinical Principles/Consultation

Tattoo Types

Tattoos can be categorized into several subtypes: professional, amateur, cosmetic, traumatic and medical.

Professional tattoos are exogenous pigment particles placed in the dermis with the moving needle of a tattoo machine. The ink of a professional tattoo is placed at a precise and consistent depth, which has shown to be at the junction of the papillary and reticular dermis extending to the mid-dermis.[5] Professional tattoos are created in an increasing range of colors, many of which are very difficult to treat with commercially available lasers. Cosmetic tattooing, or permanent makeup, is another form of professional tattoo that is becoming increasingly popular. Color can be placed in areas where makeup is ordinarily used, like eyebrows, eyeliner, lip liner, lipstick and blush.

Amateur tattoos are comprised of pigment particles more haphazardly placed with make-shift devices, like handheld needles. The pigment particles in an amateur tattoo can be found extending from the papillary dermis to the subcutaneous fat.[5] The size and shape of amateur tattoo pigment granules are more heterogeneous than those of professional tattoos.[5]

Traumatic tattoos are caused by the inadvertent deposition of pigment from foreign material, such as asphalt or graphite, into the skin. These tattoos are usually easily treated. Tattoos from explosives, like, firework debris or gunpowder should be treated cautiously as laser removal can cause combustion and pock-like scarring.[9]

Medical tattoos are most conventionally placed to mark the sites of radiation. These tattoos are best left in place and should not be removed without the consent of the treating oncologist. An increasing trend is patient imposed medical tattoos warning of medical conditions and even "do not resuscitate" orders. These tattoos are not currently advocated by physicians, but are patient directed. Additionally, flesh-colored tattoos are used to simulate the areola in breast reconstruction surgery or to camouflage scars.

Tattoo Color

The Food and Drug Administration (FDA) considers tattoo pigment to be under its jurisdiction, but admits it has not exercised its authority in this regard.[10] As such, the exact content of tattoo ink is often unknown or kept as a trade secret. Tattoo ink is pigment suspended in a carrier fluid. Most modern day tattoo pigments are made from inorganic compounds such as metal salts, metal oxides and minerals, or synthetic organic pigments such as azo dyes, phthalocyanine and anthraquinone.[11] Common carrier fluids include witch hazel, purified water, ethanol, glycerol and propylene glycol. Carrier fluids not only suspend ink for even placement into the skin, but also act as preservatives to prevent the growth of pathogens in the tattoo ink.

The pigment for amateur black tattoos is usually carbon (soot) or India ink. Professional black tattoos are made from iron oxide, carbon or logwood extract. Red pigment is traditionally mercury sulfide (cinnabar) or cadmium selenide (cadmium red). Due to toxicity, these are no longer used.[11] Alternative red inks include organic dyes (azo dyes) and hematite (ferric oxide). Red inks of all types are most likely to cause adverse inflammatory reactions. White pigment is usually made from titanium dioxide or zinc oxide. Reduction of white tattoo pigment after an initial tattoo removal treatment can cause darkening of the ink (see Table 4.1).

As an alternative to traditional inks, a removable tattoo ink was developed which can be successfully and completely removed with very few laser treatments. The inks are safe and bioremovable substances encased in polymethylmethacrylate beads with gold nanoparticles. When treated with a QS laser, the beads rupture and the ink is solubilized. Unlike traditional tattoo inks, this ink has been specifically tested for its safety and efficacy.

Contraindications

Past history of parenteral gold therapy is an absolute contraindication for treatment with a QS laser. Several case reports describe laser-induced chrysiasis creating a disfiguring hyperpigmentation.[12-14] In one case, electron microscopy demonstrated a structural change in the dermal gold deposits after treatment with a QS Ruby laser.[14] At the minimum, test spots should be done on patients with a history of gold therapy prior to treatment.

Treatment of allergic tattoos with the QS laser is a relative contraindication due to reports of systemic hypersensitivity reactions, including anaphylaxis.[1] Treatment with ablative fractional lasers may be a feasible alternative.[8]

Care should be taken when treating patients with a history of multiple sclerosis. The exact mechanism responsible for tattoo removal is not entirely known, but travel of ink and foreign material through the lymph system is likely involved. Rarely, healthy patients can experience flu-like symptoms with enlarged lymph nodes. Flaring of multiple sclerosis has been seen after tattoo removal treatment. (This has been the author's experience).

Vitiligo, or any koebnerizing dermatosis, can be precipitated by treatment with laser. In the context of tattoo removal, permanent hypopigmentation can be created in patients with vitiligo. Patients should be questioned about history or family history of vitiligo and counseled appropriately.

Treatment Details

Anesthesia

Tattoo removal is painful and anesthesia may be required for patient comfort. Topical anesthesia or local injection in the form of a ring block is the standard. Injection of anesthesia directly under the tattoo may rarely result in bleeding of ink beyond the tattoo boundary after treatment with Q-switched lasers.

Endpoint

The clinical endpoint for tattoo removal is immediate skin whitening. This corresponds to the cavitation reaction seen within pigment-laden cells. Cavitation is the formation of steam bubbles due to the evaporation of water. Pinpoint bleeding follows immediate whitening after treatment with the frequency doubled Nd:YAG (532 nm). Obvious tissue splatter or epidermal disruption is a reaction beyond the desired endpoint and indicates that the fluence should be decreased. Some advocate the use of a clear hydrogel dressing applied to the tattoo prior to treatment to prevent any aerosolized blood or tissue from reaching the treating physician. A loud snapping or sparking sound may indicate that makeup or sunscreen is overlying the tattoo on the skin. This is the sound of plasma formation with QS treatment of titanium dioxide or zinc oxide on the surface of the skin. This is not a harmful reaction, but indicates that the laser energy may not be reaching the tattoo. The skin should be cleaned thoroughly to remove any makeup or sunscreen.

Post-treatment Care

Approximately 15 minutes after treatment, tattoos no longer appear white. They can look purpuric or have pinpoint bleeding. Tattoos will crust for a week to two after the treatment. Post-treatment blistering is common and can be significant.

After treatment, tattoos require specific care. The treatment sites should be covered with petrolatum ointment and telfa bandage. This dressing should be changed daily. Friction to the treated area should be strictly avoided. Friction or repeated removal of crust with the bandage can lead to scarring. The patients should be instructed to avoid sunlight after treatment, as well as prior to treatment.

Number of Treatments Needed

Tattoo removal requires a series of treatments ideally spaced 4–8 weeks apart. Total and complete removal of ink is rare. An average of 4–6 treatments is reported for amateur tattoos and 6–10 treatments for professional tattoos.[15] Although, treatment numbers in excess of 20 are not unusual. As the tattoo fades, it usually fades unevenly with some portions of the tattoo fading faster. The rate of clearance depends on ink color and amount of ink placed by the tattoo artist. Higher color density has been associated with slower response to treatment. Other factors associated with slower clinical response include patients who smoke, colors other than red or black, large tattoos, and tattoos on the lower extremity.[16]

Treatment Complications

Post-treatment blistering occurs frequently, especially after the first treatment sessions. These correspond to subepidermal blisters seen on microscopic examination of skin after treatment with Q-switched lasers.[5] Patients should be instructed not to open or rub the blisters.

Pigmentary alterations are often seen with tattoo removal, especially with QSRL and QS 532 nm, which are more likely to cause temporary or permanent hypopigmentation. Hyperpigmentation can be treated with hydroquinone between treatment sessions.

White and flesh-colored tattoos as well as many cosmetic tattoos in red and brown may turn immediately black or gray upon treatment. It is possible to remove the darkened ink with continued treatments, but it may be more difficult than treating a standard black tattoo.[1,16] Reduction of titanium dioxide and iron oxides are responsible for this color change.[11] Patients with cosmetic, flesh-colored or white tattoos should be counseled on the risk of tattoo darkening and the possibility that the darkened ink may not be removed. White pigment may be present in lighter colored inks, as well, like pink or light blue (Figs 4.4A to C and 4.5A and B). Tattoo artists placing cosmetic tattoos may layer ink colors to achieve the desired color effect. It may be possible to fade more easy to treat colors like black, and leave behind more difficult to treat colors like orange (Figs 4.6 A and B).

Scarring is a potential complication from tattoo removal. The risk of scarring is increased with the use of higher fluences of the QS laser, with tanned skin, and with inappropriate postprocedure care. Lasers with millisecond pulse durations and intense pulsed light devices are not appropriate treatment

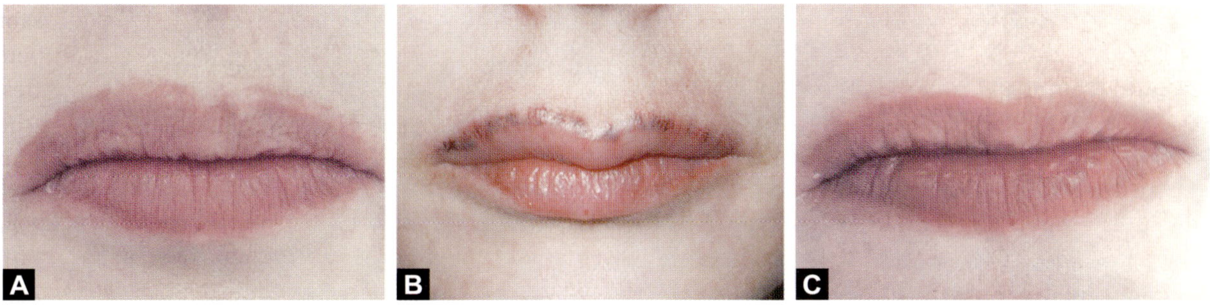

Figs 4.4A to C: Before, during and after treatment of lip liner tattoo showing darkening of ink after one treatment with Q-switched ruby laser and complete removal with one session of repeat treatments

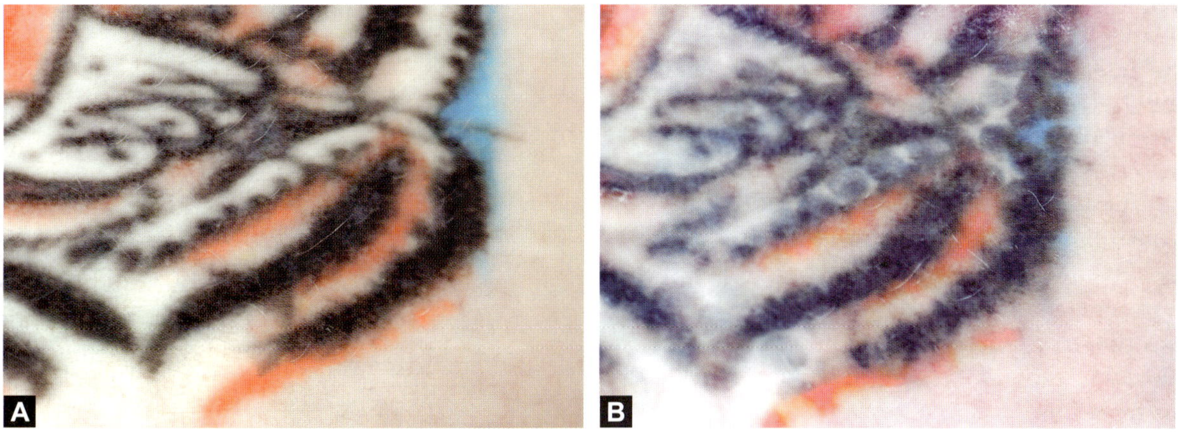

Figs 4.5A and B: Before and after. Darkening of white ink and light blue ink with one treatment with Q-switched alexandrite laser

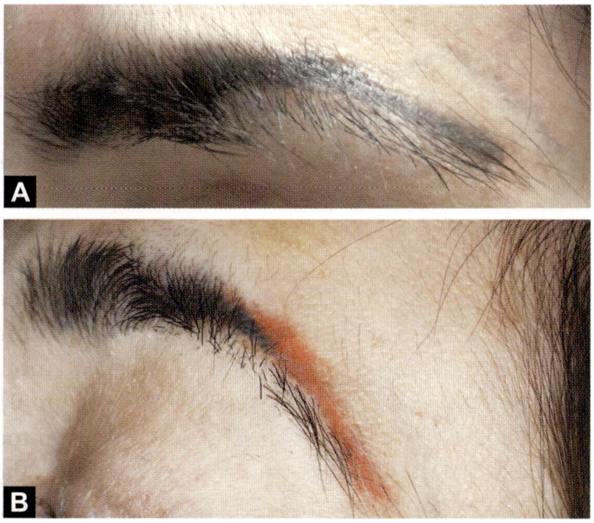

Figs 4.6A and B: Before and after. Cosmetic eyebrow tattoo treated with Q-switched ruby laser. Black ink was successfully treated revealing orange ink that is difficult to treat

options for tattoo removal due to the high potential for scarring.

Immediate and delayed hypersensitivity reactions, both local and systemic, have been reported with tattoo removal.[1,17,18] In one case report, treatment with a QS laser caused a localized urticaria, which was suppressed in subsequent treatments with prophylactic antihistamines and corticosteroids.[17] Tattoo removal treatment can rarely cause flu-like symptoms with fever and enlarged lymph nodes.

Future Directions in Tattoo Removal

Of those with tattoos, an unfortunate 17–20% are dissatisfied enough to consider removal, yet only 0–6% actually seek removal.[2,3] This discrepancy suggests that a widespread need for tattoo removal is not being met.[19] Lack of efficiency in current tattoo removal techniques is likely a major contributing factor. Although relatively effective, modern tattoo removal techniques using once monthly treatment with QS lasers are not necessarily efficient. Numerous treatments are required and complete removal of ink is usually rare, making the process time-consuming, expensive and, sometimes, disappointing. Illustrating this point, one laser center published data showing a very low rate, 1.26%, of complete tattoo clearance and cited patient compliance as a major reason.[20] On average, patients only returned for half the predicted number of treatments required, with authors postulating that patient discouragement, pain and high cost of treatments were responsible. In light of these facts, the need for enhanced tattoo removal techniques is apparent.

Since the advent of the use of QS lasers for tattoo removal approximately 25 years ago, very few advances have been made until recently. Lasers with picosecond-domain pulse durations and combination treatments have shown promising improvement in tattoo removal. According to the theory of selective photothermolysis, the laser destruction of a target is optimized when the pulse duration of the laser is matched to the thermal relaxation time of the light-absorbing targets. For the majority of tattoo particles, the optimal pulse duration is predicted to be in the picosecond domain. Studies showing improvement in tattoo removal with lasers emitting picosecond-domain pulses have been recently published.[21-23]

Combining treatments of the QS laser with either repeated QS treatments or fractional resurfacing treatments has also shown some promise. One study showed a marked improvement in tattoo clearance by repeating treatments with the QS laser on a single tattoo in the same day.[24] In this technique, the immediate whitening was allowed to resolve and the tattoo was treated again. The length of time between treatments was 20 minutes. Sixty-one percent of tattoos were completely removed in one treatment session. These extraordinary results have not yet been duplicated. Repeat treatments with the QS laser may have the most utility in treating inks displaying immediate ink darkening, like white, flesh-colored or cosmetic tattoos (Figs 4.4A to C). Combining the QS laser treatments with fractional resurfacing lasers improves treatment tolerability and may enhance tattoo clearance.[7]

DERMAL PIGMENT

Melasma

Melasma is a pigmentary disorder with an incompletely understood pathogenesis that disproportionately affects women of childbearing age, mostly with darker skin phototypes. However, patients of both sexes and all races and ages can be affected. Classically, melasma can involve the epidermis, dermis or both. Epidermal melasma appears as an ill-defined light brown patch that is accentuated by the Wood's lamp. Dermal melasma may appear more blue-gray due to the Tyndall effect and is not enhanced by the Wood's lamp. Patches appear on face and rarely the arms. Melasma corresponds histologically to enlarged melanocytes within the epidermis with prominent dendritic processes, an increase in melanin containing keratinocytes, and melanophages in the dermis.[25]

Ultraviolet light and hormonal changes are the factors most commonly implicated in melasma. Photosensitizing medications and thyroid or ovarian dysfunction have also been associated. The standards for treatment of melasma include strict sun protection, topical therapies like hydroquinone (HQ), retinoids, and combination formulas (hydroquinone, retinoid and corticosteroid combinations), as well chemical peels and microdermabrasion. Lasers and light therapies have not been the mainstay of treatment for melasma due to high incidence of recurrence and the risk for worsening of pigmentation. Ablative fractional lasers, nonablative fractional lasers, QS lasers and intense pulsed light (IPL) have all been used with varying results.

Treatment Principles

Fractional Lasers

Both ablative and nonablative fractional lasers have been used to treat melasma, with nonablative fractional treatments increasing in popularity. The FDA has approved fractional resurfacing for melasma. The mechanism of action appears to be the destruction of melanocytes and elimination of melanin through the epidermis within the microscopic treatment zones (MTZ).[25,26] Additionally, fractional lasers may serve to increase drug delivery of topical melasma treatments. A study comparing topical combination therapy (HQ, retinoic acid

0.1%, dexamethasone 0.1%) and fractional CO_2 laser treatment for melasma showed a greater improvement in the group treated with the fractional CO_2 laser together with topical combination therapy than either treatment alone.[27] Nonablative fractional laser treatments (either 1550, 1540 or 1927 nm devices) have been shown to improve melasma both with and without topical adjuncts, but the improvement is often not sustainable with recurrence at or before 6 months.[28-32] The rate of post-inflammatory hyperpigmentation and worsening of melasma with nonablative fractional treatments has been reported in some studies to be relatively high, at 28–31% of patients.[33,34] Yet another study showed identical improvement in melasma between the nonablative fractional treatment group and the group using sunscreen as monotherapy.[35] Given the potential for no improvement, the high risk for worsening pigmentation and a nonsustainable result, nonablative fractional therapy is best reserved for those with refractory melasma desiring short-term improvement.

QS Laser

QS lasers are capable of selectively destroying pigment-laden keratinocytes and melanophages and have been used as treatment for melasma. QS neodymium-doped yttrium aluminum garnet (Nd:YAG) laser at low fluences has been most frequently reported to improve melasma.[36-44] Lower fluence QS Nd:YAG laser treatments have demonstrated superiority over higher fluence treatments.[45] Mottled hypopigmentation or punctate leukoderma is a concerning potential side effect.[46] One promising treatment regimen combines low fluence, single pass treatment of QS Nd:YAG laser with microdermabrasion and a topical regimen of HQ and tretinoin. More than 80% of patients achieved greater than 75% improvement in their melasma and this improvement was sustained for up to 12 months.[47] Further studies are being done to evaluate this combination therapy.

Intense Pulsed Light

Treatment of melasma with intense pulsed light (IPL) has been reported to be successful, but has the same limitations as other laser treatments for melasma.[48-50] Recurrence and post-inflammatory hyperpigmentation complicate the treatments making IPL best for those expecting temporary improvement of melasma refractory to medical treatments.

NEVUS OF OTA AND OTHER DERMAL MELANOCYTOSES

Dermal melanocytosis includes Nevus of Ota, Nevus of Ito, acquired bilateral nevus of Ota-like macules (ABNOM), and congenital dermal melanocytosis. Nevus of Ota is a blue-gray patch consisting of coalescing macules present unilaterally on the face in the distribution of the first and second trigeminal nerve. The lesion often extends onto the sclera and can involve other structures in the eye. They are more commonly seen in those of Asian or African descent but can be found in Caucasian skin types as well. Nevus of Ota is present in 0.2–0.8% of all dermatology patients in Japan.[51] Nevus of Ota typically presents either within the first year of life or around puberty. Histologically, there are spindle-shaped dermal melanocytes distributed throughout the dermis between collagen bundles. The melanocytes can be seen around blood vessels and skin appendages as well. Nevus of Ito is a lesion identical in appearance and histology to Nevus of Ota but is seen on the posterior shoulder and scapular area. Acquired bilateral nevus of Ota-like macules (ABNOM) (Hori's macules) are another entity similar to Nevus of Ota. ABNOM are gray-brown to blue-gray macules with a bilateral distribution present on the zygomatic cheeks, mostly in Asian women. The age of onset is greater than Nevus of Ota and the eye is not involved. Histologically, ABNOM consists of spindle-shaped melanocytes that are concentrated in the upper dermis and more often around blood vessels when compared to Nevus of Ota.[52] Lastly, dermal melanocytosis is a congenital blue patch most often seen on the lumbosacral area and buttocks. Rarely, it can be found elsewhere on the body. Lesions typically regress in childhood.

Given location and persistence, Nevus of Ota and ABNOM present the greatest concern to patients, but all dermal melanocytosis can be treated with QS lasers.

Treatment Principles

The pulse duration of QS lasers is optimal for selective destruction of melanocytes making them the ideal tool for treatment of dermal melanocytoses. Nevus of Ota and ABNOM have been successfully treated with the QS ruby laser, QS alexandrite laser, and QS Nd:YAG laser, with ABNOM being more difficult to remove. Local anesthesia may be required and could include nerve blocks or topical anesthesia. The laser–skin interaction is similar to tattoo removal. Immediate whitening, followed by erythema and edema is seen. The average number of treatments needed for removal is 4–8. A significant amount of postinflammatory hyperpigmentation (PIH) can be seen with treatment and usually fades within months. For reasons unknown, treatment of ABNOM results in PIH more often than Nevus of Ota.[52] Postinflammatory hyperpigmentation appears weeks after treatment as a nonmottled hyperpigmentation. Expectations should be set prior to the treatment of ABNOM because treatment may result in more pigmentation than present at baseline.

REFERENCES

1. Bernstein EF. Laser tattoo removal. Semin Plast Surg. 2007;21(3):175-92.
2. Laumann A, Derick A. Tattoos and body piercings in the United States: A national data set. Journal of the American Academy of Dermatology. 2006; 55(3):413-21.
3. Armstrong ML, et al. Motivation for contemporary tattoo removal: a shift in identity. Arch Dermatol. 2008;144(7):879-84.
4. Kent KM,Graber EM. Laser tattoo removal: a review. Dermatol Surg. 2012; 38(1):1-13.
5. Taylor CR, Anderson RR, Gange RW, et al. Light and electron microscopic analysis of tattoos treated by Q-switched ruby laser. J Invest Dermatol. 1991; 97(1):131-6.
6. Izikson L, et al. Safety and effectiveness of black tattoo clearance in a pig model after a single treatment with a novel 758 nm 500 picosecond laser: a pilot study. Lasers Surg Med. 2010;42(7):640-6.
7. Weiss ET, Geronemus RG. Combining fractional resurfacing and Q-switched ruby laser for tattoo removal. Dermatol Surg. 2011;37(1):97-9.
8. Ibrahimi OA, et al. Treatment of tattoo allergy with ablative fractional resurfacing: a novel paradigm for tattoo removal. J Am Acad Dermatol. 2011; 64(6):1111-4.
9. Taylor CR. Laser ignition of traumatically embedded firework debris. Lasers Surg Med.1998;22(3):157-8.
10. Tattoos and Permanent Makeup. 2012 [cited 2012 07/08]; Available from: http://www.fda.gov/cosmetics/productandingredientsafety/productinformation/ucm108530.htm.
11. Ortiz AE, Alster TS. Rising concern over cosmetic tattoos. Dermatol Surg. 2012;38(3):424-9.
12. Almoallim H, et al. Laser induced chrysiasis: disfiguring hyperpigmentation following Q-switched laser therapy in a woman previously treated with gold. J Rheumatol. 2006;33(3):620-1.
13. Geist DE, Phillips TJ. Development of chrysiasis after Q-switched ruby laser treatment of solar lentigines. J Am Acad Dermatol. 2006;55(2 Suppl):S59-60.
14. Trotter MJ, et al. Localized chrysiasis induced by laser therapy. Arch Dermatol. 1995;131(12):1411-4.
15. Jow T, Brown A, Goldberg DJ. Patient compliance as a major determinant of laser tattoo removal success rates: a 10-year retrospective study. J Cosmet Laser Ther. 2010;12(4):166-9.
16. Bencini PL, et al. Removal of tattoos by Q-switched laser: variables influencing outcome and sequelae in a large cohort of treated patients. Arch Dermatol. 2012;148(12):1364-9.
17. England RW, Vogel P, Hagan L. Immediate cutaneous hypersensitivity after treatment of tattoo with Nd:YAG laser: a case report and review of the literature. Ann Allergy Asthma Immunol. 2002;89(2): 215-7.
18. Ashinoff R, Levine VJ, Soter NA. Allergic reactions to tattoo pigment after laser treatment. Dermatol Surg. 1995;21(4):291-4.
19. Anderson R. Commentary: Tattoos and body piercing. Journal of the American Academy of Dermatology. 2006;55(3):422.
20. Jow T, Brown A, Goldberg DJ. Patient compliance as a major determinant of laser tattoo removal success rates: a 10-year retrospective study. J Cosmet Laser Ther. 2010;12(4):166-9.
21. Izikson L, et al. Safety and effectiveness of black tattoo clearance in a pig model after a single treatment with a novel 758 nm 500 picosecond laser: a pilot study. Lasers in Surgery and Medicine. 2010;42(7):640-6.
22. Ross V, et al. Comparison of responses of tattoos to picosecond and nanosecond Q-switched neodymium: YAG lasers. Arch Dermatol. 1998;134(2): 167-71.
23. Brauer JA, et al. Successful and rapid treatment of blue and green tattoo pigment with a novel picosecond laser. Arch Dermatol. 2012;148(7):820-3.
24. Kossida T, et al. Optimal tattoo removal in a single laser session based on the method of repeated exposures. J Am Acad Dermatol. 2012;66(2):271-7.
25. Goldberg DJ, Berlin AL, Phelps R. Histologic and ultrastructural analysis of melasma after fractional resurfacing. Lasers Surg Med. 2008;40(2):134-8.
26. Hantash BM, et al. Laser-induced transepidermal elimination of dermal content by fractional photothermolysis. J Biomed Opt. 2006;11(4):041115.

27. Trelles MA, Velez M, Gold MH. The treatment of melasma with topical creams alone, CO_2 fractional ablative resurfacing alone, or a combination of the two: a comparative study. J Drugs Dermatol. 2010;9(4):315-22.
28. Lee HS, et al. Treatment of melasma in Asian skin using a fractional 1,550-nm laser: an open clinical study. Dermatol Surg. 2009;35(10):1499-504.
29. Katz TM, et al. Treatment of melasma using fractional photothermolysis: a report of eight cases with long-term follow-up. Dermatol Surg. 2010;36(8): 1273-80.
30. Kroon MW, et al. Nonablative 1550-nm fractional laser therapy versus triple topical therapy for the treatment of melasma: a randomized controlled pilot study. J Am Acad Dermatol. 2011;64(3):516-23.
31. Tourlaki A, et al. Combination of fractional erbium-glass laser and topical therapy in melasma resistant to triple-combination cream. J Dermatolog Treat; 2012.
32. Rokhsar CK, Fitzpatrick RE. The treatment of melasma with fractional photothermolysis: a pilot study. Dermatol Surg. 2005;31(12):1645-50.
33. Hong SP, et al. Split-face comparative study of 1550 nm fractional photothermolysis and trichloroacetic acid 15% chemical peeling for facial melasma in Asian skin. J Cosmet Laser Ther. 2012;14(2):81-6.
34. Wind BS, et al. Non-ablative 1,550 nm fractional laser therapy versus triple topical therapy for the treatment of melasma: a randomized controlled split-face study. Lasers Surg Med. 2010;42(7):607-12.
35. Karsai S, et al. Is non-ablative 1550-nm fractional photothermolysis an effective modality to treat melasma? Results from a prospective controlled single-blinded trial in 51 patients. J Eur Acad Dermatol Venereol. 2012; 26(4):470-6.
36. Cho SB, Kim JS, Kim MJ. Melasma treatment in Korean women using a 1064-nm Q-switched Nd:YAG laser with low pulse energy. Clin Exp Dermatol. 2009;34(8):e847-50.
37. Wang HW ,Liu KY. Efficacy and safety of low-energy QS Nd:YAG and QS alexandrite laser for melasma. Zhongguo Yi Xue Ke Xue Yuan Xue Bao. 2009; 31(1):45-7.
38. Choi M, et al. Low-dose 1064-nm Q-switched Nd:YAG laser for the treatment of melasma. J Dermatolog Treat. 2010;21(4):224-8.
39. Polnikorn N. Treatment of refractory melasma with the MedLite C6 Q-switched Nd:YAG laser and alpha arbutin: a prospective study. J Cosmet Laser Ther. 2010;12(3):126-31.
40. Wattanakrai P, Mornchan R, Eimpunth S. Low-fluence Q-switched neodymium-doped yttrium aluminum garnet (1,064 nm) laser for the treatment of facial melasma in Asians. Dermatol Surg. 2010;36(1):76-87.
41. Brown AS, Hussain M, Goldberg DJ. Treatment of melasma with low fluence, large spot size, 1064-nm Q-switched neodymium-doped yttrium aluminum garnet (Nd:YAG) laser for the treatment of melasma in Fitzpatrick skin types II-IV. J Cosmet Laser Ther. 2011;13(6):280-2.
42. Park KY, et al. A randomized, observer-blinded, comparison of combined 1064-nm Q-switched neodymium-doped yttrium-aluminium-garnet laser plus 30% glycolic acid peel vs. laser monotherapy to treat melasma. Clin Exp Dermatol. 2011;36(8):864-70.
43. Suh KS, et al. Efficacy of the 1064-nm Q-switched Nd:YAG laser in melasma. J Dermatolog Treat. 2011; 22(4):233-8.
44. Zhou X, et al. Efficacy and safety of Q-switched 1,064-nm neodymium-doped yttrium aluminum garnet laser treatment of melasma. Dermatol Surg. 2011; 37(7):962-70.
45. Kar HK, Gupta L, Chauhan A. A comparative study on efficacy of high and low fluence Q-switched Nd:YAG laser and glycolic acid peel in melasma. Indian J Dermatol Venereol Leprol. 2012;78(2): 165-71.
46. Chan NP, et al. A case series of facial depigmentation associated with low fluence Q-switched 1,064 nm Nd:YAG laser for skin rejuvenation and melasma. Lasers Surg Med. 2010;42(8):712-9.
47. Kauvar AN. Successful treatment of melasma using a combination of microdermabrasion and Q-switched Nd:YAG lasers. Lasers Surg Med. 2012; 44(2):117-24.
48. Li YH, et al. Efficacy and safety of intense pulsed light in treatment of melasma in Chinese patients. Dermatol Surg. 2008;34(5):693-700; discussion 700-1.
49. Zoccali G, et al. Melasma treated with intense pulsed light. Aesthetic Plast Surg. 2010;34(4):486-93.
50. Wang CC, et al. Intense pulsed light for the treatment of refractory melasma in Asian persons. Dermatol Surg. 2004;30(9):1196-200.
51. Taylor CR, et al. Treatment of nevus of Ota by Q-switched ruby laser. J Am Acad Dermatol. 1994; 30(5 Pt 1):743-51.
52. Lee B, Kim YC, Kang WH, et al. Comparison of characteristics of acquired bilateral nevus of Ota-like macules and nevus of Ota according to therapeutic outcome. J Korean Med Sci. 2004;19(4):554-9.
53. Beute TC, et al. In vitro spectral analysis of tattoo pigments. Dermatol Surg. 2008;34(4):508-15; discussion 515-6.

CHAPTER 5

Laser Hair Removal

Omar A Ibrahimi, Suzanne L Kilmer, Mathew M Avram

INTRODUCTION

The ability of lasers to nonspecifically damage hair follicles was noted nearly 50 years ago in the first reports on the use of lasers on human skin. However, it was not until the theory of selective photothermolysis was proposed by Anderson and Parrish at the Wellman Center for Photomedicine at Harvard Medical School, that the concept of selectively targeting a particular chromophore based on its absorption spectra and size was realized. Several years later, this group also reported the first successful use of a normal-mode ruby laser for long-term and permanent hair removal.

Today, removing unwanted body hair is an increasingly prevalent trend in our society, and photoepilation by laser or other light-based technology is the fastest growing procedure in cosmetic dermatology. Other methods for removing unwanted hair include bleaching, plucking, shaving, waxing and chemical depilatories. Threading is a common practice in some cultures. None of these methods provide a permanent solution to unwanted hair, and can be inconvenient and tedious. Electrolysis is a method for hair removal in which a fine needle deep into the hair follicle destroys the follicle via electrical current, thus allowing for permanent hair removal of both terminal and nonterminal hair, as well as of both pigmented and nonpigmented hair. However, this technique is extremely operator dependent and efficacy in achieving permanent hair removal is variable among patients. Thus, it is often impractical in terms of treating large areas. Eflornithine is a topical inhibitor of ornithine decarboxylase that slows the rate of hair growth and is effective for unwanted facial hair, and is currently indicated for the removal of unwanted facial hair in women. Eflornithine can be combined with lasers and intense pulsed light (IPL) for hair removal. In this chapter, we provide a detailed overview on laser hair removal (LHR) including discussion of hair follicle biology, the science behind LHR, key factors in optimizing treatment and future trends.

THE HAIR FOLLICLE

Hair Anatomy

The hair follicle is an intricate, hormonally active structure with a programmed growth pattern (Fig. 5.1). It is anatomically divided into the infundibulum (hair follicle orifice to insertion of the sebaceous gland), isthmus (insertion of the sebaceous gland to the insertion of the arrector pili muscle), and inferior (insertion of the arrector pili to the base of the hair follicle) segments. The dermal papilla, a neurovascular structure that supplies the cells of the proliferating matrix at the base of the follicle, helps form the hair shaft.

Hair Growth

Each hair follicle consists of a permanent (upper) and nonpermanent (lower) part, with the follicular bulge forming the lowermost aspect of the permanent

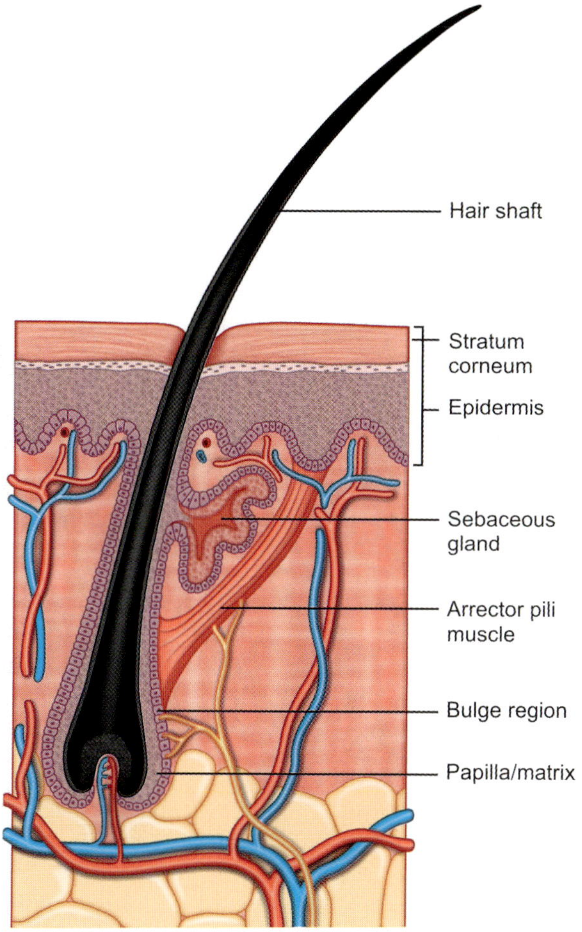

Fig. 5.1: Anatomy of the hair follicle
Source: Reproduced from Tsao SS, Hruza GJ. Laser hair removal. In: Robinson JK, Hanke CW, Sengelmann RD, Siegel DM, (Eds). Surgery of the Skin. Philadelphia: Elsevier Mosby; 2005.pp.575-88

part. In periods of active growth (anagen) the rapidly developing bulbar matrix cells differentiate into the hair shaft and the hair lengthens. A transition period follows in which the bulbar part of the hair follicle undergoes degradation through apoptosis (catagen). A resting period (telogen) phase ensues, and regrowth is started once again in early anagen. Stem cells within the hair follicle regenerate the follicle within or near the hair bulb matrix. Slow-cycling stem cells have also been found in the follicular bulge arising off the outer root sheath at the site of arrector pili muscle attachment. The duration of each growth phase is body site dependent.

Hair Types

There are three main types of hair: lanugo, vellus and terminal hairs. Lanugo hairs are fine hairs that cover a fetus and are shed in the neonatal period. Vellus hairs are nonpigmented, and have a diameter of roughly 30 μm. Terminal hair shafts range from 150 μm to 300 μm in cross-sectional diameter. The type of hair produced by an individual follicle is capable of change (e.g. vellus to terminal hair at puberty or terminal to vellus hair in androgenic alopecia).

Hair Color

Hair color is determined by the amount of pigment in the hair shaft. Melanocytes produce two types of melanin—eumelanin, a brown-black pigment; and pheomelanin, a red pigment. Melanocytes are located in the upper portion of the hair bulb and outer root sheath of the infundibulum.

Classification of Excess Hair

Excessive and unwanted body hair ranges in severity, depending on cultural mores, and can usually be classified as either hypertrichosis or hirsutism. Hirsutism is defined as the abnormal growth of terminal hair in women in male-pattern (androgen-dependent) sites, such as the face and chest. Hypertrichosis refers to excess hair growth at any body site that is not androgen-dependent. Additionally, the use of grafts and flaps in dermatologic and reconstructive skin surgery can often introduce hair to an area that causes a displeasing appearance or functional impairment.

MECHANISM OF LASER HAIR REMOVAL

The theory of selective photothermolysis enables one to selectively target pigmented hair follicles by using the melanin of the hair shaft as a chromophore. Melanin is capable of functioning as a chromophore for wavelengths in the red and near-infrared portion of the electromagnetic spectrum. However, to achieve permanent hair removal the biological "target" is likely the follicular stem cells located in the bulge region and/or dermal papilla. Based on the slight spatial separation of the chromophore and the desired target, an extended theory of selective photothermolysis was proposed which requires diffusion of heat from the chromophore to the desired target for destruction. This requires a laser pulse duration that is longer in duration than if the actual chromophore and desired target were identical.

Temporary LHR can result when the follicular stem cells are not completely destroyed, primarily through induction of a catagen-like state in pigmented hair follicles. Temporary LHR is much easier to achieve than permanent removal, using lower fluences. Long-term hair removal depends on hair color, skin color and tolerated fluence. Roughly 15–30% long-term hair loss may be observed with each treatment when optimal treatment parameters are used. A list of laser and light devices that are commercially available at the time of this publication for hair removal are summarized in Table 5.1.

Table 5.1: Commercially available lasers and light sources for hair removal*

Laser/Light Source	*Wave-length (nm)*	*System Name*	*Pulse Duration (ms)*	*Fluence (J/cm²)*	*Spot Size (mm)*	*Other Features*
Long-pulsed ruby	694	RubyStar and Ruby Star + (Aesclepion, Germany)	4	Up to 24	8, 10, 12, 18	Contact cooling
Long-pulsed alexandrite	755	Apogee (Cynosure, Westford, MA, USA)	0.5–300	25–50	5–15	Cold air or integrated cooling, can add 1064 nm Nd:YG module to form Apogee Elite
		Arion (Quantel Derma, Germany)	5–140	Up to 40	6–16	Cold air cooling
		ClearScan ALX (Sciton, Palo Alto, CA, USA)	Up to 200	Up to 140	3, 6 and 30×30	Contact cooling
		Coolglide (Cutera, Brisbane, CA, US)	0.1–300	5–300	10	Contact cooling
		Elite (Cynosure)	0.5–300	25–50	5–15	Cold air cooling, available with 1064 nm Nd:YAG, Elite MPX model can simultaneously treat with 755 nm alexandrite and 1064 nm Nd:YAG
		EpiCare LP/ LPX (Light Age, Somerset, NJ, USA)	3–300	22–40	7–46	
		GentleLASE, (Syneron-Candela, Wayland, MA, USA)	3	Up to 100	6–18	Dynamic cooling
		GentleMax (Syneron-Candela)	0.25–300	Up to 600	1.5–18	Dynamic cooling, comes with 1064 Nd:YAG
		Ultrawave 755/II/ III (AMC Aesthetics and Advance Aesthetic Concepts, Plattsburgh, NY, USA)	Up to 100	Up to 125	Up to 16	Available with 532, 1064, and 1320 nm Nd:YAG
Diode	800–810	F1 Diode (Opusmed, Canada)	15–40	Up to 40	5, 7	Chiller tip

Contd...

Contd...

	808, 980	Leda (Quantel Derma)	6–60	Up to 60	50×12, 10×12	Contact cooling
	810, 940	MeDioStar XT (Aesclepion)	5–500	Up to 90	6, 12	Integrated scanner with cold air cooling
	800	LightSheer Duet (Lumenis, Israel)	5–400	10–100, 4.5–12	9×9, 22×35	Chilltip for smaller handpiece, vacuum skin flattening for larger handpiece
	810	Soprano XL (Alma Lasers, Buffalo Grove, IL, USA)	10–1350	Up to 120	12×10	Contact cooling
Long-pulsed Nd:YAG	1064	Acclaim (Cynosure)	0.4–300	35–600	1.5–15	Cold air or integrated cooling, can add 755 nm alexandrite module to form Apogee Elite (Cynosure)
		ClearScan YAG (Sciton)	0.3–200	Up to 400	3,6 and 30×30	Contact cooling
		CoolGlide CV/XEO/Excel/Vantage (Cutera)	0.1–300	Up to 300	3–10	Contact cooling
		Cynergy (Cynosure)	0.3–300	Up to 600	1.5–15	Cold air
		SP and XP Dynamis, XP Focus, XP Max (Fotona)	0.1–50	Up to 300	2–10	N/A
		GentleYAG (Syneron-Candela, Wayland, MA)	0.25–300	Up to 600	1.5–18	Dynamic cooling
		Gemini (Cutera)	1–100	Up to 990	2, 10	Available with 532 nm KTP
		LightPod Neo (Aerolase, Tarrytown, NY, USA)	0.65–1.5	Up to 312	2	Built-in cooling system
		Lyra (Cutera)	20–100	5–900	1–5, 10	Contact cooling
		MultiFlex(Ellipse, United Kingdom)	N/A	Up to 600	1.5–5	Equipped with IPL device
		Mydon (Quante Dermal)	0.5–90	10–450	1.5–10	Integrated air cooling
		NaturaLase 1064/LP (Focus Medical, Bethel, CT, USA)	0.5–100	Up to 400	3–15	Integrated air cooling
		Profile (Sciton)	0.1–10000	Up to 75	N/A	Contact cooling, 2490 nm Er: YAG and 410–1400 nm flashlamp in same device

Contd...

Contd...

		SmartEpil (Deka, Italy)	Up to 20	11	2.5, 4, 5, 6	
		Synchro_FT (Deka)	2–30	Up to 50	2.5–13	
		Ultrawave II/III (AMC Aesthetics, and Advance Aesthetic Concepts)	Up to 300	5–500	Up to 12	Available with IPL handpiece
		Varia (CoolTouch, Roseville, CA, USA)	0.6	Up to 500	2–10	Pulsed cryogen cooling
						Dynamic cryogen cooling
Intense-pulsed light sources	520–1200	Axiom (Viora, Jersey City, NJ, USA)	25–75 and 2.2–12.5	Up to 39	50×25, 35×15, 20×10	Built-in cooling system
		BBL (Sciton)				
	420–1400	Cynergy (Cynosure)	Up to 200	Up to 30	15×45	Built-in cooling system
	560–590	Duet/SkinStation/ SpaTouch II (Radiancy	0.3–300	Up to 600	N/A	Built-in cooling system
	400–1200	Orangeburg, NY, USA)	3–10	35	22×55	
		Ellipse 12PL/ MultiFlex (Ellipse)				
	600–950	Harmony XL (Alma Lasers)	2.5–88.5	4–26	10×48	MultiFlex model with long-pulsed Nd:YAG
	650–950	iPulse (Dermavista, Birmingham, AL, USA)	30–50	Up to 40	30×30	Available with 755 nm alexandrite and 1064 and 1320 nm Nd:YAG
	530–1200	Med Flash II (General Project, Italy)	10–110	Up to 20	8.9 cm^2	Air cooling
	390–1200	Icon/StarLux, R, Rs (Palomar, Burlington, MA, USA)	Up to 100	Up to 45	N/A	
	525–1200	MiniSilk_FT (Deka)	5–500	Up to 70	28×12, 46×16	1064 Nd:YAG handpiece
	500–1200	Mistral (Radiancy)	3–8	Up to 160	48×13, 23×13	Contact cooling
	400–1200	NannoLight MP50 (Sybaritic, Minneapolis, MN, USA)	Up to 80		25×50, 13×50, 13×35, 12×12	
	640–1400		1–30	4–15	40×8	

Contd...

Contd...

		NaturaLight (Solamed, Tampa, FL, US)		2.8–50		Nd:YAG handpiece, optional cooling
	640–1200	Solera Opus (Cutera)	Up to 500	Up to 50	10×40	
	750–1100	PhotoSilk Plus (Deka)	Auto	3–24	10×30	
	550–950	ProWave (Cutera)	Up to 30	10–340	21×10, 46×10, 46×18	Nd:YAG handpiece
	770–1100	Quadra Q4 (DermaMed, Lenni, PA, USA)	Auto	5–35	10×30	
		Quantum HR (Lumenis)				
	500–1200	SmoothCool (Eclipse, Dallas, TX, USA)	48	10–20	33×15	Built-in cooling system
	695–1200		15–100	25–45	34×8	
	560–950	Trios (Viora)	1–60	10–45	8×34	Automatic temperature control system
	530–1200		25	Up to 22	15×50	
Fluorescent pulsed light	615–920	OmniLight/ NovaLight (American Medical Bio Care, Newport Beach, CA, USA)	2–500	Up to 90	7×15, 10×20, 30×30	Sapphire tip cooling
Optical energy combined with radiofrequency (RF) electrical energy	580–980	eMax//eLight (Syneron)	Up to 100	Up to 50 optical; Up to 50 J/cm^3 RF	12×15	Contact cooling
Diode combined with RF electrical energy	800	eLaser (Syneron)	Up to 100	Up to 50 optical; Up to 50 J/cm^3 RF	12×15	Contact cooling
	810	MeDioStar Effect (Aesclepion)	Up to 500	Up to 90	10, 12, 14	Acoustic wave technology, integrated scanner with cold air cooling device, 940 nm simultaneously

*This table is intended only as a reference aid. The authors have made every attempt to provide an exhaustive list of available devices for laser hair removal but do not guarantee comprehensiveness.

KEY FACTORS IN OPTIMIZING TREATMENT

The ability to selectively target hair follicles with lasers and light sources has revolutionized the ability to eliminate unwanted hair temporarily and permanently in many individuals. As laser technology advances, the ability to treat individuals of all skin types and all hair colors broadens. Proper patient selection, preoperative preparation, informed consent, understanding of the principles of laser safety, and laser and light source selection are key to the success of laser treatment. An understanding of hair anatomy, growth and physiology, together with a thorough understanding of laser–tissue interaction, in particular within the context of choosing optimal laser parameters for effective LHR, should be acquired before using lasers for hair removal.

Patient Selection

Despite the seemingly cosmetic nature of LHR, a focused medical history, physical examination and informed consent, including setting realistic patient expectations and potential risks, should be performed prior to any laser treatment. Any patient with evidence for endocrine or menstrual dysfunction should be appropriately worked up. Similarly, patients with an explosive onset of hypertrichosis should be evaluated for paraneoplastic etiologies. Treatment of a pregnant woman for nonurgent conditions is discouraged, although there is no evidence suggesting a potential risk to pregnant women undergoing LHR. The past medical history should be reviewed to identify patients with photosensitive conditions, such as the autoimmune connective tissue disorders, or disorders prone to the Koebner phenomenon. A history of recurrent cutaneous infections at or in the vicinity of treatment area might warrant the use of prophylactic medications. Any past history of keloid or hypertrophic scar formation should be elicited as well. Previous methods for hair removal, including any past laser treatments, should be reviewed. Any methods of epilation, such as waxing or tweezing, that entirely remove the target chromophore, render LHR ineffective for at least 2 weeks. Although there is little evidence for the time frame, a patient must wait after complete epilation of the hair shaft and laser treatment, the authors recommend a minimum of 6 weeks. Shaving and depilatory creams can be used up to the day of laser treatment as they do not remove the entire hair shaft.

A thorough medication history should be obtained. Any history of gold intake is a contraindication for laser therapy with Q-switched lasers. The use of any photosensitizing medications or over-the-counter supplements should also delay treatment until these medications can be safely discontinued. There is controversy as to whether patients on isotretinoin should be treated with laser, although conventionally most practitioners recommend a 6 month to 1 year washout period prior to laser treatment. Topical retinoids used in the treatment area should be discontinued 1–2 days prior to treatment.

One should evaluate the patient's Fitzpatrick skin phototype. This will help determine which lasers and light sources are safe to use for that patient (Table 5.1), because epidermal melanin in darkly pigmented patients can compete with the melanin within hair follicles as the target chromophore. Importantly, every patient should always be evaluated for the presence of a tan, and if present, laser treatment should be delayed or the treatment parameters appropriately adjusted until the tan has faded. The physical examination should also document the coarseness and quality of the hair to be treated. Finally, the patient's hair color should be noted as the chromophore for LHR is melanin. Black and brown hair contain sufficient amounts of melanin to serve as a chromophore for LHR. In contrast the lack of melanin, paucity of melanin or presence of eumelanin in the hair follicle, which clinically correlates to white, gray, or red/blonde hair, is predictive of a poor response to laser hair removal. For patients with little to no melanin in their hair follicles, attempts have been made to use an exogenous chromophore that can be topically delivered to the hair follicles, thereby making the removal of white, gray, red and blonde hair hypothetically possible. This concept was first demonstrated with a topical carbon solution dissolved in mineral oil. However, the authors have noticed very little efficacy of topical chromophores in their vast experience.

Informed Consent

An explanation of the potential risks of LHR should be reviewed as part of the informed consent process. The risks include but are not limited to temporary and permanent hypo/hyperpigmentation, blister formation, scar formation, ulceration, hive-like response, bruising, infection, acne flare and folliculitis. For those patients with Fitzpatrick skin type IV or greater or of Mediterranean, Middle Eastern, Asian or South Asian descent, the low risk of paradoxical hypertrichosis (conversion of vellus hairs to terminal hairs), especially when treating the lateral face and jaw, should be reviewed. Patients should be counseled that permanent and complete hair removal is not likely but that with multiple treatments, significant long-term reduction can be achieved. Hirsute women with hormonal abnormalities may require continued maintenance therapy and should be advised of this possibility. Procedural pain is expected with LHR but can be minimized with topical anesthetics. Erythema and edema are also expected with treatment and may last up to 1 week. Patients should be aware of the need for strict sun avoidance for a minimum of 6 weeks before and after each treatment.

Preoperative Preparation and Laser Safety

The need for topical anesthesia is variable amongst patients and particular anatomic sites. Various topical anesthetics including lidocaine, lidocaine/prilocaine and other amide/ester anesthetic combinations can be used to diminish the procedural discomfort, and should be applied 30 minutes to 1 hour before treatment under occlusion. Care should be taken when using lidocaine or prilocaine to apply these medications to a limited area to diminish the risk of lidocaine toxicity or methemoglobulinemia, respectively.

Patients should be placed in a room with a treatment chair that makes the desired treatment area easily accessible. The room should be adequately cooled to keep the laser device from overheating and be free of any hanging mirrors or uncovered windows. A fire extinguisher should be readily available, especially if oxygen is being used. Having a vacuum device on hand during treatment can minimize the plume and unpleasant odor created by each laser pulse. Because the retina contains melanin which can be damaged by all LHR devices, proper eye protection is absolutely critical for both the patient and laser surgeon. Each device requires the use of protective goggles that are unique to the device's particular wavelengths. Goggles cannot be interchangeably used with laser or IPL devices of other wavelengths. Furthermore, because of the risk of retinal damage, it is the authors' strong opinion that one should never treat a patient for LHR within the bony orbit.

Device Variables

Wavelength

The chromophore for laser hair removal is melanin. Within the hair follicle, melanin is principally located within the hair shaft, although the outer root sheath and matrix area also contain melanin. Melanin is capable of functioning as a chromophore for wavelengths in the red and near-infrared portion of the electromagnetic spectrum, and can be targeted by ruby, alexandrite, diode and Nd:YAG lasers, as well as IPL devices.

The long-pulsed ruby laser (694 nm) was the first device used to selectively target hair follicles, resulting in long-term (2 years) hair loss (6-mm spot size, 270 μs pulse duration and fluences of 30–60 J/cm^2). The long-pulsed ruby laser can be safely used in Fitzpatrick skin phototypes I–III. A large multicenter trial of nearly two hundred patients showed that the majority of patients had more than 75% hair loss at 6-month follow-up after an average of four treatments. Table 5.1 lists the long-pulsed ruby lasers that are commercially available.

The long-pulsed alexandrite (755 nm) laser has been shown to be effective for hair removal in multiple studies. The long-pulsed alexandrite laser can be safely used in Fitzpatrick skin phototypes I–IV, although some experts limit the use of the long-pulsed alexandrite laser to Fitzpatrick skin phototypes I–III. A few studies have demonstrated the safety of the long-pulsed alexandrite laser in a large cohort of patients with Fitzpatrick skin phototypes IV–VI. A randomized, investigator-blinded clinical trial of subjects with Fitzpatrick skin phototypes III–IV treated with a long-pulsed alexandrite laser (12- and 18-mm spot size, 1.5 ms pulse duration and fluences of 20 or 40 J/cm^2) for 4 sessions at 8-week interval showed 76–84% hair reduction 18 months after the last treatment and provides the best evidence for long-term hair removal efficacy with the alexandrite laser. A randomized controlled trial of 144 Asian subjects with Fitzpatrick skin types III–V with a long pulsed alexandrite laser (12.5-mm spot size, pulse duration of 40 ms, fluences of 16–24 J/cm^2) found that subjects with three treatments had 55% hair reduction compared to subjects treated two times with 44% hair reduction and subjects treated one time had 32% hair reduction at 9 months follow-up. Combination treatment of alexandrite and

Nd:YAG lasers provides no added benefit over the alexandrite laser alone. The commercially available long-pulsed alexandrite devices are summarized in Table 5.1.

The long-pulsed diode (800–810 nm) laser has also been extensively used for LHR. The diode laser can be safely used in patients with Fitzpatrick skin phototypes I–V. Two long-term nonrandomized controlled studies showed roughly 40% hair reduction at a mean follow-up of 20 months after one or two treatments (9-mm spot size, pulse duration of 5–30 ms, fluences of 15–40 J/cm^2), and 84% hair reduction at one year follow-up after 4 treatments (9-mm spot size, pulse duration of 5–30 ms, fluences of 12– 40 J/cm^2) demonstrated the efficacy of the diode laser for long-term hair removal.

The long-pulsed Nd:YAG laser has been thought to offer the best combination of safety and efficacy for Fitzpatrick skin phototype VI patients. Long-term hair reduction with 18-month followship showed 73.6% clearance following four treatments at 2-month intervals.

Intense pulsed light is composed of polychromatic, noncoherent light ranging from 400–1200 nm. Various filters can be used to target particular chromophores, including melanin. Long-term (>1 year) hair removal has not been convincingly demonstrated to date. Various reports have demonstrated short-term efficacy. One study of patients treated with a single IPL session reported 75% hair removal 1 year after treatment. Two studies providing a head-to-head comparison of IPL versus either the long-pulsed alexandrite laser, or Nd:YAG laser both found the IPL to be inferior to laser devices for hair removal. In contrast, a study of hirsute women, some with a diagnosis of polycystic ovarian syndrome, who underwent a split face treatment with six IPL or long-pulse diode laser (LPDL), show statistically equivalent reductions in hair counts at one (77% vs 68%, respectively), three (53% vs 60%, respectively) and six months (40% vs 34%, respectively) after the final treatment.

Fluence

Fluence is defined as the amount of energy delivered per unit area and is expressed as J/cm^2. Higher fluences have been correlated with greater permanent hair removal, but are also more likely to cause untoward side-effects. Recommended treatment fluences are often provided with each individual laser device for nonexperienced operators. However, a more appropriate method of determining the optimal treatment fluence for a given patient is to evaluate for the desired clinical endpoint of perifollicular erythema and edema (Fig. 5.2). The highest possible tolerated fluence which yields this endpoint, without any adverse effects, is the best fluence for treatment.

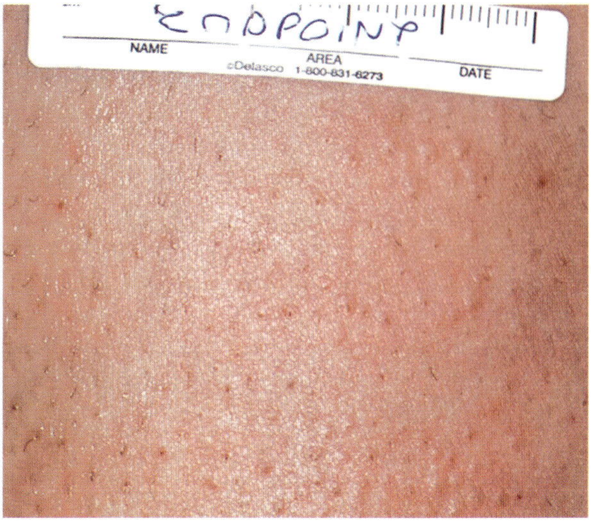

Fig. 5.2: Appropriate clinical endpoint of perifollicular erythema and edema

Pulse Duration

Pulse duration is defined as the duration in seconds of laser exposure. The theory of selective photothermolysis enables the laser surgeon to select an optimal pulse duration based on the thermal relaxation time (TRT). Terminal hairs are about 300 μm in diameter, and thus the calculated TRT of a terminal hair follicle is about 100 ms. However, unlike many other laser applications, the hair follicle is distinct in that there is a spatial separation of the chromophore (melanin) within the hair shaft and the biological "target" stem cells in the bulge and bulb areas of the follicle. The expanded theory of selective photothermolysis takes this spatial separation into account and proposes a thermal damage time (TDT), which is longer than the TRT. Shorter pulse widths are also capable of removing hair, and it is unclear which is more effective in producing permanent hair removal. Longer pulse widths are likely more selective for melanin within the hair follicle and can minimize epidermal damage as the pulse widths are greater than the TRT of the melanosomes in epidermal keratinocytes and melanocytes.

Spot Size

The spot size is the diameter in millimeters of the laser beam. As photons within a laser beam penetrate the dermis, they are scattered by collagen fibers, and those that are scattered outside the area of the laser beam are essentially wasted. Photons are more likely to be scattered outside of the beam area for smaller spot sizes, whereas in a larger spot size, the photons are likely to remain within the beam area following scatter. A double-blind, randomized controlled trial of a long-pulsed alexandrite laser for LHR of the axillary region comparing 18- and 12-mm spot sizes at otherwise identical treatment parameters showed a 10% greater reduction in hair counts with the larger spot size. Recently, a prospective study using a LPDL with a large 22 × 35 mm handpiece at low fluences and no skin cooling was shown to have similar long-term hair removal efficacy to published studies of LPDLs with smaller spot sizes using higher fluences and skin cooling. Thus, larger spot sizes are preferable to smaller spot sizes.

Skin Cooling

The presence of epidermal melanin, particularly in darker skin types, presents a competing chromophore to hair follicle melanin, which can be damaged during LHR (Figs 5.3A to D). Cooling of the skin surface is used to minimize epidermal damage, while permitting treatment with higher fluences. All of the skin cooling methods function by acting as a heat sink and removing heat from the skin surface. The least effective type of cooling is the use of an aqueous cold gel which passively extracts heat from the skin and then is not capable of further skin cooling. Alternatively, cooling with forced chilled air can provide cooling to the skin before, during and after a laser pulse. Currently, most of the available LHR devices have a built-in skin cooling system, which either consists of contact cooling or dynamic cooling with a cryogen spray. Contact cooling, usually with a sapphire tip, provides skin cooling just before and during a laser pulse. It is most useful for treatments with longer pulse durations (>10 ms). Dynamic cooling with cryogen liquid spray precools the skin with a millisecond spray of cryogen just before the laser pulse. A second spray can be delivered just after the laser pulse for post-cooling, but parallel cooling during the laser pulse is not possible as the cryogen spray interferes with the laser beam. Dynamic cooling is best suited for use with pulse durations shorter than 5 ms.

Postprocedure Care

It is expected for the patient to have perifollicular erythema and edema in the treatment area following LHR. This generally persists for 2 days but can last for up to 1 week. Ice and application of a topical corticosteroid can be used to shorten the duration of these desired clinical findings. Patients will often find that a single treatment of LHR with shorter pulse durations results in nearly total epilation of the hair follicles in the treatment area. It is important to counsel the patient that a majority of these hairs will likely regrow, and this is not considered a treatment failure. Generally, only about 15% of hairs are permanently removed with each laser treatment. On the other hand, LHR treatments with longer pulse durations may leave behind many hairs which appear to "grow" following treatment. It is important to reassure the patient that these "growing" hairs are dislodged from the hair follicle and require 1–2 weeks to be completely shed. Nearly any method of epilation can be used to hasten their removal.

The importance of strict sun precaution following LHR treatments cannot be overemphasized. This can be achieved by the use of topical sunscreens, ultraviolet light impermeable garments and sun avoidance.

Long-term Efficacy

Evidence of permanent hair removal was evident as early as the seminal hair removal trial from the Wellman Center involving a single treatment with the normal mode ruby laser. Seven of the 13 original subjects were evaluated at 2-year follow-up. Of the 7 subjects, 4 had evidence of persistent permanent hair reduction at 2-year follow-up, whereas 3 subjects experienced complete regrowth. Follow-up of 18 out of the 50 original study subjects treated with a LPDL, showed a 25–33% and 36–46% hair reduction at a mean follow-up of 20 months after one or two treatments (9-mm spot size, pulse duration of 5–20 ms, fluences of 15–40 J/cm^2, single or triple pulsed), respectively. A head-to-head trial comparing a LPDL to a long-pulsed alexandrite laser found a 49–94% hair reduction at 1-year follow-up after 4 treatments (9-mm spot size, pulse duration of 20 ms, fluences of 12–40 J/cm^2) with the LPDL in 15 subjects.

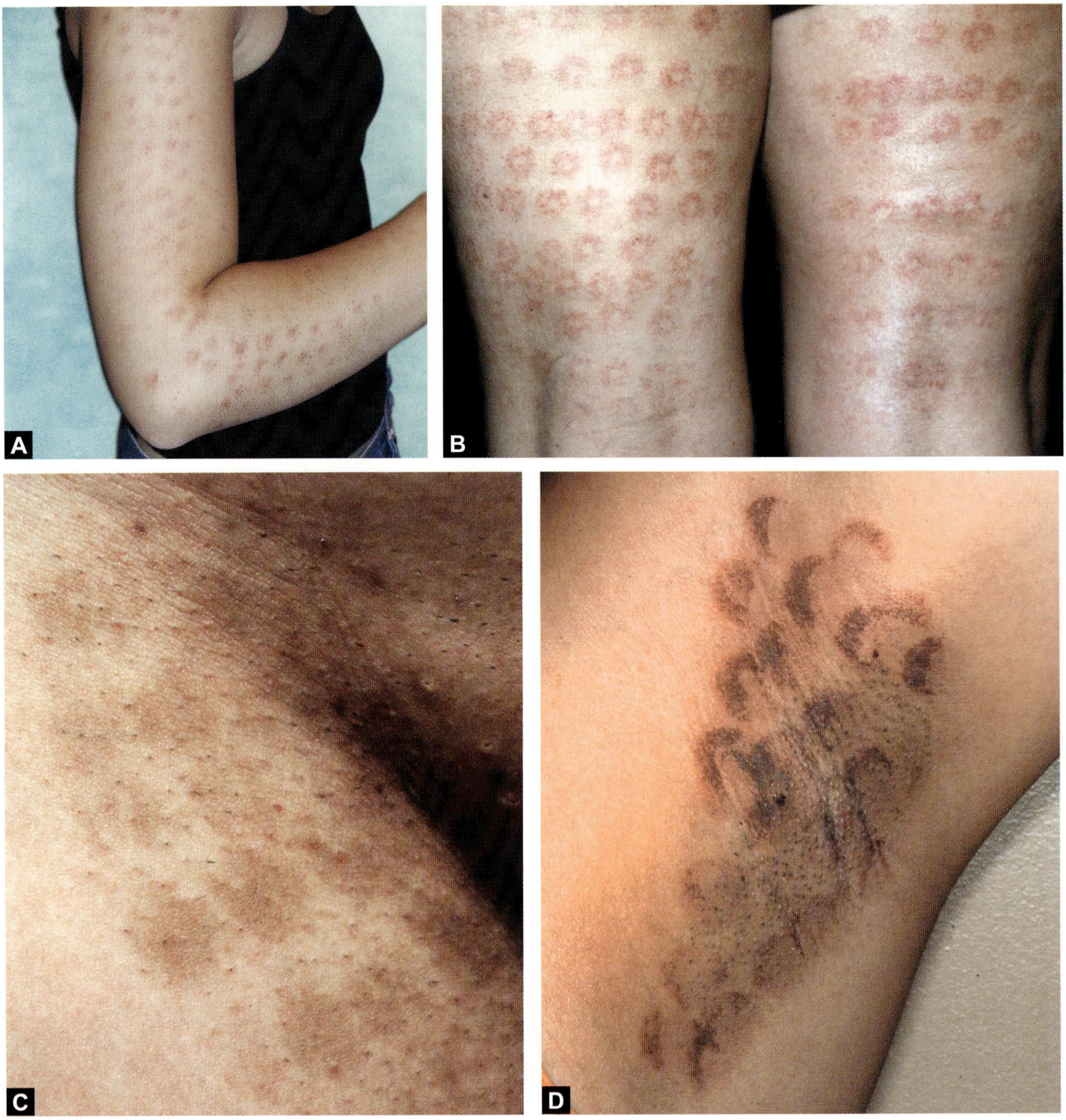

Figs 5.3A to D: Examples of LHR-induced hyperpigmentation

Similar results were achieved with the alexandrite laser used in this study. Fifteen of 20 subjects with Fitzpatrick skin phototypes III–IV treated with a long-pulsed alexandrite laser (12- and 18-mm spot size, 3 ms pulse duration and fluences of 20 or 40 J/cm^2) or a long-pulsed Nd:YAG laser (12-mm spot size, 3 ms pulse duration and fluence of 40 J/cm^2) for 4 sessions at 8-week interval showed 76–84% and 74%, hair reduction 18 months after the last treatment, respectively. Another head-to-head trial of a high fluence LPDL (9-mm spot size, pulse duration of 30 ms, fluences of 20–50 J/cm^2) versus a low fluence LPDL (12 x 10 mm spot size, pulse duration of 20 ms, fluences of 5–10 J/cm^2) in 22 subjects showed similar, 94% and 90% hair reduction at 18-month follow-up following 5 treatments spaced 6–8 weeks apart, respectively. Finally, the authors recently reported statistically significant hair clearance, 54% and

42%, at 6- and 15-month follow-up visits following three monthly treatments using a LPDL with a large handpiece in the largest prospective trial to date. Remaining hairs were found to also grow back less thick and lighter.

Complications

The most common complication of LHR is pigmentary alteration, including hyper- and hypopigmentation (Figs 5.3A to D and 5.4A to D). This may result either from selecting a nonoptimal wavelength, pulse duration, fluence, nonfunctional epidermal cooling, or by treating a tanned patient. Pigmentary alterations may also occur even when optimal treatment parameters are used. These changes are often transient and improve with time, although permanent hypopigmentation can occur (Figs 5.4A to D). Zones of untreated hairs can result from a lack of overlapping between laser pulses (Fig. 5.5). Scarring is an exceedingly rare complication but can occur when excessive fluences are used.

Treatment of vellus hairs, especially of the lateral cheeks and chin area, may result in the induction of terminal hairs, a phenomenon known as paradoxical hypertrichosis (Figs 5.6A and B). This has been reported to occur more commonly in females of Mediterranean, Middle Eastern, Asian and South Asian descent.

CONCLUSION

Future Directions

Advances in Pain Control

A novel technique to reduce LHR associated pain is pneumatic skin flattening (PSF). This technique works by coupling a vacuum chamber to generate

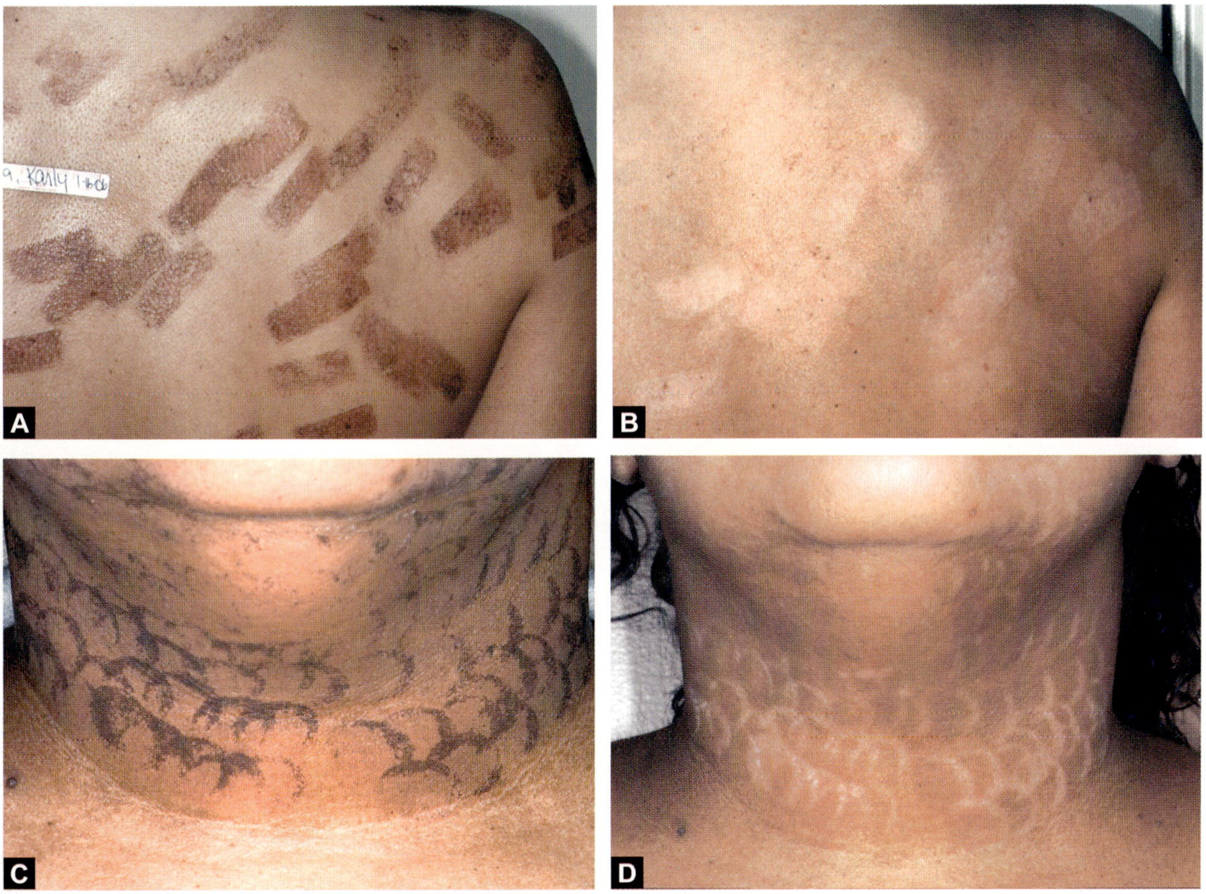

Figs 5.4A to D: Permanent hypopigmentation resulting from LHR. (A) Temporary hyperpigmentation in a Fitzpatrick skin phototype IV treated with an IPL device for hair removal; (B) One month later, the hyperpigmented patches were replaced with persisting hypopigmented patches; (C) Temporary hyperpigmentation in a Fitzpatrick skin phototype VI patient treated with an Nd:YAG device; (D) Two weeks later, the annular hyperpigmented patches were replaced with persisting hypopigmented patches

negative pressure and to flatten the skin against the handpiece treatment window. Based on the gate theory of pain transmission, it stimulates pressure receptors in the skin immediately prior to firing of the laser pulse, thereby blocking activation of pain fibers. Pneumatic skin flattening is just beginning to be incorporated into commercially available lasers (Table 5.1). A recent study of LHR using a LPDL with a large spot size and vacuum-assisted suction showed that the majority of subjects reported feeling no pain at all or up to moderate pain without the use of skin cooling or topical anesthetics. Notably, none of the subjects in the study reported experiencing severe or intolerable pain.

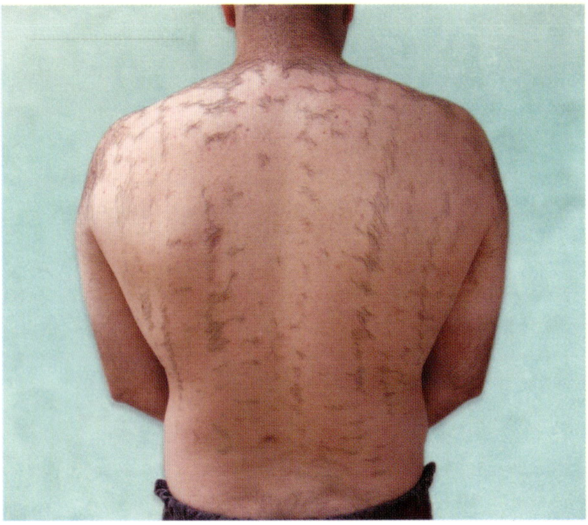

Fig. 5.5: Zones of untreated skin resulting from poor operator technique

Home Use Laser and Light Source Devices for Hair Removal

In recent years, a number of devices have been developed that seek to provide patients with the ability to achieve energy-based hair removal at home. These devices are based on intense pulsed light (IPL), laser and thermal technologies that target the hair follicle for destruction. Devices that have 510(k) clearance by the Federal Drug Administration (FDA) in the United States include: (1) Thermal-based devices [no!no!hair (Radiancy, Orangeburg, NY)]; (2) IPL-based devices including Silk'n SensEpil (Skinnovations, Israel) and Viss IPL (Viss Beauty, Korea); (3) Laser-based devices [Tria Laser 3.0 (Tria Beauty, Pleasanton, CA)]; and (4) Combined IPL/thermal-based devices including the SpaTouch Elite and Kona (Radiancy). Similar technologies are also being utilized by a variety of other home use devices that do not currently have FDA 510(k) clearance.

The evidence behind such devices is scant and limited to small noncontrolled studies. In addition, the risk for devastating eye injuries with improper use of laser- and IPL-based devices and lack of medical training raises a dilemma of how much autonomy a patient should have with potentially harmful devices. Nonetheless, the appeal of having a personal device to remove unwanted hair in the privacy of one's home without the expense and inconvenience of

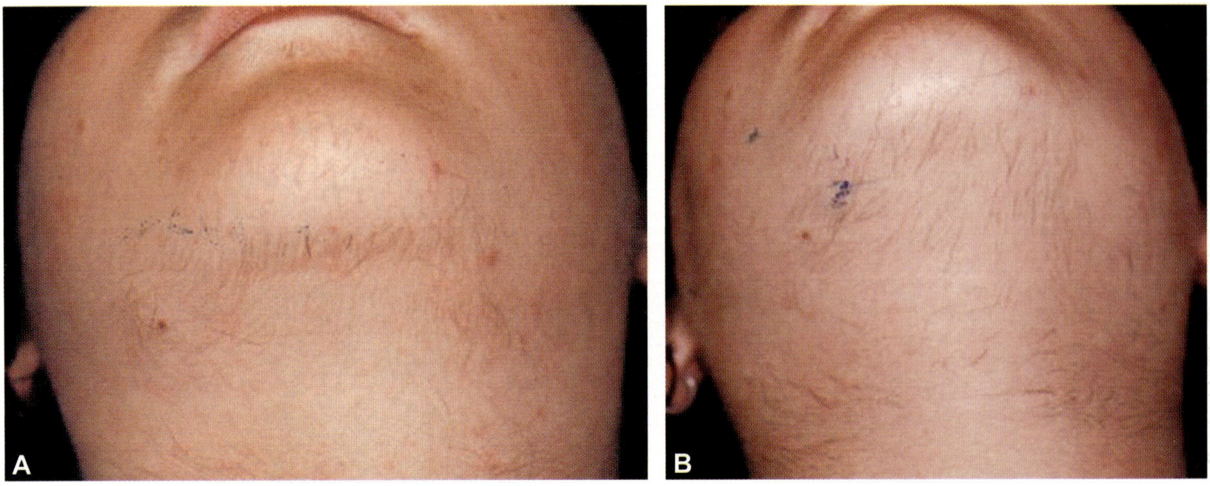

Figs 5.6A and B: Paradoxical hypertrichosis. (A) Baseline appearance of chin and neck; (B) Apparent increase in pigmented hair density following treatment with a long-pulsed alexandrite laser
Courtesy: Images provided by Andrea Willey and Nerea Landa

multiple dermatologist or spa visits will likely drive the development of additional home use devices.

Alternative Technologies for Hair Removal

Photodynamic therapy (PDT) with aminolevulinic acid (ALA) has been shown in a small pilot study to result in up to 40% hair reduction with a single treatment, although wax epilation was performed prior to treatment in this study.

Electro-Optical Synergy (ELOS) technology combines electrical (conducted radiofrequency) and optical (laser/light) energies. A handful of devices based on this technology have been produced (Table 5.1). The theory behind ELOS is based on the optical component (laser or IPL) heating the hair shaft, which then is thought to concentrate the bipolar radiofrequency (RF) energy to the surrounding hair follicle. Based on this combination, lower fluences are needed for the optical component, thereby suggesting it might be well tolerated in all Fitzpatrick skin phototypes, and potentially effective in the removal of white and poorly pigmented hair. A study of forty patients (Fitzpatrick skin phenotypes II–V) with varied facial and nonfacial hair colors were treated with combined IPL/RF ELOS technology. An average clearance of 75% was observed at 18 months following four treatments. No significant adverse sequelae were noted and there were no treatment differences between patients of varying skin types or hair color. Pretreatment with ALA prior to use of a combined IPL and radiofrequency device has been shown to further augment the removal of terminal white hairs.

In conclusion, hair removal has made a dramatic shift from an art to science based on the theory of selective photothermolysis. Since the first reports of selective hair removal in 1996 by Anderson and colleagues, there has been a tremendous explosion in the number of devices used for LHR; making LHR the most commonly requested cosmetic procedure in the world. This chapter provides the reader with the fundamentals of hair follicle anatomy and physiology, pearls for patient selection and preoperative preparation, principles of laser safety, an introduction to the various laser/light devices and a discussion of laser–tissue interactions that are vital to optimizing treatment efficacy while minimizing complications and side-effects.

Acknowledgments

This chapter is modified and updated with permission from Ibrahimi OA, Avram MM, Hanke CW, Kilmer SL, Anderson RR. Laser hair removal. Dermatol Ther. 2011;24(1):94-107.

FURTHER READING

1. Alster TS, Bryan H, Williams CM. Long-pulsed Nd:YAG laser-assisted hair removal in pigmented skin: a clinical and histological evaluation. Arch Dermatol. 2001;137(7):885-9.
2. Altshuler GB, Anderson RR, Manstein D, et al. Extended theory of selective photothermolysis. Lasers Surg Med. 2001;29(5):416-32.
3. Anderson RR, Parrish JA. Selective photothermolysis: precise microsurgery by selective absorption of pulsed radiation. Science.1983;220(4596):524-7.
4. Bernstein EF. Hair growth induced by diode laser treatment. Dermatol Surg. 2005;31(5):584-6.
5. Braun M. Comparison of high-fluence, single-pass diode laser to low-fluence, multiple-pass diode laser for laser hair reduction with 18 months of follow up. J Drugs Dermatol. 2011;10(1):62-5.
6. Campos VB, Dierickx CC, Farinelli WA, et al. Hair removal with an 800-nm pulsed diode laser. J Am Acad Dermatol. 2000;43(3):442-7.
7. Davoudi SM, Behnia F, Gorouhi F, et al. Comparison of long-pulsed alexandrite and Nd:YAG lasers, individually and in combination, for leg hair reduction: an assessor-blinded, randomized trial with 18 months of follow-up. Arch Dermatol. 2008;144(10):1323-7.
8. Dierickx CC, Grossman MC, Farinelli WA, et al. Permanent hair removal by normal-mode ruby laser. Arch Dermatol. 1998;134(7):837-42.
9. Eremia S, Li C, Newman N. Laser hair removal with alexandrite versus diode laser using four treatment sessions: 1-year results. Dermatol Surg. 2001;27(11):925-9; discussion 929-30.
10. Garcia C, Alamoudi H, Nakib M, et al. Alexandrite laser hair removal is safe for Fitzpatrick skin types IV-VI. Dermatol Surg. 2000;26(2):130-4.
11. Gold MH, Bell MW, Foster TD, et al. One-year follow-up using an intense pulsed light source for long-term hair removal. J Cutan Laser Ther. 1999;1(3):167-71.
12. Goldberg DJ, Littler CM, Wheeland RG. Topical suspension-assisted Q-switched Nd:YAG laser hair removal. Dermatol Surg.1997;23(9):741-5.
13. Grossman MC, Dierickx C, Farinelli W, et al. Damage to hair follicles by normal-mode ruby laser pulses. J Am Acad Dermatol.1996;35(6):889-94.
14. Haak CS, Nymann P, Pedersen AT, et al. Hair removal in hirsute women with normal testosterone levels: a randomized controlled trial of long-pulsed

diode laser vs. intense pulsed light. Br J Dermatol. 2010;163(5):1007-13.
15. Hussain M, Polnikorn N, Goldberg DJ. Laser-assisted hair removal in Asian skin: efficacy, complications, and the effect of single versus multiple treatments. Dermatol Surg. 2003;29(3):249-54.
16. Ibrahimi OA, Avram MM, Hanke CW, et al. Laser hair removal. Dermatol Ther. 2011;24(1):94-107.
17. Ibrahimi OA, Kilmer SL. Long-term clinical evaluation of an 800nm long-pulsed diode laser with a large spot size and vacuum-assisted suction for hair removal. Manuscript under review.
18. Khoury JG, Saluja R, Goldman MP. Comparative evaluation of long-pulse alexandrite and long-pulse Nd:YAG laser systems used individually and in combination for axillary hair removal. Dermatol Surg. 2008;34(5):665-70; discussion 670-71.
19. Lask G, Friedman D, Elman M, et al. Pneumatic skin flattening (PSF): a novel technology for marked pain reduction in hair removal with high energy density lasers and IPLs. J Cosmet Laser Ther. 2006;8(2):76-81.
20. Lou WW, Quintana AT, Geronemus RG, et al. Prospective study of hair reduction by diode laser (800 nm) with long-term follow-up. Dermatol Surg. 2000;26(5):428-32.
21. Nouri K, Chen H, Saghari S, et al. Comparing 18- versus 12-mm spot size in hair removal using a gentlease 755-nm alexandrite laser. Dermatol Surg. 2004;30(4 Pt 1):494-7.
22. Rao J, Goldman MP. Prospective, comparative evaluation of three laser systems used individually and in combination for axillary hair removal. Dermatol Surg. 2005;31(12):1671-6; discussion 1677.
23. Richards RN, Meharg GE. Electrolysis: observations from 13 years and 140,000 hours of experience. J Am Acad Dermatol. 1995;33(4):662-6.
24. Rohrer TE, Chatrath V, Yamauchi P, et al. Can patients treat themselves with a small novel light based hair removal system? Lasers Surg Med. 2003;33(1):25-9.
25. Zenzie HH, Altshuler GB, Smirnov MZ, et al. Evaluation of cooling methods for laser dermatology. Lasers Surg Med. 2000;26(2):130-44.

HAPTER

6

Laser and Light Therapy for Acne Vulgaris

H Ray Jalian, Fernanda H Sakamoto

INTRODUCTION

Acne vulgaris is the most common cutaneous disease in the United States.[1,2] Over 60% of the population will at some point have acne, and 20% of these individuals will develop severe acne that results in scarring. While usually not life threatening, acne can cause severe psychosocial impairment and is associated with decreased quality of life, depression, and suicide.[3] Despite its ubiquity, the pathogenesis of acne remains largely unknown. What we do understand is that the disease is multifactorial and involves aberrant follicular keratinization, excess sebum production, overgrowth of *Propionibacterium acnes*, and a host inflammatory response. While we have some insight into the nuances of these individual factors and how they contribute to the evolution of disease, the complex interplay and sequence of events is yet to be clarified.

There are a variety of agents available for the treatment of acne. Used alone or in combination, these treatments exert their effect on one or more of the pathogenic factors. Currently, the main therapeutic targets are aimed at: (1) correcting the altered pattern of follicular keratinization; (2) decreasing sebaceous gland activity and sebum production; (3) decreasing follicular *P. acnes* population, and subsequent inflammatory mediators; (4) producing an anti-inflammatory effect and (5) hormonal treatments. Topical agents are often used first-line in mild to moderate acne with the systemic agents used in more severe cases. While effective in some, long-term sustained improvement after discontinuation of therapy is suboptimal. Despite advances in research, the armamentarium of medical treatments for acne vulgaris has not significantly changed in the last decade. This is largely attributed to the relative success of isotretinoin—a systemic retinoid. Isotretinoin is the only medication capable of long-term, often permanent reduction in acne severity. However, despite its efficacy, the medication is a potent teratogen and is cumbersome to prescribe due to a federally mandated regulatory program. Despite governmental efforts, the number of birth defects related to the use of oral retinoids has not decreased. Moreover, recent litigations involving suicidality and a potential link to inflammatory bowel disease has made patients and some prescribers weary of the medication.

Given the limited medical therapies for acne, rise in antibiotic resistance, and the increasing pitfalls of isotretinoin use, laser and light-based sources are increasingly being used in the management of acne. These treatments are varied, but with similar aims to medical therapy in that they are hypothesized to target various aspects of the pathogenesis of acne. These device-based treatments can largely be classified into either photothermal and/or photochemical treatments. Unlike other popular, clinically relevant lasers and light sources, to date, no approved device uses an optimal chromophore for selective targeting of sebaceous glands for the treatment of acne. Currently only vascular lasers (targeting hemoglobin), mid-infrared lasers (targeting water) and broad-spectrum flash-lamps (somewhat targeting hemoglobin, melanin and water) have been used for photothermal treatment of acne. While there is promising laboratory data to suggest that photothermal treatment of acne by the selective targeting of sebaceous glands is possible, studies to demonstrate the efficacy of these lipid-selective wavelengths of light are forthcoming. In addition, intense blue or red light exposure in combination with a photosensitizer is effective for treatment of inflammatory acne, by photochemical mechanisms.

LASERS

Vascular Selective Lasers

Pulsed-dye lasers (PDL) cause selective photothermal damage to cutaneous microvessels throughout the dermis. Pulsed-dye laser treatment has had variable results when used as a treatment for acne. An initial study found a statistically and clinically significant reduction in acne as measured by a validated measure of acne severity and lesion counts 12 weeks after a single PDL treatment using a 585-nm PDL at 1.5–3.0 J/cm^2 and 0.35 ms pulse durations.[4] While these results seemed promising, a subsequent study, near identical in design and dosimetry, did not show any significant improvement.[5] A recent trial investigating the utility of PDL treatment demonstrated no substantial benefit for this modality in the treatment of acne vulgaris.[6] Other published randomized controlled trials compared the pulsed-dye laser to other light-based therapies or in combination with photosensitizers, making it difficult to determine the efficacy of PDL as a monotherapy. One such study comparing 585-nm PDL at 8–10 J/cm^2 and 40 ms pulse duration to a flash-lamp intense pulsed light source showed improvement in patient satisfaction, lesion count, and standardized acne scoring scale.[7] While there is evidence in the literature to support its efficacy, reports remain inconsistent and very few well-controlled studies comparing it to standard topical regimens have been conducted. Moreover, the wide variety of parameters utilized in these studies makes it difficult to draw a conclusive comparison. Despite its questionable efficacy, the pulsed-dye laser can have a role in the treatment of inflammatory acne, especially when combined with conventional topical therapies (Figs 6.1A to C). In addition, the literature strongly supports the safety of PDL and from this standpoint it has an excellent track record.

Efficacy of pulsed-dye laser is hypothesized to be related to its photothermal effects on tissue, perhaps by targeting dilated vasculature associated with the hyperemic nature of inflammatory acne. There is no demonstrable decrease in *P. acnes* counts or sebum excretion rate following pulsed-dye laser treatments.[8] Some have suggested expression of soluble mediators such as transforming growth factor (TGF)-β which is upregulated in tissue 24 hours after nonablative pulsed-dye laser treatment. TGF-β is an important cytokine involved in wound healing and neocollagenesis, and the mechanism of action of PDL for acne may be related to this soluble factor. Moreover, the expression of a soluble mediator could explain the global improvement seen in subjects in these studies and the lack of statistically significant difference between treatment and nontreatment side.[8]

Mid-infrared Lasers

Initial excitement for the use of a 1450-nm diode laser stemmed from demonstration that this device damaged sebaceous glands in an in vivo rabbit ear model as well as ex vivo in human skin. This observation led to a clinical trial assessing the use of a 1450-nm diode laser with dynamic cryogen spray for the treatment of acne. A preliminary study performed four treatments separated by a period of 3 weeks on the back of 27 patients. Treatment was performed at various dosimetries ranging from 14–22 J/cm^2. Study design was split-back with randomization to treatment and control site, which was treated with cryogen spray alone. In the 15 patients that completed the study (24 weeks after final treatment) there was a statistically significant reduction in lesion counts between the treated and control sites. In one biopsy specimen obtained immediately after treatment there was evidence of photothermal coagulation of the pilosebaceous unit, though specimens taken later, including from the same subject, showed normal sebaceous gland and skin adnexal architecture.[9] With these encouraging results, follow-up studies with the same device confirmed utility for this treatment for inflammatory acne on the face.[10] Dose response studies have shown longevity of this treatment up to 12 months as well as safety in use with darker skin phenotypes.[11] While these studies were encouraging,

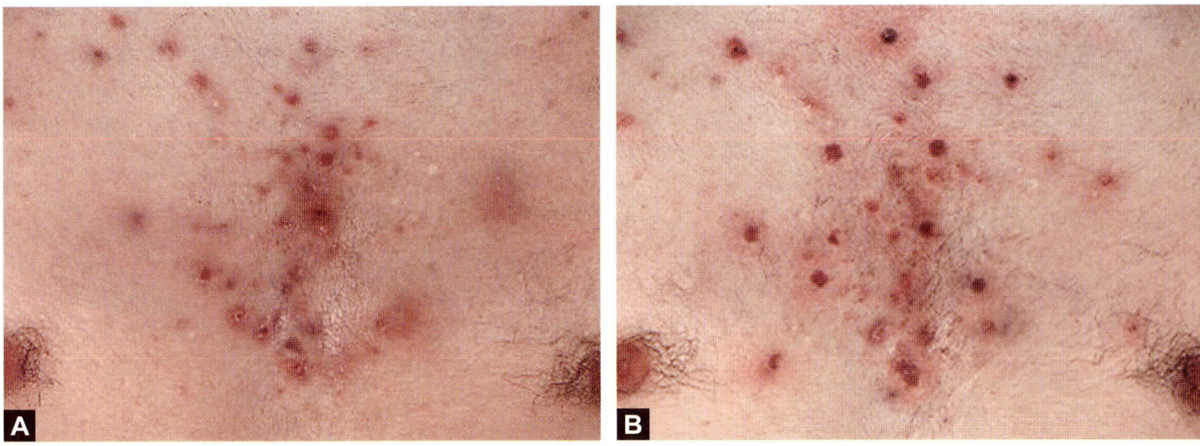

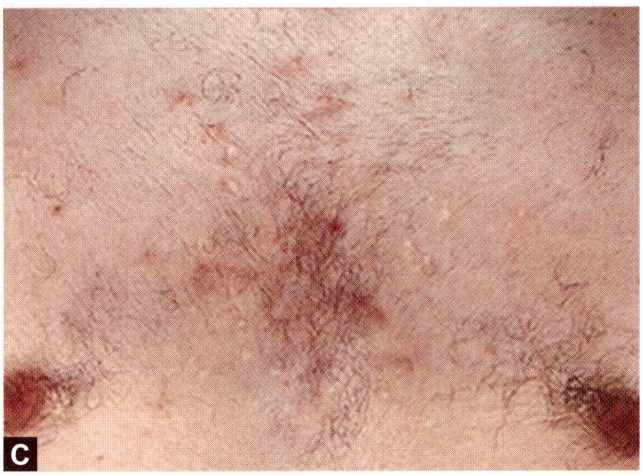

Figs 6.1A to C: Pulsed-dye laser (PDL) treatment of nodule-cystic acne. (A) Before treatment; (B) Immediately after treatment (4th session). Note immediate endpoint with spotted erythema and bruising on laser treated lesions; (C) After 5 sessions 1–3 months apart. PDL was used with 7-mm spot size, 3–6 ms, 8–9 J/cm^2. This patient continued conventional topical treatment; however, significant improvement of his acne and scars was noticed only after initiation of laser therapy
Source: Photographs obtained at the Wellman Center for Photomedicine, Massachusetts General Hospital, Harvard Medical School, Boston

flaws in study design limit their impact. None of the initial studies utilized standardized acne scores but relied on lesion counts alone. Moreover, the degree of blinding of investigators is not disclosed in these studies. Finally, in one of the studies subjects were allowed to continue their current topical or oral acne regimens, with all but one subject on some form of oral and/or topical therapy.

In the largest, and perhaps the best-designed study, 38 subjects were enrolled in a split-face double-blinded randomized control trial. Subjects enrolled in the study were allowed to continue oral or topical regimens as they were deemed to affect both sides of the face equally. A double pass technique utilizing fluences of 8–9 J/cm^2 was performed monthly for a total of three treatment sessions. Lesion counts and blinded observer assessment using the Leeds Revised Acne Grading Scale failed to demonstrate a statistically significant reduction between treatment and control sites with subjects followed up to 12 months.[12] There was, however, an improvement in both the treatment and control sites again suggesting there may be a systemic effect of acne treatments mediated by a soluble factor. This has been suggested by others who failed to show a statistically significant difference between treated and untreated side, in the setting of an overall improvement in acne severity.[8]

Despite the lack of definitive evidence regarding clinical efficacy, the 1450-nm diode laser can be a useful adjuvant treatment in combination with other topical and systemic agents. Adverse effects of the treatment are limited to transient erythema, and pigmentary alteration in darker skin phenotypes. Given the relatively painful nature of the procedure, topical anesthetic is invariably utilized. Multiple pass, lower fluence protocols are effective for improving acne lesion counts and are reportedly more tolerable, often not requiring anesthesia.[13] This approach may also be helpful in darker skin phototypes for minimizing post inflammatory hyperpigmentation.[14] Given the narrow therapeutic window of this device, the practice of pulse-stacking should be avoided due to the risk of bulk heating and subsequent scar formation.

Another mid-infrared laser with a wavelength of 1320 nm demonstrated a transient, although statistically significant improvement in absolute comedone count. This split-face, blinded trial failed to show improvement in inflammatory lesion count or blinded investigator assessment using the Leeds criteria.[15]

The mechanism of action related to the efficacy of these mid-infrared lasers is likely related to the photothermal effects on the sebaceous gland. By heating the superficial dermis enveloping the sebaceous gland, investigators hypothesize a transient alteration in sebaceous gland architecture and function. This is supported by both objective and subjective evidence for decreased sebum production after treatment with these devices.[11,16] Despite this suggestive evidence in support of mechanism, one should keep in mind that permanent destruction of sebaceous glands has never been demonstrated with either device. Moreover, conflicting data on its effect on sebum production[17] point to alternate methods for its effect on acne. Perhaps the damage of more superficially located components of the pilosebaceous unit alter follicular keratinization, resulting in decreased microcomedo formation and the resultant clinical improvement. Valid theories, concrete evidence of the efficacy of these devices and their mechanism of action are lacking and further studies are needed at this time.

NONCOHERENT LIGHT SOURCES

Noncoherent light sources have variable efficacy in the treatment of acne. The use of broadband light sources is not a new practice, with both sunlight and ultraviolet light used to treat acne. The efficacy of noncoherent, low-energy light sources is related to its photochemical effects. Photoactivating endogenous bacterial porphyrins with visible or ultraviolet light causes the formation of free radicals and reactive oxygen species (ROS), inducing membrane damage and subsequent decrease in *P. acnes* counts.[18] This is independent of antibiotic resistance, and does not affect the remainder of the epithelium or follicle, as these cells do not contain porphyrins. The action spectrum for killing *P. acnes* is within the ultraviolet A (UVA) and blue light region, with a relative peak from 400 nm to 420 nm, corresponding to blue light.[19] This is supported by absorption spectrum of sebaceous glands that have an absorption peak from 381 nm to 405 nm.[20] Given the potential for carcinogenesis and photodamage, the use of UVA has been abandoned. Additional peaks can be extrapolated from the action spectrum of protoporphyrin IX, the main endogenous porphyrin produced by *P. acnes*, corresponding to green, yellow and red light.

Narrow-Band Light Sources

Narrow-band blue light continuous wave (CW) light sources have been extensively studied for the treatment of acne. Results from studies are variable but suggest some modest efficacy for acne after a series of treatments, though long-term improvement is unlikely. Several studies have demonstrated reductions in lesions using variable narrow-band blue light sources (400–420 nm). Elman and colleagues demonstrated a significant reduction in inflammatory lesions that was sustained 8 weeks after therapy.[21] This was the seminal paper that led to the Food and Drug Administration (FDA) approval of blue light for acne treatment. Kawada et al. showed similar results in an open-label prospective study in 30 subjects with mild to moderate acne in which there was 64% reduction in lesion count after twice weekly treatment with a 407–420 nm blue light device.[22] Others have demonstrated the efficacy of blue light in comparison to 1% topical clindamycin solution.[23] Overall, blue light therapy appears to be effective for a subset of patients with acne, predominantly for those with inflammatory lesions. There is minimal to no effects on comedonal lesions.

Others have demonstrated efficacy with different spectrums of light. Sigurdsson et al. demonstrated improvement in acne lesions on the face and trunk without significant side-effects after treatment with broad-spectrum, green and violet light.[24] Combination of blue light (414 nm) and red light (660 nm) appears to be superior to blue light, or benzoyl peroxide alone for the treatment of inflammatory lesions.[25] This may be related to the fact that red light therapy limits *P. acnes* viability, alters macrophage activity, and may penetrate the epidermis deeper than blue light.[26]

Overall, CW visible light sources appear to be effective for a subset of patients with acne, predominantly for those with inflammatory lesions. There is minimal to no effect on comedonal lesions, and some have suggested it is best when combined with a topical keratolytic.[24] Moreover, relapse rate seems to be high after cessation of therapy. The devices are uniformly safe with adverse effects related to post-treatment erythema and dryness. It is the authors' opinion that low-energy CW visible light sources can be an adjunct to topical or oral medical regimen, and can be an appropriate choice for those patients who wish to take an "active" role in the management of their acne. Moreover, with the recent FDA clearance of home versions of these devices, it improves accessibility and cost effectiveness of this treatment.

Intense Pulsed Light Sources

Longer wavelengths than blue light have been postulated to provide more porphyrin activation by being able to penetrate deeper into the follicle. Flashlamp light sources (intense pulsed light or IPL) administers broad spectrum, noncoherent pulses of visible light. One study demonstrated the efficacy of such a device with up to 68–87% clearance of both inflammatory and noninflammatory lesions.[27] Other studies have offered contradictory information regarding efficacy for IPL in improving inflammatory acne.[28] In addition, newer devices combining suction apparatus with light sources, so called photopneumatic devices, are modestly effective for acne.[29,30] However, these studies were not well controlled for the pneumatic effect alone, which should be beneficial for comedonal lesions as well as enhanced penetration of topical medications.

Photodynamic Therapy

Photodynamic therapy (PDT) uses a combination of a photosensitizer, light and oxygen, triggering a cascade of photochemical reactions that will finally result in the formation of reactive oxygen species (ROS), especially singlet oxygen ($^1O_2$), other subproducts and free radicals. The production and accumulation of ROS causes damage by oxidation of proteins and lipids in the target tissue.

Many photosensitizers and light sources have been described over the past decades for a variety of medical applications including non-skin cancers, macular degeneration and Barrett's esophagus. In dermatology, PDT using topical porphyrin precursors was introduced by Kennedy et al. for the treatment of nonmelanoma skin cancers and actinic keratoses, using a natural porphyrin precursor, aminolevulinic acid.[31]

Today, different porphyrin-precursor drugs are approved for dermatological applications in various countries. In the US, however, aminolevulinic-acid, ALA (aka 5-ALA or δ-ALA) and its methyl-ester, the methyl-aminolevulinate (M-ALA or MAL) are FDA approved only for treatment of actinic keratosis, not for acne. Other photosensitizers for acne treatment are still under investigation at an early stage.

Porphyrins are naturally occurring photosensitizers that are precursors of heme. In the complex heme synthesis pathway, four molecules of ALA combine to form the porphyrin ring structure. Iron is inserted into the ultimate porphyrin, protoporphyrin IX (PpIX). After uptake into a cell, both ALA and MAL follow this metabolic pathway resulting in the formation of excess protoporphyrin IX (PpIX), which is synthesized inside the mitochondria. When exogenously applied, ALA and MAL will overdrive the metabolic pathway, increasing heme synthesis until intracellular iron stores are depleted, and then the PpIX will accumulate.

The photodynamic effect occurs when PpIX absorbs a photon, causing an excited electronic singlet state from which the energy can be released as fluorescence, or by transformation into a triplet excited state. From this triplet state, PpIX can transfer energy to oxygen (which is also a triplet state molecule), resulting in the formation of singlet oxygen—a potent oxidizing agent.

Interestingly, in a preclinical study, Divaris et al. observed that after intraperitoneal injection, porphyrins accumulated preferentially in sebaceous glands in a murine model.[32] However, it was not until the year 2000 that ALA-PDT was studied for the treatment of acne by Hongcharu et al.[33] The same year, Itoh and colleagues in Japan also published a case report using ALA-PDT for acne treatment.[34]

Given the complexity of the photochemical reactions combined with the presence of multiple variables affecting PDT, it is not surprising that over a decade later there are still mechanistic questions, as well as a range of opinion on treatment guidelines, resulting in a broad range of efficacy rates of PDT for acne.[35]

Most clinical studies have varied the incubation time (time between drug application and light irradiation); type of activating light—wavelength (nm), dosimetry (J/cm^2), irradiance (W/cm^2), types of light sources(pulsed or continuous), among other variables,[35] rendering it hard to compare results. In fact, PDT has not been optimized for the treatment of acne and in the US remains an "off-label", though frequently used, application. It is clear that long-term remission of acne can be achieved by ALA-PDT or MAL-PDT, based on the partial destruction of sebaceous glands. Although blue light or red light activation of ALA-PDT is appropriate for treating superficial actinic keratosis, the anatomical depth of sebaceous glands is such that red light activation but not blue light, reaches this target. Due to scattering, longer wavelengths penetrate deeper into the skin.[36] Although the strongest porphyrin light absorption is the "Soret" band in the blue spectrum (405–415 nm), this short wavelength does not penetrate deeply enough to reach the sebaceous glands at about 500–1000 μm.[37] Fortunately, PpIX also has absorption peaks at the green (~506–540 nm), yellow (~572–582 nm) and red (~628–635 nm) spectrum, called the "Q bands".

While tempting to reduce the time of incubation, when using porphyrin-precursor drugs, a lag of time to allow drug absorption and penetration, and drug metabolism from the prodrug to porphyrin should be considered. In preclinical studies, sebaceous gland porphyrin fluorescence was only observed after 70–90 minutes after topical application of ALA,[37] while the maximum peak of porphyrin accumulation is only reached after 12 hours.

In general, there are basically two modalities of treatment: (1) a "high-dose PDT" that maximizes the treatment parameters for sebaceous gland inhibition, with better clinical results but more side-effects; and (2) various "low-dose PDT" approaches that compromises the parameters in order to make the treatment faster and to avoid side-effects.[35] To date, even though the low-dose techniques have been more popular in clinical practice, only the high-dose treatments have shown reliable and significant clinical results.[33,34,38-42] High-dose PDT studies have in common the use of a CW light source emitting in the red spectrum at an absorption band of PpIX (~633 nm) and a relatively long incubation time between drug application and light exposure (≥ 3 hours). Generally, the maximized PDT modality shows clinical clearance of ~40–70% of the inflammatory lesions, in ~50–100% of subjects for 3–6 months. Recurrence starts in about 1 month of one treatment session. Increasing the number of treatment sessions (4 vs 1) produces greater longevity of acne clearance.[33] Even though these results are extremely promising and similar in effectiveness to oral isotretinoin, inflammatory side-effects related to high-dose PDT discourages many clinicians and patients to opt for this modality of treatment. Side-effects include intense pain during treatment, 48h post-treatment photosensitivity, intense phototoxic reactions such as edema, erythema, folliculitis, sterile pustulation, crusting, exfoliation and blistering, forcing patients to avoid social interactions for a week after treatment (Fig. 6.2). An acne flare-up is also often observed about 2–3 weeks after treatment. For the so called "low-dose" PDT, a wide range of light sources and incubation times have been used. Even with modest, but positive results, the majority of publications using low-dose PDT regimens are poorly controlled and limited short-term follow-up (weeks). Interestingly, a single paper comparing the use of IPL plus ALA vs IPL alone vs control, showed no statistical difference among the groups.[43]

In terms of mechanism of action, high-dose PDT seems to be associated to direct gland damage. It is also possible that PDT changes local inflammatory reaction,[44] resulting in decrease of keratinization, increase of metalloproteinases (MMP-1 and MMP-3) among other unknown mechanisms. There is little evidence to support that PDT acts as an antibiotic, since most studies have shown little or no, transient reduction of *P.acnes.*[38,45-48]

Clinically, high-dose ALA or MAL-PDT is a useful alternative to systemic retinoid therapy for moderate to severe acne, in selected patients. This

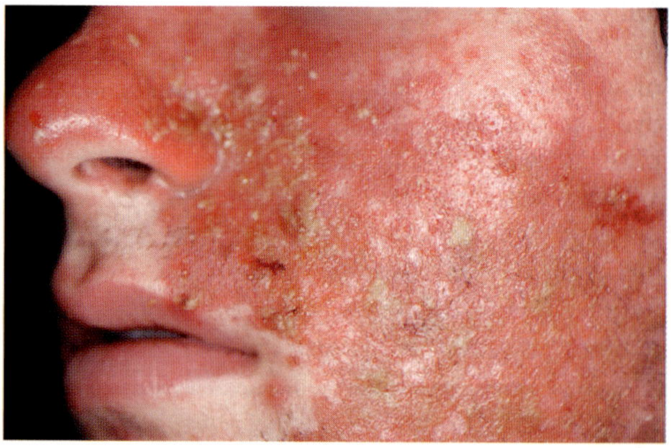

Fig. 6.2: Severe inflammatory side-effects of high dose photodynamic therapy (PDT) for acne treatment. Twenty percent aminolevulinic acid (ALA) was applied followed by 3h of incubation and 200 J/cm^2 red (633 nm) continuous wave (CW) light irradiation at 100 mW/ cm^2. Even with intense reaction 2–3 days after treatment, patients usually recover in 7–10 days with no long-term severe side-effects or scarring. Acne clearance is very high, similar to oral isotretinoin

Source: Photograph obtained at the Wellman Center for Photomedicine, Massachusetts General Hospital, Harvard Medical School, Boston includes people who have absolute or relative contraindications for use of isotretinoin, who have failed to respond to isotretinoin or other conventional therapies, who do not want to practice birth control or are planning to become pregnant, who prefer an office-based procedure and can accept significant side-effects for 7–10 days after treatment. Based on present evidence, 3–5 high-dose ALA or MAL-PDT treatments given at approximately one-month intervals are typically needed to achieve long-term remission of inflammatory acne. There is no evidence that PDT improves comedonal acne.

LIPID SELECTIVE LIGHT: TOWARDS A TRUE SEBACEOUS GLAND SELECTIVE LASER

Selective photothermolysis involves the selection of a wavelength of light and pulse duration that sufficiently heats a specific target without damage to the surrounding tissue. This confinement of heat allows for the targeting of individual chromophores without disruption of adjacent tissue. Recently, infrared vibrational bands have been found to be useful for the selective targeting of lipid-rich tissues, such as fat. Lipids are rich in copious C-H bonds that could be specifically stimulated at this spectrum. Anderson et al. measured the absorption spectrum of fat, identifying peaks at 1210 nm and 1720 nm where the absorption coefficient of lipid is greater than that of water.[49] Indeed, in vitro exposure of fresh, intact, full-thickness porcine tissue samples at wavelengths near 1,210 nm reproducibly caused thermal damage of subcutaneous fat with little or no injury to the overlying skin.[49] These results were later tested in a pilot clinical study for subcutaneous fat removal.[50]

Similarly, because acne sebum contain about 30% of lipids,[51] investigators hypothesized that sebum also has a characteristic absorption spectrum. Using both natural and artificially prepared sebum, absorption peaks near 1,210, 1,728, 1,760, 2,306 and 2,346 nm were observed[52] (Fig. 6.3). The results suggested the use of sebum as a new chromophore for selective photothermolysis. Ex vivo samples exposed to 1700 nm at 100–135 ms pulse durations confirmed selective photothermolysis of sebaceous glands without epidermal or dermal damage. While there is no clinical data supporting efficacy of lipid-selective wavelengths of light for the treatment of acne, medical therapies which reduce sebaceous gland volume or sebum secretion have a proven track record for efficacy.[53]

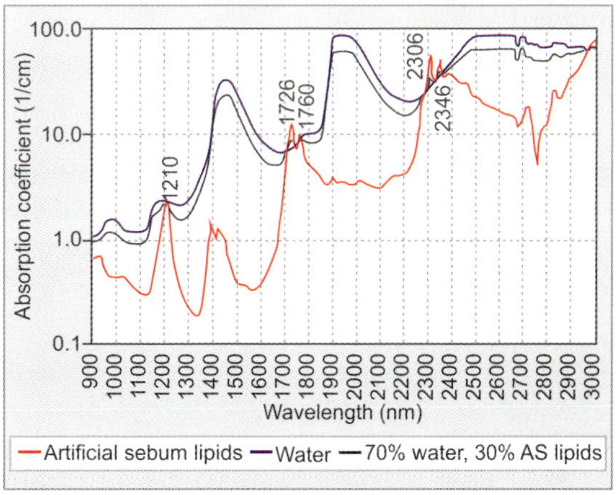

Fig. 6.3. Sebum absorption coefficient. Note sebum higher absorption than water at ~1210 nm and ~1726 nm

Source: Reprinted with permission from Sakamoto, et al. Selective photothermolysis to target sebaceous glands: theoretical estimation of parameters and preliminary results using a free electron laser. Lasers Surg Med. 2012.44(2):175-83

CONCLUSIONS

A critical appraisal of laser and light-based therapies leaves many questions unanswered. First, many of the aforementioned studies were limited in both number and severity of subjects enrolled. Few trials included patients with severe acne, and many trials failed to disclose exclusion and inclusion criteria making comparison difficult. Very few trials compared acne to standard, accepted topical therapies, and of those that did few found superiority to standard topical monotherapy.

Indeed, acne clinical trials are difficult to perform. The disease alone can suffer enormous variation over the course of time, with seasonal variation and a well-defined placebo effect. Therefore only large, controlled, blinded, long-term studies would really translate the results into real clinical improvement. Unfortunately, most of the studies using light sources as a treatment followed the subjects over a relatively short period of time.

Nevertheless, it is the authors' opinion that laser-based therapies can be an important addition to topical and oral regimens. It is clear from the evidence presented that laser treatment should not be used as a monotherapy. This is supported by national consensus data.[54] Development of novel therapeutic options for acne is a popular topic; an alternative, reliable, and "user-friendly" treatment with fever side effects would benefit billions of people worldwide and is the main goal for those who study acne.

REFERENCES

1. Stern RS. The prevalence of acne on the basis of physical examination. Journal of the American Academy of Dermatology. 1992;26(6):931-5.
2. Stern RS. Dermatologists and office-based care of dermatologic disease in the 21st century. Journal of Investigative Dermatology Symposium Proceedings. 2004;9(2):126-30.
3. Kellett S, Gilbert P. Acne: a biopsychosocial and evolutionary perspective with a focus on shame. Br J Health Psychol. 2001;6(Pt 1):1-24.
4. Seaton ED, et al. Pulsed-dye laser treatment for inflammatory acne vulgaris: randomised controlled trial. Lancet. 2003;362(9393):1347-52.
5. Orringer JS, et al. Treatment of acne vulgaris with a pulsed dye laser: a randomized controlled trial. JAMA. 2004;291(23):2834-9.
6. Karsai S, Schmitt L, Raulin C. The pulsed-dye laser as an adjuvant treatment modality in acne vulgaris: a randomized controlled single-blinded trial. Br J Dermatol. 2010;163(2): 395-401.
7. Choi YS, et al. Intense pulsed light vs. pulsed-dye laser in the treatment of facial acne: a randomized split-face trial. J Eur Acad Dermatol Venereol. 2010;24(7):773-80.
8. Seaton ED, et al. Investigation of the mechanism of action of nonablative pulsed-dye laser therapy in photorejuvenation and inflammatory acne vulgaris. Br J Dermatol. 2006; 155(4):748-55.
9. Paithankar DY, et al. Acne treatment with a 1,450 nm wavelength laser and cryogen spray cooling. Lasers Surg Med. 2002;31(2):106-14.
10. Friedman PM, et al. Treatment of inflammatory facial acne vulgaris with the 1450-nm diode laser: a pilot study. Dermatol Surg. 2004;30(2 Pt 1):147-51.
11. Jih MH, et al. The 1450-nm diode laser for facial inflammatory acne vulgaris: dose-response and 12-month follow-up study. J Am Acad Dermatol. 2006;55(1):80-7.
12. Darne S, Hiscutt EL, Seukeran DC. Evaluation of the clinical efficacy of the 1,450 nm laser in acne vulgaris: a randomized split-face, investigator-blinded clinical trial. Br J Dermatol. 2011;165(6):1256-62.
13. Bernstein EF. A pilot investigation comparing low-energy, double pass 1,450 nm laser treatment of acne to conventional single-pass, high-energy treatment. Lasers Surg Med. 2007;39(2):193-8.
14. Yeung CK, et al. Treatment of inflammatory facial acne with 1,450-nm diode laser in type IV to V Asian skin using an optimal combination of laser parameters. Dermatol Surg. 2009;35(4):593-600.
15. Orringer JS, et al. A randomized, controlled, split-face clinical trial of 1320-nm Nd:YAG laser therapy in the treatment of acne vulgaris. J Am Acad Dermatol. 2007;56(3):432-8.
16. Perez-Maldonado A, Runger TM, Krejci-Papa N. The 1,450-nm diode laser reduces sebum production in facial skin: a possible mode of action of its effectiveness for the treatment of acne vulgaris. Lasers Surg Med. 2007;39(2):189-92.
17. Laubach HJ, et al. Effects of a 1,450 nm diode laser on facial sebum excretion. Lasers Surg Med. 2009;41(2):110-5.
18. Arakane K, et al. Singlet oxygen (1 delta g) generation from coproporphyrin in Propionibacterium acnes on irradiation. Biochem Biophys Res Commun. 1996;223(3): 578-82.
19. Kjeldstad B, Johnsson A. An action spectrum for blue and near ultraviolet inactivation of Propionibacterium acnes; with emphasis on a possible porphyrin photosensitization. Photochem Photobiol. 1986;43(1):67-70.
20. Johnsson A, Kjeldstad B, Melo TB. Fluorescence from pilosebaceous follicles. Arch Dermatol Res. 1987;279(3):190-3.
21. Elman M, Slatkine M, Harth Y. The effective treatment of acne vulgaris by a high-intensity, narrow band 405-420 nm light source. J Cosmet Laser Ther. 2003;5(2):111-7.
22. Kawada A, et al. Acne phototherapy with a high-intensity, enhanced, narrow-band, blue light source: an open study and in vitro investigation. J Dermatol Sci. 2002;30(2):129-35.
23. Gold MH, et al. A multicenter clinical evaluation of the treatment of mild to moderate inflammatory acne vulgaris of the face with visible blue light in comparison to topical 1% clindamycin antibiotic solution. J Drugs Dermatol. 2005;4(1):64-70.
24. Sigurdsson V, Knulst AC, van Weelden H. Phototherapy of acne vulgaris with visible light. Dermatology. 1997;194(3):256-60.
25. Papageorgiou P, Katsambas A, Chu A. Phototherapy with blue (415 nm) and red (660 nm) light in the treatment of acne vulgaris. Br J Dermatol. 2000;142(5):973-8.
26. Konig K, et al. Red light kills bacteria via photodynamic action. Cell Mol Biol (Noisy-le-grand). 2000;46(7):1297-303.
27. Elman M, Lask G. The role of pulsed light and heat energy (LHE) in acne clearance. J Cosmet Laser Ther. 2004;6(2):91-5.
28. Rojanamatin J, Choawawanich P. Treatment of inflammatory facial acne vulgaris with intense pulsed light and short contact of topical 5-aminolevulinic acid: a pilot study. Dermatol Surg. 2006;32(8):991-6; discussion 996-7.
29. Gold MH, Biron J. Efficacy of a novel combination of pneumatic energy and broadband light for the treatment of acne. J Drugs Dermatol. 2008;7(7):639-42.
30. Wanitphakdeedecha R, Tanzi EL, Alster TS. Photopneumatic therapy for the treatment of acne. J Drugs Dermatol. 2009;8(3):239-41.

31. Kennedy JC, Pottier RH, Pross DC. Photodynamic therapy with endogenous protoporphyrin IX: basic principles and present clinical experience. J Photochem Photobiol B. 1990;6(1-2):143-8.
32. Divaris DX, Kennedy JC, Pottier RH. Phototoxic damage to sebaceous glands and hair follicles of mice after systemic administration of 5-aminolevulinic acid correlates with localized protoporphyrin IX fluorescence. Am J Pathol. 1990;136(4):891-7.
33. Hongcharu W, et al. Topical ALA-photodynamic therapy for the treatment of acne vulgaris. J Invest Dermatol. 2000;115(2):183-92.
34. Itoh Y, et al. Photodynamic therapy for acne vulgaris with topical 5-aminolevulinic acid. Arch Dermatol. 2000;136(9):1093-5.
35. Sakamoto FH, Lopes JD, Anderson RR. Photodynamic therapy for acne vulgaris: a critical review from basics to clinical practice: part I. Acne vulgaris: when and why consider photodynamic therapy? J Am Acad Dermatol. 2010;63(2):183-93; quiz 193-4.
36. Anderson RR, Parrish JA. The optics of human skin. J Invest Dermatol. 1981;77(1):13-9.
37. Sakamoto FH, et al. Porphyrin distribution after topical aminolevulinic acid in a novel porcine model of sebaceous skin. Lasers Surg Med. 2009;41(2):154-60.
38. Hong SB, Lee MH. Topical aminolevulinic acid-photodynamic therapy for the treatment of acne vulgaris. Photodermatol Photoimmunol Photomed. 2005;21(6):322-5.
39. Horfelt C, et al. Topical methyl aminolaevulinate photodynamic therapy for treatment of facial acne vulgaris: results of a randomized, controlled study. Br J Dermatol. 2006; 155(3):608-13.
40. Itoh Y, et al. Photodynamic therapy of acne vulgaris with topical delta-aminolaevulinic acid and incoherent light in Japanese patients. Br J Dermatol. 2001;144(3):575-9.
41. Wiegell SR, Wulf HC. Photodynamic therapy of acne vulgaris using methyl aminolaevulinate: a blinded, randomized, controlled trial. Br J Dermatol. 2006; 154(5):969-76.
42. Wiegell SR, Wulf HC. Photodynamic therapy of acne vulgaris using 5-aminolevulinic acid versus methyl aminolevulinate. J Am Acad Dermatol. 2006;54(4):647-51.
43. Yeung CK, et al. A comparative study of intense pulsed light alone and its combination with photodynamic therapy for the treatment of facial acne in Asian skin. Lasers Surg Med. 2007;39(1):1-6.
44. Akamatsu H, Horio T. The possible role of reactive oxygen species generated by neutrophils in mediating acne inflammation. Dermatology. 1998;196(1):82-5.
45. Pollock B, et al. Topical aminolaevulinic acid-photodynamic therapy for the treatment of acne vulgaris: a study of clinical efficacy and mechanism of action. Br J Dermatol. 2004; 151(3):616-22.
46. Horfelt C, et al. Photodynamic therapy for acne vulgaris: a pilot study of the dose-response and mechanism of action. Acta Derm Venereol. 2007;87(4):325-9.
47. Yung A, et al. Microbiological effect of photodynamic therapy (PDT) in healthy volunteers: a comparative study using methyl aminolaevulinate and hexyl aminolaevulinate cream. Clin Exp Dermatol. 2007;32(6):716-21.
48. Bryld LE, Jemec GB. The bacterial flora of the skin surface following routine MAL-PDT. J Dermatolog Treat. 2006;17(4):222-3.
49. Anderson RR, et al. Selective photothermolysis of lipid-rich tissues: a free electron laser study. Lasers Surg Med. 2006;38(10):913-9.
50. Wanner M, et al. Effects of non-invasive, 1,210 nm laser exposure on adipose tissue: results of a human pilot study. Lasers Surg Med. 2009;41(6):401-7.
51. Nordstrom KM, et al. Measurement of sebum output using a lipid absorbent tape. J Invest Dermatol. 1986;87(2):260-3.
52. Sakamoto FH, et al. Selective photothermolysis to target sebaceous glands: theoretical estimation of parameters and preliminary results using a free electron laser. Lasers Surg Med. 2012;44(2):175-83.
53. Janiczek-Dolphin N, et al. Can sebum reduction predict acne outcome? Br J Dermatol. 2010;163(4): 683-8.
54. Gollnick H, et al. Management of acne: a report from a Global Alliance to Improve Outcomes in Acne. J Am Acad Dermatol. 2003;49(1 Suppl):S1-37.

CHAPTER

7

Introduction to Laser Skin Resurfacing

Tina S Alster, Jennifer L MacGregor

INTRODUCTION TO LASER RESURFACING

The spectrum of nonfractionated laser skin resurfacing procedures ranges from traditional ablative resurfacing with carbon dioxide (CO_2) and erbium: yttrium-aluminum-garnet (Er:YAG) lasers to newer nonablative infrared and fractional laser devices (Table 7.1). The devices and techniques used must be tailored to the skin type, goals and lifestyle of each individual patient and the type and depth of the photoaging, rhytides, scars, or epidermal lesions being treated. Attention to basic principles related to preoperative evaluation, intraoperative technique and postoperative care lead to consistent clinical results and a low risk of complications.

RESURFACING LASERS: EVOLUTION AND MECHANISM OF ACTION

Ablative Resurfacing

The earliest resurfacing devices used for laser skin resurfacing involved continuous-wave (CW) argon, neodymium:yttrium-aluminum-garnet (Nd:YAG), and carbon dioxide (CO_2) lasers. The infrared 10,600-nm CO_2 laser is absorbed by water in the superficial layers of the skin leading to vaporization of tissue. The vaporized tissue is surrounded by denatured collagen, coagulated debris and cauterized small cutaneous blood vessels.[1] The destructive and hemostatic capabilities of the early CO_2 lasers made them useful tools for removal of epithelial lesions and neoplasms as well as for cutting.[1-3] These same CW devices; however, also produced excess thermal damage to tissue and an unacceptably high risk of skin necrosis and scarring due to their long tissue dwell times.[4-6]

Pulsed- or rapidly scanned CO_2 laser systems were subsequently developed for selective absorption of laser light by the target chromophore in the skin (water) to induce temperature-controlled, target-specific injury without damage to surrounding healthy tissue.[7] Initial attempts to accomplish this involved "superpulsed" high peak power devices that produced rapid-repetition ultra-short pulses (200–1,000 pulses per second) or shuttering of the continuous beam to produce a 0.1–1 second burst of laser energy.[8,9] Modern devices emit either a high-energy pulse of 1 millisecond (ms) or shorter (pulsed CO_2) or rapidly scan a CW laser beam so that the dwell time on any individual spot is less than 1 ms (scanned CO_2).[10] With delivery of high energy, the laser light penetrates 20–30 μm into the skin in a single pass and the short pulses ensure that exposure is shorter than the thermal relaxation time of the cutaneous tissue that absorbs this wavelength, thus limiting thermal damage to surrounding structures.[11-17] Additional passes with the CO_2 wavelength produce deeper residual thermal damage (RTD) that extends approximately 100–150 μm into the dermis and stimulates collagen contracture, remodeling and skin tightening.[10,13,17] Clinically, this translates into significant improvement of cutaneous photoaging, rhytides and scars. Carbon dioxide laser resurfacing remains the gold standard resurfacing device to which other systems are compared.

Table 7.1: Spectrum of nonfractional lasers for skin resurfacing

Ablative		*Nonablative*	
Laser	**Wavelength**	**Laser**	**Wavelength(s)**
CO_2	10,600 nm	PDL	585–595 nm
Erbium:YAG	2940 nm	KTP	532 nm
Erbium:YSGG	2790 nm	Nd:YAG (Q-switched, long-pulsed)	1064 nm
		Nd:YAG (long-pulsed)	1320 nm
		Diode (long-pulsed)	1450 nm
		Erbium:glass	1540 nm
		Non-Laser	
		Intense pulsed light (IPL)	515–1200 nm
		Photodynamic therapy with 5-ALA or MAL	Activation with blue or red light, IPL, PDL

CO_2: Carbon dioxide; YAG: Yttrium-aluminum-garnet; YSGG: Yttrium-scandium-gallium-garnet; PDL: Pulsed-dye laser; KTP: Potassium-titanyl-phosphate; Nd: Neodymium; Q-switched: Quality-switched; 5-ALA: 5-aminolevulinic acid; MAL: Methyl aminolevulinate

The 2940-nm Er:YAG laser has an absorption coefficient that is 16 times that of the CO_2 laser, a shorter pulse duration, narrower depth of vaporization and smaller zone of RTD. While Er:YAG resurfacing is associated with shorter recovery times, it is less clinically effective than is the CO_2 laser for treatment of rhytides and scars.[11,17-22] The multiple-pass CO_2 laser resurfacing procedure has the greatest efficacy, but a longer postoperative recovery and higher complication risk than either single-pass CO_2 or multiple-pass Er:YAG laser.[18,20] A variety of combination treatments using ablative lasers and traditional excisional surgery have been described in an effort to enhance results and minimize recovery for patients.[23-27] The erbium:yttrium-scandium-gallium-garnet (Er:YSGG) system's unique 2790-nm wavelength has been shown to exhibit better coagulation and shorter recovery times than Er:YAG due to an absorption coefficient roughly five times that of the CO_2 laser.[28]

Nonablative Resurfacing

Most nonablative laser systems used for skin resurfacing were developed to deliver heat to the dermis without creating an external wound in an effort to stimulate neocollagenesis and improve skin surface texture with minimal postoperative recovery.[17,29-31] Some lasers that were originally developed for other clinical applications (e.g. pulsed-dye lasers for vascular lesions) have also been shown to remodel collagen and smooth the texture of photodamaged and scarred skin.[32-34] The systems most frequently used for nonablative laser skin resurfacing include infrared wavelengths (1064-nm Nd:YAG, 1320-nm Nd:YAG, 1450-nm diode, 1540-nm erbium:glass) which penetrate deeper into the dermis to provide more uniform dermal heating for increased collagen effect.[29-31,35-45] While some differences have been demonstrated between these systems, they each essentially provide noticeable (albeit, mild) clinical improvement of rhytides and scars with minimal side-effects and recovery profiles.[29]

Fractionated Resurfacing

The introduction of fractional technology in 2004 revolutionized the field of laser skin resurfacing with devices that deliver microscopic columns of energy to treat a fraction of the skin surface.[46] The microscopic, intervening areas of untreated skin serves as a reservoir for faster wound healing. As such, fractionated laser technology permits deeper delivery of laser energy and improves the recovery time and side-effect profile over pulsed and scanned laser systems and has been used successfully to treat a variety of the same cutaneous lesions as these older systems.[47-50] Fractionated laser skin resurfacing is discussed separately in Chapters 8 and 9.

Table 7.2: Indications for laser skin resurfacing
Actinic cheilitis
Actinic damage/photoaging with rhytides and/or skin laxity
Adnexal tumors
Angiofibroma
Epidermal nevi
Lymphangioma circumscriptum (microcystic)
Rhinophyma
Scars
Sebaceous hyperplasia
Seborrheic keratosis
Xanthelasma
Squamous cell carcinoma in situ
Superficial basal cell carcinoma

CLINICAL INDICATIONS

Ablative and nonablative laser resurfacing techniques are used to address a variety of skin conditions (Table 7.2). With the ongoing development of new devices, the list of clinical indications for which they can be utilized continues to expand. Nonablative wavelengths and fractional devices provide safer treatment alternatives in areas of higher risk (nonfacial sites) and in patients with darker skin phototypes.[50-52]

Facial Aging

Photoaged skin is characterized by dyschromia, rhytides, fragility, laxity and dull tone. Histologically, the epidermis appears thickened with variable increase in melanocytes (correlating clinically with dyschromia) and the healthy mature collagen and elastic fibers in the dermis are replaced by clumped, fragmented and amorphous material (solar elastosis). Carbon dioxide laser resurfacing physically removes the entire epidermis in a single pass and, depending on the system used and the number of laser passes delivered, a variable thickness of the dermis is vaporized.[13] Dyschromia and superficial lesions are removed. The residual thermal damage (RTD) that extends into the dermis induces wound healing, neocollagenesis, tissue tightening and a smoothing effect.[10,13] Histological comparisons of two high-energy pulsed systems (Coherent Ultrapulse vs Sharplan SilkTouch) showed roughly equivalent epidermal ablation and RTD of 20–30 μm after one pass with either system. Mild differences between systems were observed with additional passes, but both yielded less tissue vaporization and additional RTD— 40 μm and 70 μm, respectively, for the second and third passes with the Ultrapulse and 80 μm and 150 μm, respectively, for the SilkTouch.[13]

In the first few days after CO_2 laser treatment, a portion of the denatured collagen sloughs, followed by re-epithelialization over 5–7 days. Granulation tissue formation and the wound healing cascade ensues over the next 3–6 months, resulting in a final zone of fibroplasia that is roughly proportional to the RTD produced in the dermis.[10] After CO_2 laser vaporization, the amorphous layer of solar elastosis markedly decreases and is replaced with an increased thickness and density of collagen fibers. This translates into dramatic and durable rhytide reduction and overall improvement in skin tone and texture[11,12,53-57] (Figs 7.1A and B). Patients with deeply etched rhytides and skin laxity may elect to endure the longer recovery associated with this procedure, but the prolonged recovery (discussed in detail below) makes it a less attractive option for many.

With its stronger absorption coefficient for water, each Er:YAG pulse yields a brisk audible "pop" as tissue is ablated and heat dissipates from the skin surface. With limited penetration of 2–5 μm/J/cm^2, approximately three Er:YAG passes are typically required to ablate the epidermis.[21] Intraoperative bleeding is more significant than that seen with CO_2 laser treatment because of the diminished residual thermal damage and coagulation produced with Er:YAG laser irradiation.[58] Given the laser–tissue interaction, the Er:YAG is best suited for skin requiring less contouring and rhytide reduction and/or for those patients who desire a shorter recovery[22,30,31,59-62] (Figs 7.2A and B). Single pass CO_2 laser resurfacing is another less aggressive resurfacing option and is nearly comparable to multiple pass Er:YAG procedures.[18,20,63]

The use of nonablative lasers for photodamaged skin became popularized due to their ability to effect clinical improvement without significant postoperative recovery or morbidity. A distinct advantage of nonablative laser skin treatment is its application to nonfacial sites without undue risk of side-effects and complications.[30,31,60,61] Multiple monthly treatments are typically prescribed and clinical improvement is slow and progressive [35,36] (Figs 7.3A and B).

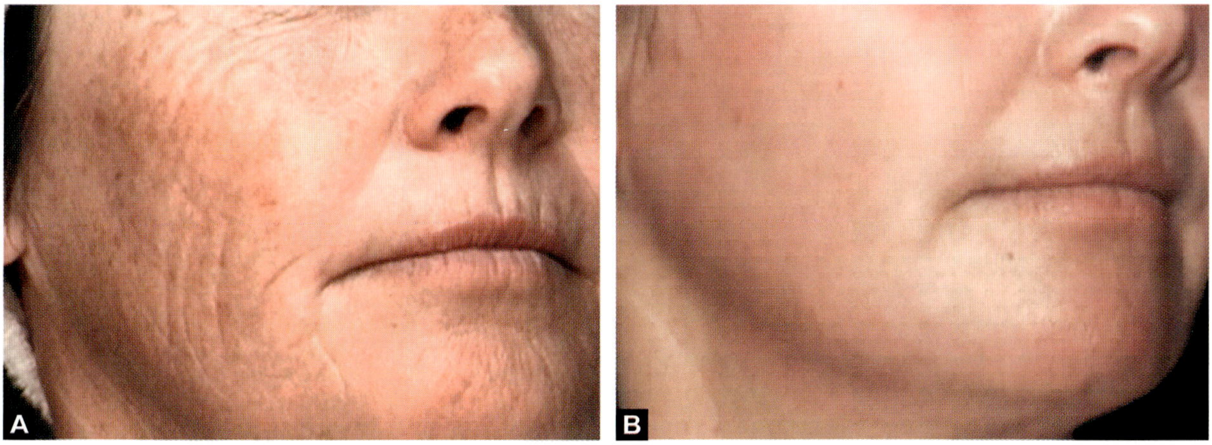

Figs 7.1A and B: Photodamaged skin before (A) and 6 months after multiple pass CO_2 laser skin resurfacing (B)

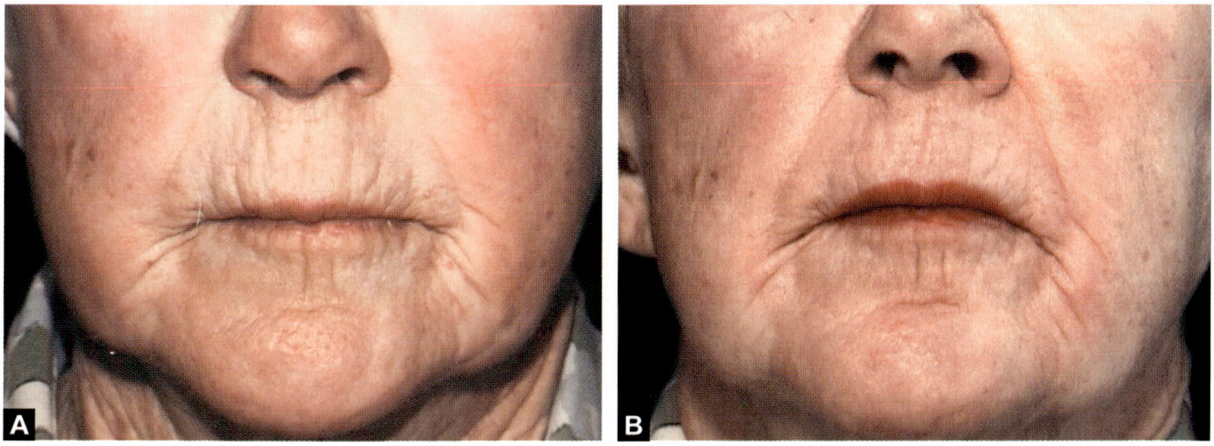

Figs 7.2A and B: Photoaged skin before (A) and 6 months after multiple pass Er:YAG laser skin resurfacing (B)

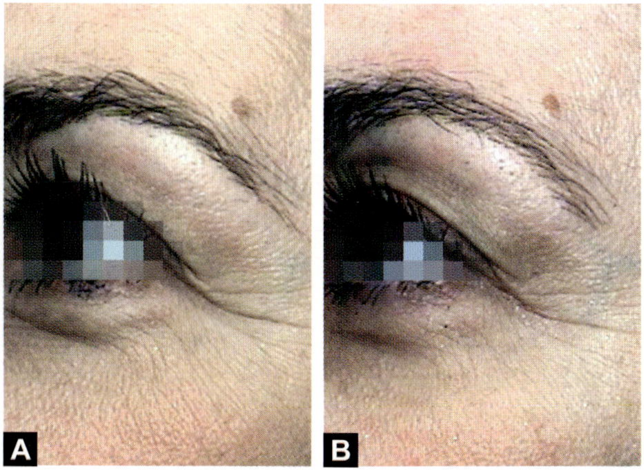

Figs 7.3A and B: Photodamaged skin before (A) and 6 months after three consecutive monthly nonablative infrared laser treatments (B)

Atrophic Scars

Atrophic scars appear as depressions in the skin and result from inadequate collagen replacement during the remodeling phase of wound healing.[64] Atrophic acne scars are often classified into three types: rolling, boxcar and icepick.[65] Rolling scars are wide, undulating depressions with sloping borders where the depression is often associated with deep fibrous tethering. Boxcar scars have sharply marginated borders with marked "step-offs" and icepick scars are 1–2 mm diameter narrow, tapered pits. Ablative skin resurfacing with CO_2 or Er:YAG lasers leads to a smooth skin surface by tissue vaporization and dermal recontouring through neocollagenesis.[66-68] As a consequence, scar borders become less distinct and surface texture becomes more uniform.

Clinical improvement of scars after ablative laser skin resurfacing averages 50–80% with the most dramatic results seen after multiple pass CO_2 laser resurfacing.[66,69] Sustained and even continued scar improvement has been observed after a single CO_2 laser procedure.[70] Short-pulsed Er:YAG laser treatment yields mild to moderate improvement

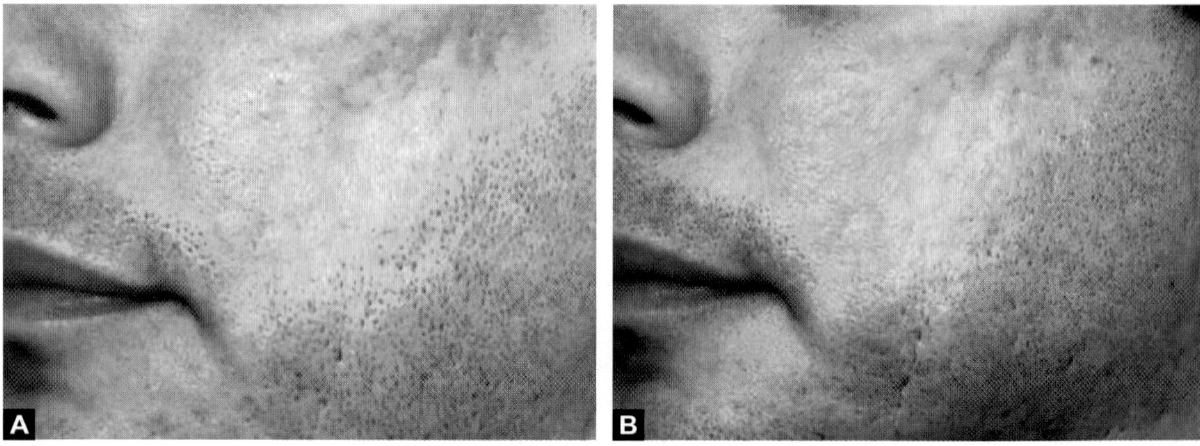

Figs 7.4A and B: Atrophic acne scars before (A) and after ablative laser skin resurfacing treatment (B)

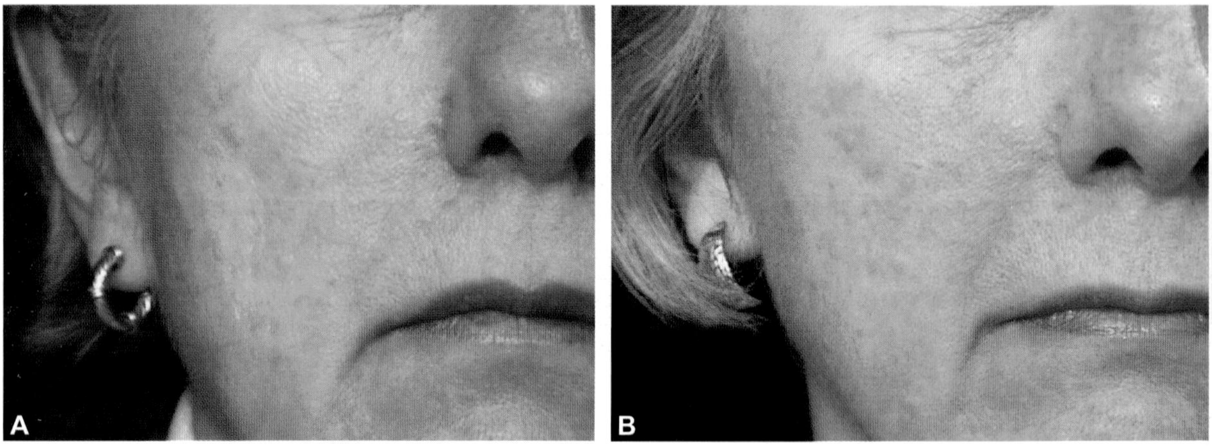

Figs 7.5A and B: Atrophic facial scars before (A) and after three consecutive monthly nonablative laser treatments (B)

of scars,[71] but a longer-pulsed (dual mode) Er:YAG system has been shown to be a better treatment alternative for more severe scars[22] (Figs 7.4A and B).

Nonablative lasers have also been used successfully to treat a variety of atrophic scars due to their ability to deliver energy to the papillary and mid-dermis and effect neocollagenesis.[38-40,43-45] A series of three or more treatments are typically delivered on a monthly basis with gradual improvement of scars in most patients over the ensuing 6 months. Nonablative laser treatment is particularly useful for those individuals who do not have time for postoperative recovery or have dark skin tones and/or scars in nonfacial body regions[66] (Figs 7.5A and B).

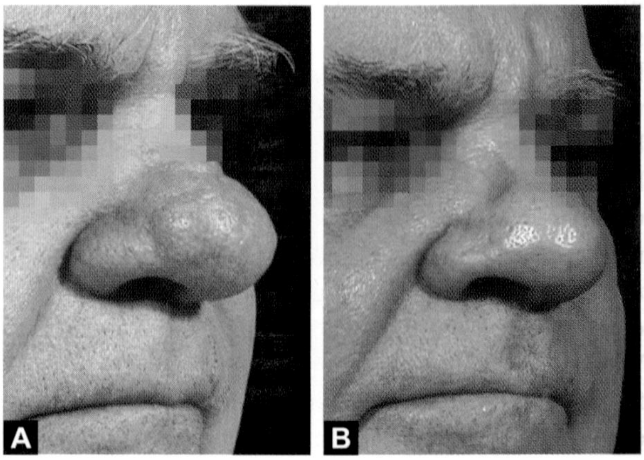

Figs 7.6A and B: Rhinophyma before (A) and 6 months after one ablative laser skin resurfacing treatment (B)

Epidermal and Dermal Lesions

Ablative lasers are particularly useful for vaporization of a wide variety of benign epidermal and dermal lesions including seborrheic keratoses, epidermal nevi, xanthelasma, lymphangioma circumscriptum (microcystic) and sebaceous hyperplasia[72-78] (Figs 7.6A and B). Initial enthusiasm for CO_2 laser treatment of verrucae[73,79] has been dampened by

Table 7.3: Preoperative considerations and management

Preoperative Consideration	*Management*
Darker skin phototype	Proper wavelength selection, caution regarding postinflammatory pigmentation risk, consider test area
History of herpes simplex virus (HSV)	Antiviral prophylaxis*
Anticoagulant use	Discontinue 2 weeks prior to treatment for pulsed dye and ablative resurfacing
Acne prone	Empiric systemic therapy if recent history of inflammatory lesions
Smoking	Avoid or reduce smoking pre- and postablative resurfacing
Dermatographism	Consider pretreatment with antihistamines
Rosacea	Consider vascular laser treatment in combination, anticipate flare
Atopic history	Anticipate and control dermatitis
Psoriasis or vitiligo	Consider potential for Koebner phenomenon
Pregnancy/nursing	Delay procedure
Isotretinoin use	Delay treatment 6 months
Concurrent infection	Avoid laser treatment to affected area
Ectropion	Avoid ablative infraorbital treatment, caution in patients with prior lower blepharoplasty
Previous dermabrasion or phenol chemical peel	Greater risk for poor healing and postoperative hypopigmentation, consider nonablative therapies
Seizures or migraine headache	Possible laser-induced trigger, avoid treatment with visible light wavelengths
Keloids or abnormal scarring	Greater scar risk, avoid ablative resurfacing (exceptions possible)
Radiation history or scleroderma	Greater risk for poor healing, avoid ablative resurfacing (exceptions possible)

*All patients (regardless of HSV history) receive oral antiviral prophylaxis with perioral or full face ablative laser resurfacing

the aerosolization of human papilloma virus and its potential inhalation by health care practitioners and staff. Hyperplastic conditions (rhinophyma) and adnexal tumors such as trichoepitheliomas, syringomas, papillomas, and angiofibromas can be substantially reduced with CO_2 or Er:YAG laser treatment,[80-90] but serial treatments every few years may be required to smooth new and expanding residual lesions particularly when underlying syndromes (e.g. Cowden's, Brook-Spiegler) exist. There are multiple reports also supporting the use of ablative lasers for the treatment of actinic chelitis, superficial basal cell carcinoma, and squamous cell carcinoma in situ.[91-96] While ablative lasers have proven most successful for these epidermal and dermal lesions, nonablative devices are not useful except as adjunct treatment to improve the cosmesis of results.

PATIENT SELECTION AND PREPARATION

Patients should be carefully screened as to their health and lifestyle factors during the preoperative consultation. Their goals, expectations of the procedure and its recovery as well as their tolerance for potential risks should be assessed.[97] The patient must be able to strictly adhere to pre- and postoperative instructions. Patients that elect to undergo ablative resurfacing must also prepare mentally for a low mood or "lull" in the immediate postoperative period followed by improved perspective and satisfaction as healing is completed and results become evident.[98] Nonablative treatments are better suited to those who are unwilling or unable to tolerate a significant recovery, for those with darker skin types, and for resurfacing of nonfacial skin. If choosing a nonablative approach, the patient should be willing to undergo a series of multiple treatment sessions and accept modest incremental improvement in exchange for a shorter and less risky recovery period. Table 7.3 summarizes the components of the preoperative evaluation and management.

Traditional ablative resurfacing of the face can be safely performed on patients who have Fitzpatrick skin phototypes I–II and are in good general health. Fractional ablative resurfacing can be performed on those with darker Fitzpatrick skin phototypes III–VI; however, there is a higher risk of postinflammatory hyperpigmentation. A variety of pretreatment regimens including hydroquinone, glycolic acid and tretinoin, have not been shown to reduce the postoperative pigmentation associated with ablative laser resurfacing.[99] Prior to full face ablative resurfacing, particularly if general anesthesia is planned, an age-appropriate preoperative medical clearance is required. The patient must be prepared with postoperative transportation and adequate home-care assistance and skin care supplies. Patients must provide consent for the procedure and clinical photography, have had all their questions answered to their complete satisfaction, and have prescriptions verified prior to the procedure.

LASER SAFETY AND OPERATIVE TECHNIQUE

The discomfort associated with nonablative resurfacing is typically mild to moderate, depending on wavelength. Commercially-available anesthetic cream (4% or 5% lidocaine) or compounded higher concentrations are safe to use prior to nonablative resurfacing procedures when limited to small areas. Ablative resurfacing is associated with significant discomfort during and immediately after treatment. At a minimum, patients will require anxiolytics, pain medication, and sensory nerve blockade with tumescent anesthesia to the lateral face, mandible and eyelids. Most physicians and patients prefer intravenous (twilight) anesthesia for ablative resurfacing of the face. This necessitates the skills of an anesthesiologist or certified nurse anesthetist for intravenous access, appropriate intraoperative monitoring and emergency equipment.

Safety

The treatment room should have the appropriate physical eye protection for intraoperative personnel. Internal metal eye shields should be inserted for any laser or light procedure that involves treatment of skin within the orbital rim and cutaneous laser surgeons should be accomplished at applying and removing such shields. There should be no flammable solutions or materials in the laser field. Alcohol and aluminum chloride are particularly dangerous.

Technique

Topical anesthetic cream should be removed and the skin dried thoroughly prior to laser irradiation. Nonablative resurfacing procedures and techniques generally involve a series of full-facial treatments delivered monthly for 3–6 months, with follow-up assessments occurring at 3 months, 6 months and 1 year.

For ablative procedures, the hair is secured with a headband and the patient is positioned supine with adequate lighting. Intravenous or local anesthesia is administered and the skin is prepped with chlorhexidine or similar surgical preparation and then completely dried. Test pulses of the laser should be fired on a dampened tongue depressor (or other inanimate object) prior to proceeding. A collimated spot handpiece may be used first to sculpt scar edges and papular lesions. The scanning handpiece can then be used to deliver nonoverlapping laser passes over the cutaneous surface. Deeper rhytides and concavities are stretched to ensure smooth treatment. A tongue depressor or Jaeger bone plate can be used to protect the lashes and brows while treating periorbital skin. Lower energy and/or fewer passes are recommended when treating the thin periorbital skin and extreme caution should be used in patients with previous blepharoplasty surgery. The perioral area should be treated over the vermillion border while covering the teeth with moist gauze to protect from laser-induced etching of dental enamel. The transition of the mandible to the neck should be feathered with lower fluence and/or fewer passes to prevent a sharp demarcation line between treated and untreated skin. If the patient has had previous face and neck lifting, the neck skin may be transposed over the mandible, necessitating very low density treatment.

In multiple pass procedures, partially desiccated tissue is removed with saline-soaked gauze and dried prior to placement of additional passes. A third- or fourth pass is useful in areas of fibrotic acne scars, deep rhytides, or papular lesions. The Er:YAG laser vaporizes less tissue per pass and may require additional passes, depending on the energy, to ablate the epidermis or epidermal lesions. Moderately overlapping pulses should be applied until rhytides/scars are effaced. Partially desiccated tissue from the final pass is left intact to serve as a wound dressing. At the completion of the procedure, moist gauze and ice packs are applied for 10–20 minutes. Petrolatum-based ointment (or short-term occlusive dressing) is applied, vital signs are documented, and the patient is escorted to the lavoratory to ensure they are oriented and ambulatory prior to discharge home.

Table 7.4: Side-effects and complications of ablative laser skin resurfacing

Mild/Transient	*Moderate*	*Severe/Prolonged*
Prolonged erythema	Localized infection	True hypopigmentation
Postinflammatory hyperpigmentation	Topical anesthesia toxicity	Disseminated infection
Relative hypopigmentation	Eruptive keratoacanthomas	Scarring
Milia and/or acne exacerbation		Ectropion
Dermatitis		

POSTOPERATIVE MANAGEMENT

Nonablative laser skin resurfacing requires minimal postoperative care. Patients are simply prescribed gentle cleanser, sun protection and noncomedogenic moisturizer after the procedure. Transient erythema and edema generally resolves within a few days.

Ablative laser skin resurfacing involves a more significant recovery period. Postoperative pain and swelling is diminished with application of ice packs and oral analgesics. Anxiolytics and antihistamines can be prescribed for insomnia and pruritis, respectively. Bio-occlusive dressings may be used in the first 24–72 hours to speed re-epithelialization, but there is no consensus regarding their use and daily examination of the patient during the initial postoperative period is necessary to assess for signs of infection. The authors use dilute 0.25% acetic acid-soaked compresses with ice packs to the treated skin for 15–20 minutes every 2–4 hours followed by application of bland petrolatum-based ointment. Head elevation with extra pillows also helps to minimize edema, but if severe periorbital swelling is anticipated such that it threatens to impair vision, a short course (3–5 days) of systemic corticosteroids can be prescribed.

The skin should be completely protected from the sun until epithelialization is complete, followed by aggressive sun avoidance and sunscreen use. Botulinum toxin injections are often recommended to soften dynamic rhytides (e.g. brow, lateral canthi) during the most active phase of collagen remodeling following laser resurfacing.[100] Following ablative laser resurfacing of the full face, patients are seen in the office the next day. Depending on the procedure performed, surface area treated, and patient needs, several visits are required in the first postoperative week. Since most infections occur during the re-epithelialization process, very close monitoring during the initial postoperative period is essential for early detection and management of potential complications.[101,102]

COMPLICATIONS

Nonablative laser resurfacing can be complicated by prolonged erythema, edema, pigmentation, acne flare or herpes simplex outbreak. Those with history of labial herpes simplex are given empiric antiviral prophylaxis. Scarring and textural changes are rare using modern nonablative devices and correct technique. Patients are able to apply makeup and return to their regular activities within 1–3 days following treatment.

Recovery, side-effects and complications following ablative laser resurfacing are well documented.[103-109] Although patients do not generally report pain after the first few hours following treatment, they experience some discomfort associated with subsequent healing, serosanguinous discharge and edema. This evolution of the healing process should be expected and managed. True complications from ablative laser resurfacing range from mild acne flares and prolonged erythema to devastating infection and hypertrophic scarring. Reported complications of ablative laser resurfacing are listed in Table 7.4. Fractional ablative laser resurfacing is associated with a much lower incidence of these side-effects.[110] Faster recovery and lower risk profile along with a greater diversity in treatment settings and applications have popularized fractional devices beyond that of the nonfractional laser resurfacing techniques described herein.

The skin after multiple-pass CO_2 laser resurfacing will re-epithelialize in approximately 1 week. Postoperative erythema may last for several weeks to months and is an expected side-effect of treatment. Single-pass CO_2 and multiple-pass Er:YAG treatment is associated with a faster re-epithelialization process (5–7 days) and less severe and prolonged erythema (approximately 1 month).[18] Individuals with underlying atopic dermatitis or rosacea may be predisposed to more significant erythema. Management techniques include aggressive sun protection, green-tinted facial makeup, light-emitting diode (LED) treatment,[111] and topical corticosteroids for associated pruritis.

Approximately one third of patients treated with CO_2 or erbium laser will develop some degree of post-inflammatory hyperpigmentation, with a higher incidence typical in darker skin phototypes (Fitzpatrick III–VI).[22,103,109] The pigmentation first appears as areas of intense erythema resolve. The discoloration can last for several months, but faster resolution can be achieved with the use of topical skin lighteners (e.g. hydroquinone, lignin peroxidase, retinoic acid, azelaic acid, ascorbic acid, and glycolic acid) as well as office-based chemical peels and aggressive sun protection.

Laser resurfacing removes lentigines and actinic bronzing to yield a lighter, more even skin tone. Treated skin may appear hypopigmented relative to adjacent skin with actinic bronzing and photodamage. Lines of demarcation along the mandible and lateral neck are typical and can easily be blended by treating the neck and chest with intense pulsed light, vascular and pigment-specific lasers, nonablative or fractional laser resurfacing, or chemical peels. Delayed hypopigmentation, appearing as a pale glassy skin tone, is a rare complication of multiple pass CO_2 laser resurfacing that appears 6–12 months after treatment.[107-109] Feathering at the mandible with lower energy and/or fewer passes minimizes this undesirable effect. Repigmentation has been attempted with topical psoralen and ultraviolet exposure and with the use of an excimer laser with variable results.[109]

Acne and milia are thought to be related to the use of occlusive ointments and/or aberrant follicular epithelialization during the healing process.[109] Although mild lesions resolve spontaneously without treatment, those with significant involvement should be treated with systemic antibiotics to prevent scarring. Milia also resolve spontaneously, but can be manually extracted to improve clinical appearance. Patients with recent acne or inflammatory lesions should receive oral antibiotics prior to and after resurfacing.

Dermatitis occurs after laser resurfacing due to barrier compromise with increased sensitivity to allergens or irritants. Bland emollient ointment should be used exclusively in the postoperative period and medicated topicals, home remedies, fragrance and preservative-containing products must be avoided.[106-109] Dermatitis typically resolves as the offending agent is discontinued, but application of topical corticosteroids are useful to prevent excoriations and potential damage to resurfaced skin.

Viral, bacterial and fungal infections can be devastating in newly resurfaced skin. In the absence of cutaneous epithelium, signs of infection are atypical and must be recognized even if they are subtle. Symptoms and signs of concern include localized pain, erosions, focal areas of delayed healing, increased erythema, and excessive crusting.[105-109] Frequent early postoperative visits, very high suspicion, and a low threshold to culture and empirically treatment of patients is required until a firm diagnosis is made. All facial resurfacing patients should receive oral antiviral medication, starting on the day of (or prior to) treatment and continuing for at least 7–10 days (longer if viral infection is suspected). Despite prophylaxis, 2–7% of patients will still develop herpes simplex infection.[112] Dissemination of the herpes virus should be treated aggressively with hospital admission for intravenous acyclovir because of the associated risk of atrophic scarring. The use of prophylactic antibiotics for laser resurfacing is not considered "standard" and is not supported by medical literature; however, since bacterial infection in this setting can be devastating, many laser surgeons routinely prescribe empiric antibiotic therapy for 7–10 days.

Scarring and textural changes are rare. Poor operator technique involving overlapping pulses and use of high energy densities can lead to excessive tissue heating and scar formation. Failure to uncover important preoperative history can also have grave consequences. Scarring may occur when aggressive settings are used in the periorbital area in patients with previous lower blepharoplasty or over the mandible in patients with history of face and neck lifting. Poor wound care, missed postoperative appointments, untreated infections, severe acne flares, pruritis and excoriation may also lead to scarring. Impending scar formation should be considered if focal tenderness or induration develops in a high-risk location. Early institution of potent topical corticosteroids and pulsed-dye laser treatment can improve the appearance and symptoms of laser-induced scars.[106,109]

CONCLUSION

Laser surgeons will continue to combine, modify and individualize treatments to maximize efficacy and minimize morbidity for their patients. Technical advances, including the development of fractional technology, have expanded the clinical applications for laser skin resurfacing. The development of new devices with improved safety profiles is exciting, but the potential for complications still exists. Laser surgeons must adhere to the same set of principles and complete meticulous pre-, intra- and postoperative care in order to achieve success as new devices become available.

REFERENCES

1. Tanzi EL, Alster TS. Ablative lasers, chemical peels and dermabrasion. In: Goldsmith L, et al (Eds). Fitzpatrick's Dermatology in General Medicine,8th edition. New York: McGraw-Hill Companies, Inc.;2012.pp.3021-31.
2. Shapshay SM, Strong MS, Anastasi GW, et al. Removal of rhinophyma with the CO_2 laser: a preliminary report. Arch Otolaryng. 1980;106:257-9.
3. Dufresne RG, Garrett AB, Balin PL, et al. CO_2 laser treatment of chronic actinic chelitis. J Am Acad Dermatol. 1988;19:876-8.
4. Labandter H, Kaplan I. Experience with a "continuous" laser in the treatment of suitable cutaneous conditions: preliminary report. J Dermatol Surg Oncol. 1977;3:527-30.
5. Haina D, Landthaler M, Braun-Falco O, et al. Comparison of the maximum coagulation depth in human skin for different types of medical lasers. Lasers Surg Med. 1987;7:355-62.
6. Lanzafame RJ, Naim JO, Rogers DW, et al. Comparisons of continuous-wave, chop wave, and superpulsed laser wounds. Lasers Surg Med. 1988;8:119-24.
7. Anderson RR, Parrish JA. Selective photothermolysis: precise microsurgery by selective absorption of pulsed radiation. Science. 1983;220:524-7.
8. Olbricht SM. Use of the carbon dioxide laser in dermatologic surgery: a clinically relevant update for 1993. J Dermatol Surg Oncol. 1993;19:364-9.
9. Fitzpatrick RE, Ruiz-Esparaza J, Goldman MP. The depth of thermal necrosis using the CO_2 laser: a comparison of the superpulsed mode and conventional mode. J Dermatol Surg Oncol;1991.pp.340-4.
10. Ross EV, McKinlay JR, Anderson RR. Why does carbon dioxide resurfacing work? Arch Dermatol. 1999;135:444-54.
11. Alster TS. Cutaneous resurfacing with CO_2 and erbium:YAG lasers: preoperative, intraoperative, and postoperative considerations. Plast Reconstr Surg. 1999;103:619-32.
12. Alster TS, Nanni CA, Williams CM. Comparison of four carbon dioxide resurfacing lasers: a clinical and histopathologic evaluation. Dermatol Surg. 1999;25:153-9.
13. Alster TS, Kauvar ANB, Geronemus RG. Histology of high-energy pulsed CO_2 laser resurfacing. Semin Cutan Med Surg. 1996;15:189-93.
14. Tanzi ET, Lupton JR, Alster TS. Review of lasers in dermatology: four decades of progress. J Am Acad Dermatol. 2003;49:1-31.
15. Walsh JT, Flotte TJ, Anderson RR, et al. Pulsed CO_2 laser tissue ablation: Effect of tissue type and pulse duration of thermal damage. Lasers Surg Med. 1988;8:108-18.
16. Walsh JJ, Deutsch TF. Pulsed CO_2 laser tissue ablation: measurement of the ablation rate. Lasers Surg Med. 1988;8:264-75.
17. Alexiades-Armenakas, Dover JS, Arndt KA. The spectrum of laser skin resurfacing: nonablative, fractional, and ablative laser resurfacing. J Am Acad Dermatol. 2008;58: 719-37.
18. Tanzi EL, Alster TS. Single-pass carbon dioxide versus multiple-pass Er:YAG laser skin resurfacing: a comparison of postoperative wound healing and side effect rates. Dermatol Surg. 2003;29:80-4.
19. Alster TS, Lupton JR. Erbium:YAG cutaneous laser resurfacing. Dermatol Clin. 2001;19:453-66.
20. Ross EV, Miller C, Meehan K, et al. One-pass CO_2 versus multiple-pass Er:YAG laser resurfacing in the treatment of rhytides: a comparison side-by-side study of pulsed CO_2 and Er:YAG lasers. Dermatol Surg. 2001;27:709-15.
21. Alster TS. Clinical and histologic evaluation of six erbium:YAG lasers for cutaneous resurfacing. Lasers Surg Med. 1999;24:87-92.
22. Tanzi EL, Alster TS. Side effects and complications of variable-pulsed erbium:yttrium-aluminum-garnet laser skin resurfacing: extended experience with 50 patients. Plast Reconstr Surg. 2003;111:1524-9; discussion 1530-2.
23. Goon PK, Dalal M, Peart FC. The gold standard for decortication of rhinophyma: combined erbium-YAG/CO_2 laser.Aesthetic Plast Surg. 2004;28:456-60.
24. Alster TS, Doshi SN, Hopping SB. Combination surgical lifting with ablative laser skin resurfacing of facial skin: a retrospective analysis. Dermatol Surg. 2004;30:1191-5.
25. McDaniel DH, Lord J, Ash K, et al. Combined CO_2/erbium:YAG laser resurfacing of perioral rhytides and side-by-side comparison with carbon dioxide laser alone. Dermatol Surg. 1999;25:285-93.
26. Trelles MA, Allones I, Luna R. One-pass resurfacing with a combined-mode erbium: YAG/CO_2 laser system: a study in 102 patients. Br J Dermatol. 2002;146: 473-80.

27. Collawn SS. Combination therapy: utilization of CO_2 and erbium:YAG lasers for skin resurfacing. Ann Plast Surg. 1999;42:21-6.
28. Ross EV, Swann M, Soon S, et al. Full-face treatments with the 2790-nm erbium:YSGG laser system. J Drugs Dermatol. 2009;8:248-52.
29. Alster TS, Lupton JR. Are all infrared lasers equally effective in skin rejuvenation. Semin Cutan Med Surg. 2002;21:274-9.
30. Alster TS, Tanzi EL. Laser skin resurfacing: ablative and nonablative. In: Robinson J, Sengelman R, Siegel DM, Hanke CM (Eds). Surgery of the Skin. Philadelphia: Elsevier; 2005.pp.611-24.
31. Alster TS, Doshi S. Ablative and non-ablative laser skin resurfacing. In: Burgess C (Ed). Cosmetic Dermatology. Heidelberg: Springer-Verlag; 2005. pp.111-26.
32. Alster TS, Kurban AK, Grove GL, et al. Alteration of argon laser-induced scars by the pulsed dye laser. Lasers Surg Med. 1993;13:368-73.
33. Goldberg D, Tan M, Dale Sarradet M, et al. Nonablative dermal remodeling with a 585-nm, 350-microsec, flashlamp pulsed dye laser: clinical and ultrastructural analysis. Dermatol Surg. 2003;29:161-3.
34. Goldberg DJ, Sarradet D, Hussain M, et al. Clinical, histologic, and ultrastructural changes after nonablative treatment with a 595-nm flashlamp-pumped pulsed dye laser: comparison of varying settings. Dermatol Surg. 2004;30:979-82.
35. Lupton JR, Alster TS. Nonablative cutaneous laser resurfacing using a 1.54 um erbium glass laser: a clinical and histologic analysis. Dermatol Surg. 2002;28:833-5.
36. Tanzi EL, Williams CM, Alster TS. Treatment of facial rhytides with a nonablative 1450nm diode laser: a controlled clinical and histologic study. Dermatol Surg. 2003;29: 124-8.
37. Rogachefsky AS, Hussain M, Goldberg DJ. Atrophic and a mixed pattern of acne scars improved with a 1,320-nm Nd:YAG laser. Dermatol Surg. 2003;29:904-8.
38. Tanzi EL, Alster TS. Comparison of a 1450-nm diode laser and a 1320-nm Nd:YAG laser in the treatment of atrophic facial scars: a prospective clinical and histologic study. Dermatol Surg. 2004;30:152-7.
39. Sadick NS, Schecter AK. A preliminary study of utilization of the 1320-nm Nd:YAG laser for the treatment of acne scarring. Dermatol Surg. 2004;30:995-1000.
40. Chua SH, Ang P, Khoo LS, et al. Nonablative 1450-nm diode laser in the treatment of facial atrophic acne scars in type IV to V Asian skin: a prospective clinical study. Dermatol Surg. 2004;30:1287-91.
41. Doshi SN, Alster TS. 1,450nm long-pulsed diode laser for non-ablative skin rejuvenation. Dermatol Surg. 2005;31:1223-6.
42. Fournier N, Mordon S. Nonablative remodeling with a 1,540 nm erbium: glass laser. Dermatol Surg. 2005;31:1227-36.
43. Bhatia AC, Dover JS, Arndt KA, et al. Patient satisfaction and reported long-term therapeutic efficacy associated with 1,320 nm Nd:YAG laser treatment of acne scarring and photoaging. Dermatol Surg. 2006;32:346-52.
44. Lipper GM, Perez M. Nonablative acne scar reduction after a series of treatments with a short-pulsed 1,064-nm neodymium:YAG laser. Dermatol Surg. 2006;32:998-1006.
45. Keller R, Junior WB, Valente NYS, et al. Nonablative 1,064-nm Nd:YAG laser for treating atrophic facial acne scars: histologic and clinical analysis. Dermatol Surg. 2007;33:1470-6.
46. Manstein D, Herron GS, Sink RK, et al. Fractional photothermolysis: a new concept for cutaneous remodeling using microscopic patterns of thermal injury. Lasers Surg Med. 2004;34:426-38.
47. Wanner M, Tanzi EL, Alster TS. Fractional photothermolysis: treatment of facial and non-facial cutaneous photodamage with a 1550 nm erbium-doped fiber laser. Dermatol Surg. 2007;33:23-8.
48. Alster TS, Tanzi EL, Lazarus M. The use of fractional photothermolysis in the treatment of atrophic acne scars. Dermatol Surg. 2007;33:295-9.
49. Tanzi EL, Wanitphakdeedecha R, Alster TS. Fraxel laser indications and long-term follow-up. Aesth Surg J. 2008;28;6:1-4.
50. MacGregor JL, Alster TS. Fractional resurfacing lasers: ablative and non-ablative. In: Nouri K (Ed). Dermatologic Surgery: Step by Step. Blackwell Publishing Ltd;2013.pp.349-58.
51. Bhatt N, Alster TS. Laser surgery in dark skin. Dermatol Surg. 2008;34:184-95.
52. Shah S, Alster TS. Laser treatment of dark skin: an updated review. Am J Clin Dermatol. 2010;11:1-10.
53. Lask G, Keller G, Lowe NJ, et al. Laser skin resurfacing with the SilkTouch flashscanner for facial rhytides. Dermatol Surg. 1995;21:1021-4.
54. Lowe NJ, Lask G, Griffin ME, et al. Skin resurfacing with the ultrapulse carbon dioxide laser: observations on 100 patients. Dermatol Surg. 1995;21:1025-9.
55. Waldorf HA, Kauvar ANB, Geronemus RG. Skin resurfacing of fine to deep rhytides using a char-free carbon dioxide laser in 47 patients. Dermatol Surg. 1995;21:940-6.
56. Alster TS, Garg S. Treatment of facial rhytides with a high-energy pulsed carbon dioxide laser. Plast Reconstr Surg. 1996;98:791-4.
57. Alster TS. Comparison of two high-energy, pulsed CO_2 lasers in the treatment of periorbital rhytides. Dermatol Surg. 1996;22:541-5.
58. Hohenleutner U, Hohenleutner S, Baumler W, et al. Fast and effective skin ablation with an Er:YAG laser: determination of ablation rates and thermal damage zones. Lasers Surg Med. 1997;20:242-7.

59. Khatri KA, Ross EV, Grevelink JM, et al. Comparison of erbium:YAG and carbon dioxide laser skin resufacing of facial rhytides. Arch Dermatol. 1999;135:391-7.
60. Kauvar ANB. Laser skin resurfacing: perspectives at the millennium. Dermatol Surg. 2000;26:174-7.
61. Alster TS, Lupton JR. An overview of cutaneous laser resurfacing. Clin Plast Surg. 2001;28:37-52.
62. Zachary CB. Modulating the Er:YAG laser. Lasers Surg Med. 2002;26:223-6.
63. Alster TS, Hirsch RJ. Single-pass CO_2 laser skin resurfacing of light and dark skin: extended experience with 52 patients. J Cosmet Laser Ther. 2003;5:39-42.
64. Alster TS, Tanzi EL. Hypertrophic scars and keloids: a review of etiology and management. Am J Clin Dermatol. 2003;4:235-43.
65. Jacob CI, Dover JS, Kaminer MS. Acne scarring: a classification system and review of treatment options. J Am Acad Dermatol. 2001;45:109-17.
66. Alster TS, Zaulyanov-Scanlon L. Laser scar revision: a review. Dermatol Surg. 2007;33: 131-40.
67. Jordan R, Cummins C, Burls A. Laser resurfacing of the skin for the improvement of facial acne scarring: a systematic review of the evidence. Br J Dermatol. 2000;142:413-23.
68. Sobanko JF, Alster TS. Laser treatment for improvement and minimization of facial scars. Plast Surg Clin N Am. 2011;19:527-42.
69. Alster TS, West TB. Resurfacing of atrophic facial scars with a high-energy, pulsed carbon dioxide laser. Dermatol Surg. 1996;22:151-5.
70. Walia S, Alster RS. Prolonged clinical and histological effects from CO_2 laser resurfacing of atrophic acne scars. Dermatol Surg. 999;25:926-30.
71. Woo SH, Park JH, Kye YC. Resurfacing of different types of facial acne scar with short-pulsed, variable-pulsed, and dual-mode Er:YAG laser. Dermatol Surg. 2004;30:488-93.
72. Hruza GJ. Laser treatment of epidermal and dermal lesions. Dermatol Clin. 2002;20:147-64.
73. Fitzpatrick RE, Goldman MP, Ruiz-Esparza J. Clinical advantage of the CO_2 laser superpulsed mode: treatment of verruca vulgaris, seborrheic keratoses, lentigines, and actinic cheilitis. J Dermatol Surg Oncol. 1994;20:449-56.
74. Ratz JL, Bailin PL, Lakeland RF. Carbon dioxide laser treatment of epidermal nevi. J Dermatol Surg Oncol. 1986;12:567-70.
75. Boyce S, Alster TS. CO_2 laser treatment of epidermal nevi: long-term success. Dermatol Surg. 2002;28:611-4.
76. Alster TS, West TB. Ultrapulse CO_2 laser ablation of xanthelasma. J Am Acad Dermatol. 1997;34:848-9.
77. Bailin PL, Kantor GR, Wheeland RG. Carbon dioxide laser vaporization of lymphangioma circumscriptum. J Am Acad Dermatol. 1986;14:257-62.
78. Huilgol SC, Neill S, Barlow RJ. CO_2 laser therapy of vulvar lymphangiectasia and hymphangioma circumscriptum. Dermatol Surg. 2002;28:575-7.
79. McBurney EI, Rosen DA. Carbon dioxide laser treatment of verruca vulgaris. J Dermatol Surg Oncol. 1984;10:45-8.
80. Haas A, Wheeland RG. Treatment of massive rhinophyma with the carbon dioxide laser. J Dermatol Surg Oncol. 1990;16:645-9.
81. Rosenbach A, Alster TS. Multiple trichoepitheliomas successfully treated with a high-energy, pulsed carbon dioxide laser. Dermatol Surg. 1997;23: 708-10.
82. Wang JI, Roenigk HH. Treatment of multiple facial syringomas with the carbon dioxide (CO_2) laser. Dermatol Surg. 1999;25:136-9.
83. Song MG, Park KB, Lee ES. Resurfacing of facial angiofibromas in tuberous sclerosis patients using CO_2 laser with flashscanner. Dermatol Surg. 1999;25:970-3.
84. Sajben FP, Ross EV. The use of the 1.0mm handpiece in high energy, pulsed CO_2 laser destruction of facial adnexal tumors. Dermatol Surg. 1999;25:41-4.
85. Martins C, Bartolo E. Brooke-Spiegler syndrome: treatment of cylindromas with CO_2 laser. Dermatol Surg. 2000;26:877-82.
86. Wheeland RG, McGillis ST. Cowden's disease: treatment of cutaneous lesions using carbon dioxide laser vaporization: a comparison of conventional and superpulsed techniques. J Dermatol Surg Oncol. 1989;15:1055-9.
87. Bickley LK, Goldberg DJ, Imaeda S, et al. Treatment of multiple apocrine hidrocystomas with the carbon dioxide (CO_2) laser. J Dermatol Surg Oncol. 1989;15:599-602.
88. Lane JE, Peterson CM, Ratz JL. Treatment of pearly penile papules with CO_2 laser. Dermatol Surg. 2002;28:617-8.
89. Berlin AL, Billick RC. Use of CO_2 laser in the treatment of periungual fibromas associated with tuberous sclerosis. Dermatol Surg. 2002;28:434-6.
90. Ammirati CT, Giancola JM, Hruza GJ. Adult-onset facial colloid milium successfully treated with the long-pulsed Er:YAG laser. Dermatol Surg. 2002;28:215-9.
91. Dufresne RG, Garrett AB, Bailin PL, et al. Carbon dioxide laser treatment of chronic actinic cheilitis. J Am Acad Dermatol. 1988;19:876-8.
92. Johnson TM, Sebastien TS, Lowe L, et al. Carbon dioxide laser treatment of actinic cheilitis: clinic histopathologic correlation to determine the optimal depth of destruction. J Am Acad Dermatol. 1992;27:737-40.
93. Wheeland RG, Bailin PL, Ratz JL, et al. Carbon dioxide laser vaporization and curettage in the treatment of large or multiple superficial basal cell carcinomas. J Dermatol Surg Oncol. 1987;13:119-25.

94. Humphreys TR, Malhotra R, Scharf MJ, et al. Treatment of superficial basal cell carcinomas and squamous cell carcinoma in situ with a high-energy pulsed carbon dioxide laser. Arch Dermatol. 1998;134:1247-52.
95. Nouri K, Chang A, Trent JT, et al. Ultrapulse CO_2 used for the successful treatment of basal cell carcinomas found in patients with basal cell nevus syndrome. Dermatol Surg. 2002;28:287-90.
96. Landthaler M, Haina D, Brunner R, et al. Laser therapy of Bowenoid papulosis and Bowen's disease. J Dermatol Surg Oncol. 1986;12:1253-7.
97. Horton S, Alster TS. Preoperative and postoperative considerations for cutaneous laser resurfacing. Cutis. 1999;64:399-406.
98. Batra RS, Jacob CI, Hobbs L, et al. A prospective survey of patient experiences after laser skin resurfacing: results from 2 1/2 years of follow-up. Arch Dermatol. 2003;139:1295-9.
99. West TB, Alster TS. Effect of pretreatment on the incidence of hyperpigmentation following cutaneous CO_2 laser resurfacing. Dermatol Surg. 1999;25:15-7.
100. West TB, Alster TS. Effect of botulinum toxin type A on movement-associated rhytides following CO_2 laser resurfacing. Dermatol Surg. 1999;25:259-61.
101. Walia S, Alster TS. Cutaneous CO_2 laser resurfacing infection rate with and without prophylactic antibiotics. Dermatol Surg. 1999;25:857-61.
102. Fitzpatrick RE. Maximizing benefits and minimizing risk with CO_2 laser resurfacing. Dermatol Clin. 2002;20:77-86.
103. Nanni CA, Alster TS. Complications of CO_2 laser resurfacing: an evaluation of 500 patients. Dermatol Surg. 1998;24:315-20.
104. Manuskiatti W, Fitzpatrick RE, Goldman MP. Long-term effectiveness and side effects of carbon dioxide laser resurfacing for photoaged facial skin. J Am Acad Dermatol. 1999;40:401-11.
105. Alster TS, Lupton JR. Complications of laser skin resurfacing. Facial Plast Surg Clin N Am. 2000;8:163-72.
106. Alster TS, Lupton JR. Treatment of complications of laser skin resurfacing. Arch Facial Plast Surg. 2000;2:279-84.
107. Tanzi EL, Alster TS. Complications of ablative and nonablative lasers and light sources. In: Gloster HM (Ed). New York: Springer Science + Business Media, LLC; 2008.pp.167-82.
108. Alster TS, Tanzi EL. Complications in laser and light surgery. In: Goldberg DJ (Ed). Lasers and Lights (Vol II). Philadelphia: Saunders Elsevier; 2008.pp. 99-112.
109. Alster TS, Khoury R. Treatment of laser complications. Facial Plast Surg. 2009; 25:316-23.
110. Metelitsa AI, Alster TS. Fractionated laser skin resurfacing treatment complications: a review. Dermatol Surg. 2010;36:299-306.
111. Alster TS, Wanitphakdeedecha R. Improvement of post-fractional laser erythema with light-emitting diode (LED) photomodulation. Dermatol Surg. 2009;35:813-5.
112. Alster TS, Nanni CA. Famciclovir prophylaxis of herpes simplex virus reactivation after cutaneous laser resurfacing. Dermatol Surg. 1999;25:242-6.

CHAPTER

8

Nonablative Fractional Resurfacing

Elizabeth R Geddes, Parisa Ravanfar, Paul M Friedman

INTRODUCTION

There are an ever expanding number of laser devices available to the dermatologic laser surgeon to achieve rejuvenation of photoaged skin, correction of pigmentary alteration, treatment of rhytides and revision of scars. The spectrum of clinical disorders for which these devices may be useful is increasing at a rapid pace as well. The traditional ablative lasers, carbon dioxide and erbium-YAG, target epidermal water content and create an often large confluent surface defect. This obtains excellent results, but requires significant recovery time and has potential for infection, dyschromia and scarring. Nonablative devices such as intense pulsed light and mid-infrared lasers became popular in response to the aforementioned side-effects and were nicknamed "lunchtime rejuvenation" due to their minimal or no downtime.[1] This is possible because they utilize epidermal cooling and target dermal chromophores for collagen remodeling, which poses little risk for scarring, but produces subtle clinical improvement.

Fractional nonablative lasers may be considered the best of both worlds. By using microscopic columns of thermal injury and sparing the surrounding tissue they bridge the gap between conventional ablative and nonablative therapies and generate satisfactory results with faster healing and minimal unwanted secondary effects. The concept of fractional photothermolysis was first described in 2004 by Manstein et al. as a novel method of skin restoration using a 1500-nm fractionated laser that was both safe and effective in treating photoaged skin on forearms and periorbital wrinkles.[2] Further studies have supported these findings and extended the potential clinical indications. Fractional photothermolysis can also be performed on anatomic areas that were previously considered high risk for scarring due to their relatively low number of pilosebaceous units, such as the neck, chest and hands.[3-5] Unlike many of the other devices used for photorejuvenation and acne scarring, nonablative fractional lasers can be safely used in darker skin types, although the risk of postinflammatory hyperpigmentation necessitates doing so carefully.[6] Despite these benefits, a potential downfall is that there is a need for multiple treatments to achieve the desired outcome, usually four to five sessions spaced 4–6 weeks apart. This is because each session may target only 20% of the skin.[7] A single resurfacing treatment utilizing an ablative laser produces greater effects.

Fractional nonablative photothermolysis works using a near-infrared fractionated laser that targets water as its chromophore and delivers energy in microbeams, creating an adjustable dense pattern of microscopic treatment zones of thermal injury (MTZ) with surrounding tissue spared.[2] A density of 1000–2000 MTZs per square centimeter is commonly used.[7] The depth of penetration of each zone is energy dependent and initially ranged from 300 μm to 700 μm.[7] Newer generations of devices allow for the varying of parameters to reach depths of 1 mm or greater. Because the created wounds are small, often less than the diameter of a hair, re-epithelialization occurs quickly. In fact, repopulation with melanocytes and keratinocytes and a continuous basal layer have been demonstrated histologically by one day post treatment.[8] Corresponding with the MTZs are discrete areas of inviable dermal coagulation, an impaired dermal-epidermal junction, and subcorneal collections of microepidermal necrotic debris (MEND).[2,8] MENDs are damaged keratinocytes and have been shown to contain both melanin pigment and components of the dermis demonstrated by antihuman elastin antibody staining.[2,8] The post-procedure bronzing seen clinically correlates with the MEND formation.[9] The stratum corneum is uncompromised allowing for preserved barrier function until transepidermal elimination of the MEND occurs at approximately 1–2 weeks. At 3 months post procedure, there is enhanced mucin deposition in the papillary and superficial reticular dermis and an increased undulating rete ridge pattern observed.[2] Figures 8.1A and B show microscopic images of transepidermal elimination of dermal content one day post procedure.

Histologic studies have found evidence of an induced wound healing response in skin treated with fractional photothermolysis. There is a transient increase in heat shock protein (HSP) 70 expression, which is known to induce transforming growth factor beta, a key component of fibrogenesis, as well as temporary increased collagen III production and alpha smooth muscle actin staining, indicating the presence of myofibroblasts.[9,10] Another important molecule in dermal remodeling, metalloproteinases (MMP-1) or collagenase is also transiently elevated at one day post procedure prior to returning to baseline levels.[10] Dermal fibrosis has been seen histologically in biopsies taken 3 months after ablative, but not nonablative, fractionated laser therapy, which may reflect collagen remodeling or subclinical scar formation.[11] Similar histologic changes have been demonstrated on biopsied tissue up to 18 months after CO_2 laser resurfacing of moderate to severe atrophic facial scars, suggesting that postoperative assessment for repeat therapy should be delayed for at least 1 year.[12]

These findings support our current understanding of how fractional photothermolysis works and helps

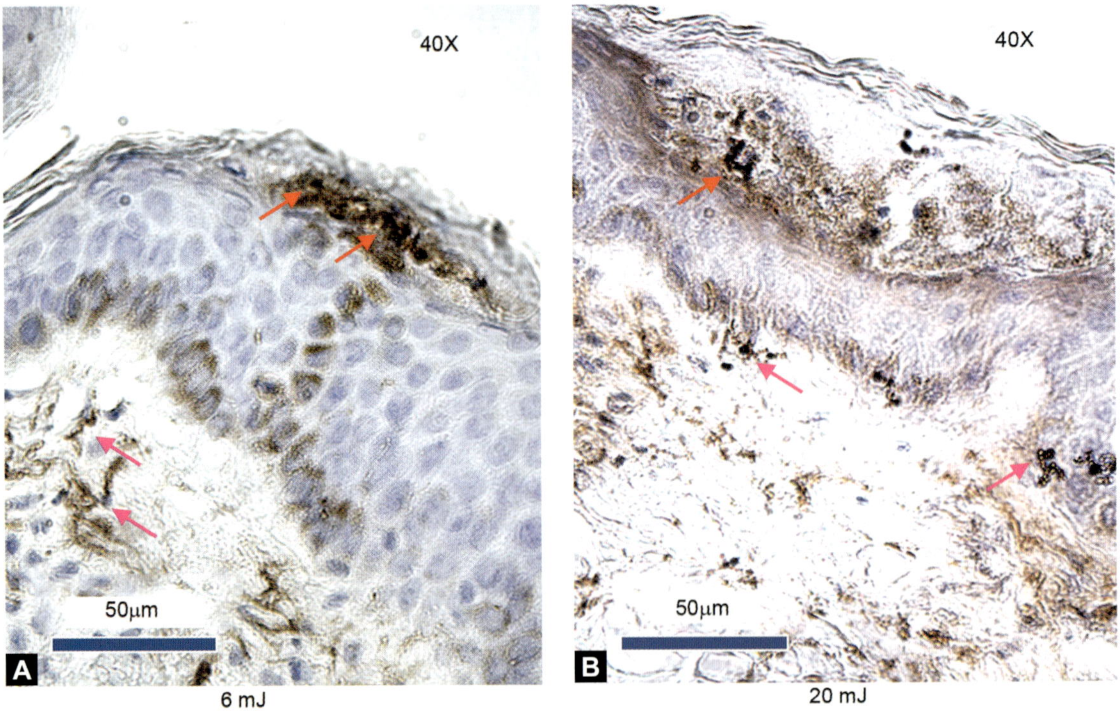

Figs 8.1A and B: Microscopic images of transepidermal elimination of dermal content one day post procedure. Red arrows: Exfoliating elastin, Pink arrows: Dermal elastin

Source: Reprinted with permission from Hantash BM, et al. Laser-induced transepidermal elimination of dermal content by fractional photothermolysis. J Biomed Opt. 2006;11(4):041115

to inspire potential applications in the clinical setting. As mentioned earlier, these indications continue to expand rapidly, despite a lagging body of published scientific evidence regarding overall efficacy, optimal regimens and recurrence rates. This is an all-to-common challenge encountered in a fast evolving field.

PATIENT SELECTION AND PREPROCEDURE INSTRUCTIONS

Nonablative fractional photothermolysis can be easily performed on adult patients of all skin types with a wide range of photodamage, bearing in mind that the degree of disease limits the perceptible response. Patients with severe photodamage in need of dramatic resurfacing may be served best with ablative therapy, while those with very mild dermatoheliosis may not experience easily detectable improvement. This is why obtaining high quality "before" photographs is crucial in helping the patient appreciate the outcome.

There are a few contraindications to undergoing fractional photothermolysis, including those with actively koebnerizing cutaneous disorders, like psoriasis or vitiligo. Those with active facial or severe systemic infections should postpone treatment until fully healed. It is also best to be avoided in pregnant or lactating women and in those with an immunodeficiency or impaired wound healing. Patients with underlying psychiatric conditions, such as body dysmorphic disorder will never be satisfied with the results and those with unrealistic expectations should not be treated. Relative contraindications include recent sun exposure or tanned skin, history of keloid formation, and prior isotretinoin therapy within the last 6–12 months due to a theoretical higher risk of scarring.[13] Neuromodulators and soft-tissue fillers can be safely and effectively used in patients undergoing fractional laser therapy. All three procedures can be performed on the same day and in the authors' experience are best done in the following order: filler, fractional laser therapy and neurotoxin. These procedures compliment one another and help to achieve the desired cosmetic outcome.

Prior to the procedure it is important to define the target areas and discuss in detail the patient's goals, realistic expectations, as well as the risks, benefits and alternatives to therapy. The anticipated number and duration of treatment sessions should be addressed as well. It takes approximately 20–30 minutes to treat the entire face and a series of treatment sessions is often necessary. Informed written consent should be obtained. A prior history of herpes simplex virus (HSV) facial outbreak should prompt the prescription of prophylactic antivirals, which are usually started 1 day prior and continued for 3 days after the procedure. Patients receiving treatment for melasma, or those with a history of postinflammatory hyperpigmentation, benefit from twice daily application of a bleaching cream a few weeks prior to the procedure, as well as a daily full ultraviolet (UV) spectrum blocking sunscreen. We also recommend low-potency topical corticosteroids for 2-days post treatment to minimize the risk of PIH for these patients.

All make-up and potentially interfering jewellery should be removed prior to therapy. The intended area of treatment is washed with a mild cleanser and then prepped with alcohol to remove surface oils. This is then followed by application of a topical anesthetic agent for approximately 60 minutes prior to treatment. One should remain aware of the potential for lidocaine toxicity if larger areas are being treated. The topical anesthetic should be thoroughly removed prior to the procedure. The average pain score was 4.6 on a scale from 1 to 10 when topical anesthesia was used in combination with a hand-held cooling device.[7] The Zimmer® machines are examples of such devices.

Table 8.1 is not meant to be an all-inclusive list of available devices, but rather a quick review of a few commercial products' specific characteristics and adjustable parameters. The most important settings are the energy level, which determines the depth of penetration and radial thermal damage, and the microbeam treatment zone density, as well as the total energy used for the procedure.[14] Increasing the pulse energy leads to increases in MTZ characteristics; high energies of 40 mJ causes zones exceeding 1 mm in depth and approaching 200 μm in width.[15] The patient's skin type and clinical indication determines the optimal choice of laser parameters. Superficial processes, like lentigines and pigmentary alteration need lower fluences (6–10 mJ) to target the epidermis, while deeper targets such as collagen for the treatment of rhytides or acne scars require higher fluences (50–70 mJ).[19] To avoid bulk heating it is best to use a lower density setting with higher energies and compensate by carefully performing multiple passes

Table 8.1: Device selection and key parameters

Company	*Device*	*Laser*	*Wavelength (nm)*	*Mode*	*Spot size (mm)*	*Max energy*	*MTZ density*	*Depth (microns)*
Cynosure	Affirm	Nd:YAG	1440±1320	Stamp	10	8/14 mJ/cm^2	1000	300–450
Lutronic	Moasic	Er:Glass	1540	Stamp/ Scan	Variable	120 mJ	50–500 spots/cm^2	
Palomar	Lux1540	Er:Glass	1540	Stamp	10/15	100/15	100/320	600–900
Sellas	1550	Erbium fiber	1550	Stamp/ Scan	0.1	1–120 mJ 1–30 mJ	25–3025 PPA	
Solta	Fraxel DUAL	Erbium fiber/ Thulium	1550/1927	Scan	7/15	70 mJ 20 mJ	5–45% 20–70%	Up to 1400 200

MTZ: Microscopic treatment zones of thermal injury

with adequate cooling time in between.[13] In addition to longer treatment intervals, these techniques may help decrease the incidence of postinflammatory hyperpigmentation in those with darker skin types.[16]

The fractionated laser is delivered to the surface using one or a combination of methods, usually stamping or scanning/gliding. Stamping allows the simultaneous delivery of a preprogrammed arrangement of treatment zones, while scanning creates microscopic columns of injury in a sequential fashion as the device is glided across the skin. A novel portable diode laser combining the two modes has been developed, which is effective at treating facial rhytides and dyschromia, and improves coverage uniformity.[17]

CLINICAL INDICATIONS AND OUTCOMES

A few of the current United States Food and Drug Administration (FDA) approved applications for nonablative fractional photothermolysis include the treatment of periorbital rhytides, pigmented lesions, melasma, skin resurfacing/texture improvement, soft tissue coagulation, acne and surgical scarring, and actinic keratoses.[19,20] There are also a number of non-FDA approved clinical indications with favorable outcomes. The following section will address these specific applications, including consensus recommendations for treatment parameters and reviews of select published literature.

RHYTIDES

One of the first indications for nonablative fractional photothermolysis was for the improvement of superficial periorbital rhytides.[2] In this landmark study, 30 subjects with skin types II–III were randomly divided into groups and treated with varying wavelengths (1480, 1535, 1550 nm) and energies (6–12 mJ/MTZ) to the lateral periorbital region. They underwent a total of four sessions using 10 passes to create a final MTZ density of 2,500/cm^2. At 3 months, 34% showed at least moderate improvement in the appearance of their wrinkles, 47% had moderate or better improvement in skin texture, and microtattoo placement confirmed small, but mentionable linear skin shrinkage.[2] These findings have since been replicated in a number of other clinical studies, most of which have utilized a 1550-nm wavelength laser for their evaluations. A split-face comparison trial using a 1565-nm Er:glass laser, and therefore deeper penetration, found a slight trend toward better results, but no statistically significant difference from the effects achieved by the 1550-nm Er:glass laser in the treatment of periorbital rhytides; both showed around 8–9% reduction in wrinkles of the lower eyelid, similar patient satisfaction rates, and histologic evidence of increased epidermal thickening and decreased solar elastosis at 3 months.[18] Consensus recommendations regarding the best parameters for treating moderate to severe periorbital rhytides using a 1550-nm erbium-doped fractionated laser are energy 30 to 70 mJ, treatment level 7 to 11, 8 passes, and 3 to 5 treatments spaced 1 month apart.[19] Figures 8.2A and B show clinical photographs of periorbital rhytids treated successfully with nonablative fractional resurfacing (NAFR).

It is not just periorbital rhytides that are improved with fractionated lasers, but also perioral rhytides. However, ablative methods are usually more effective, especially for the deep vertical lines above the upper lip.[20] Interestingly, when used in combination with/

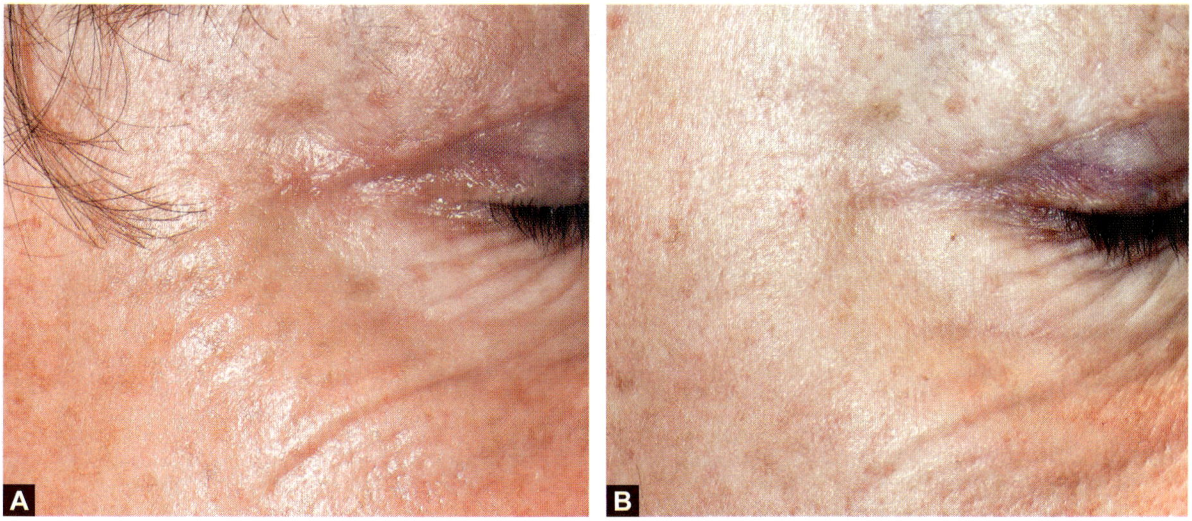

Figs 8.2A and B: Clinical photographs of periorbital rhytides treated successfully with NAFR

prior to photodynamic therapy, investigators noted greater clinical improvement in perioral rhytides than the areas treated with fractionated laser alone, suggesting a synergistic response.[21]

PHOTOAGING: DYSCHROMIA, LENTIGINES, SKIN TEXTURE RESURFACING AND TIGHTENING

Photoaging is an all-encompassing description of the cosmetically displeasing changes that accompany aging skin, much of which has been attributed to excess sun exposure. Most studies focus on one measurable aspect of photoaging, such as fine rhytides, to evaluate their results. However, a number of published reports grade all aspects, which provides a useful assessment of a tool to be used in the clinical setting where most patients have multiple concerns to address.

In one early trial, 50 patients with mild to moderate facial or nonfacial photodamage, rhytides, and dyspigmentation received three approximately monthly treatments with a 1550-nm erbium-doped fiber laser at 8 mJ with 6–8 passes and density of 250 MTZs/cm^2.[3] The subjects were evaluated at baseline, 3, 6, and 9 months post treatment and at least 51–75% improvement was seen at final follow-up in 73% of facial and 55% of nonfacial skin. While this might suggest that the face responds better than the neck and chest, the authors acknowledged that the nonfacial sites were treated less aggressively, with fewer passes.[3] The greatest clinical improvement was seen at 3 months, possibly secondary to improved dyspigmentation, which may have recurred over time from progressive UV exposure.[3]

The fractionated 1440-nm Nd:YAG and 1320/1440-nm multiplex Nd:YAG lasers were compared in a study of 19 women with mild to moderate photodamage and both were found to improve rhytides, dyschromia, texture, tightening, erythema, and overall appearance, with no significant difference between the two instruments despite the 1320-nm device's ability to create deeper dermal heating.[22] These findings were supported by histologic evaluation at 3 months that revealed significant neocollagenesis.[22]

Consensus recommendations for skin types I–III with dyschromia treated with the fractionated 1550-nm laser are energy level of 10–20 mJ with a treatment level of 7–11 and variable number of passes, noting that the extent of damage should dictate exact settings with higher treatment levels and more passes needed for severe photodamage.[19] When treating the chest and hands, settings of 10–40 mJ with treatment level of 7–11 and eight passes may be used.[19]

Besides correcting pigmentary dyschromia, the improvement in fine lines, as well as skin texture and laxity are the goals of rejuvenation and therefore are prospective targets for nonablative fractional photothermolysis. Pore size, count and skin texture were improved in twenty patients representing all skin types who underwent three full face treatments, 2 weeks apart, with a 1440-nm fractionated device and

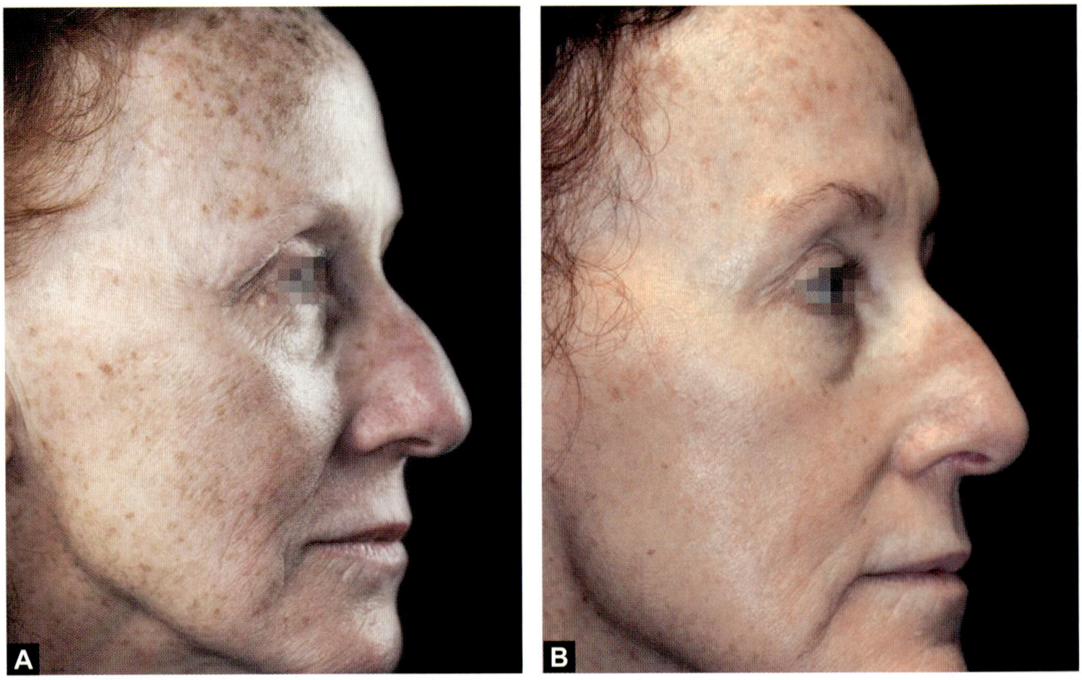

Figs 8.3A and B: Clinical photographs of photodamage treated successfully with NAFR

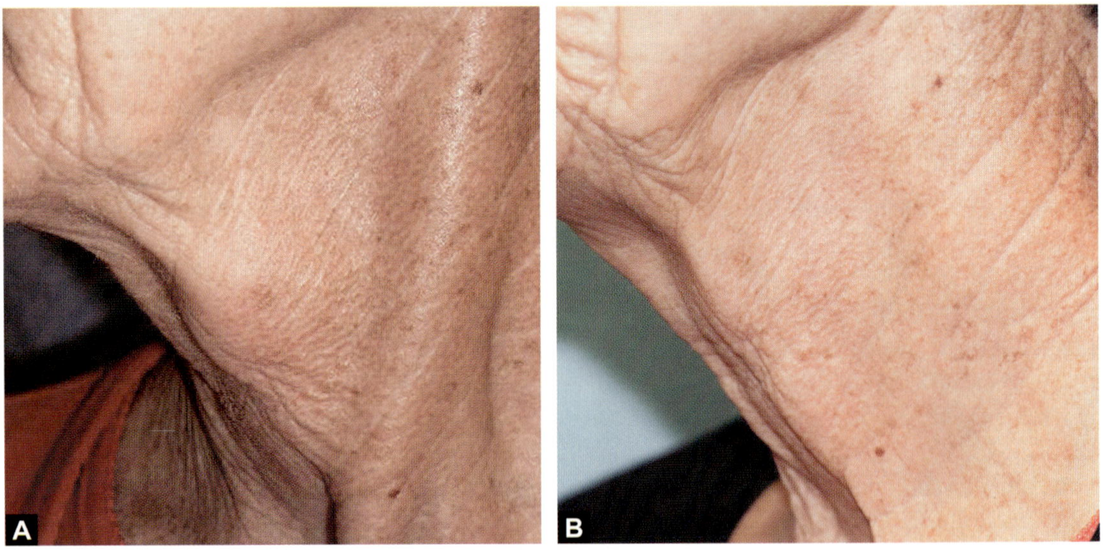

Figs 8.4A and B: Clinical photographs of photodamage treated successfully with NAFR

eight passes at 4–9 mJ.[23] Utilizing microcompression optics and pulse-stacking is a method that allows safe deep heating of the reticular dermis and subcutis, potentially stimulating skin tightening. This was demonstrated clinically and histologically in twenty-seven subjects treated after 2–3 monthly sessions with one pass of triple-stacked pulses at 70 mJ and 15 mJ, using a 1540-nm fractionated laser with point-array compression tip.[24] Figures 8.3 and 8.4 show clinical photographs of photodamage treated successfully with NAFR.

MELASMA

Clinical and histologic improvement of epidermal facial melasma has been reported in a study of ten patients with skin types III and IV who were treated with four sessions, every 2 weeks, with a 1550-nm fractionated erbium:glass laser.[25] Pre- and postprocedure biopsies were taken from all subjects and revealed a relative decrease in the number of melanocytes on light microscopy, and reduction or absence of melanin granules in the surrounding keratinocytes on electron microscopy.[25] These findings are consistent with the "melanin shuttle" theory, which is the elimination process of MENDs following fractional photothermolysis. Interestingly, there was no correlation between the degree of clinical improvement (all had fair or good improvement, none were completely cleared) with the treatment-induced changes seen histologically.[25]

Greater than 50% improvement in previously therapy-resistant melasma was seen in five of eight patients with skin types II–IV who underwent 2–7 treatments with a 1550-nm fractionated laser with energies ranging from 6 mJ to 40 mJ, treatment levels of 3–10, and 8–10 passes per treatment.[26] At follow-up, which ranged from 7 months to 36 months (average 13.5 months), five patients were satisfied and had little to no recurrence, while three patients who initially had improvement experienced recurrence. None of the patients developed postinflammatory hyperpigmentation.[26]

The appropriate settings depend on the location of the melasma, which can be difficult to judge clinically. In general, epidermal melasma should be targeted with shallower energies ranging from 6 mJ to 10 mJ and dermal involvement may require 12 to 20 mJ. Treatment level should be altered based on experience, in accordance to skin type.[19]

In a randomized controlled observer-blinded study comparing nonablative fractional photothermolysis to triple topical therapy (hydroquinone 5%, tretinoin 0.05%, triamcinolone 0.1%) for the treatment of melasma, there was no difference in the physician assessment between the two groups, although patients in the laser group were significantly more satisfied at 3 weeks despite short-term side-effects. Recurrence was seen in both groups at 6 months.[27]

OTHER PIGMENTARY AND VASCULAR DISORDERS

Poikiloderma of Civatte, Nevus of Ota/Ito, Minocycline-Induced, Postinflammatory Erythema and Hyperpigmentation

A number of pigmentary disorders have been targeted with the use of FLT as well. Dramatic improvement of Poikiloderma of Civatte has been achieved likely through microvascular destruction by the targeting of water in blood vessels, as well as direct damage to vascular structures in the MTZs.[28] For example, one case report demonstrated a 46-year-old Japanese man with a nevus of Ota that was previously resistant to standard Quality-switched (Q-switched) laser therapy was successfully treated after two sessions with a fractionated 1440-nm Nd:YAG using a fluence of 3.5 J/cm^2, then 4 J/cm^2, one pass with a 20% overlap between pulses, and 1 cm spot size.[29] The interval between sessions was 4 weeks, the lesion resolved within 6 weeks of the second treatment, and no postinflammatory hyperpigmentation was seen.[29]

Minocycline-induced blue pigmentation of the central face in a woman receiving treatment for rosacea almost completely resolved after four sessions of 1550-nm diode fractionated laser therapy, combined with strict photoprotection and discontinuation of the medication.[30] She had previously been treated with Q-switched ND:YAG 10 months earlier with only slight improvement.

Fractional photothermolysis may be useful in treating postinflammatory hyperpigmentation (PIH), as was seen in a 50-year-old Caucasian woman who developed a brown patch on her lateral neck at the site where her seatbelt rubbed against her skin. She was previously unresponsive to a chemical peel and a 2-month course of bleaching creams, but had greater than 95% improvement after three sessions using a 1550-nm fractionated laser combined with Triluma and sun protection. The settings used were fluence of 15 mJ, treatment level 6 (17% coverage), and 8–10 passes using density of 110 MTZs/cm^2/pass.[31] It was also used to treat reticulate PIH in a 42-year-old woman after carbon dioxide laser resurfacing for photorejuvenation, a long lasting complication seen in 5–10% of patients, that was previously refractive to bleaching agents, serial chemical peels, and multiple IPL and Sciton peel treatments.[32]

SCARS: ACNE SCARRING, HYPOPIGMENTED, HYPERTROPHIC, BURN, SURGICAL

The majority of the published literature on the use of nonablative fractional photothermolysis for treatment of scars focuses on atrophic acne scarring. According to a recent published review of 13 studies, one can expect an approximate improvement in the range of 26–50% after treatment.[33] One randomized controlled trial investigating the efficacy and adverse effects of 3 monthly treatments with a 1540-nm nonablative fractionated laser versus an untreated area on ten subjects with atrophic acne scarring found improved texture (median improvement of 1.5 points on a 4-point scale), minimal side-effects, and patient satisfaction at 4- and 12-week follow-up evaluations.[34] Similar findings were seen in a study with sixteen Korean subjects with type III–IV skin who experienced mild to moderate clinical improvement of their acne scarring after three sessions of 1540-nm fractionated laser with spot size 10 mm, pulse energy 70 mJ, 100 MTZ/cm^2/pass, and three passes.[35] All experienced a statistically significant mild to moderate improvement in their quality of life, as determined by comparison of pre- and post-questionnaires.[35] Histologic studies revealed an increase in collagen bundles and the elastic fiber network in the papillary dermis at 12 weeks.[35]

Ablative fractional photothermolysis produces superior results to nonablative techniques, as evidenced by a randomized split-face, evaluator-blinded comparison in eight male patients with mild to severe acne scarring.[36] However, only one treatment session was performed and the study authors recognized that multiple sequential treatments of nonablative photothermolysis are usually required to obtain optimal results. There was no statistically significant difference between overall levels of patient satisfaction.[36]

Consensus recommendations with a 1550-nm fractionated laser for treating acne scarring depend on the patient's skin type with lower treatment levels and fewer passes used in those with darker skin.[19] For skin types I–III, 30 to 70 mJ of energy with treatment level of 7 to 11, and 8 to 10 passes has been recommended, while for types IV–V, energy of 30 to 70 mJ, level of 4 to 5, and eight passes are used. Skin type VI should only be treated by experienced laser surgeons given the risk of PIH.[19] However, in a prospective trial of 15 patients with acne scarring and skin types IV–VI who were randomized to 5 monthly sessions of 10 mJ or 40 mJ, there was no significant difference in the clinical improvement or incidence of PIH between the two groups; pain levels were significantly higher in those treated with 40 mJ and in those with darker skin types.[6] One theory to explain this is that the more melanin in the skin, the more laser absorption and heat formation, which leads to pain and perhaps the development of PIH.[6] Therefore, additional consideration of pain control in this population may be prudent.

Nonablative fractional photothermolysis has also been studied in the treatment of thermal burn scars in a randomized trial comparing side-by-side treatments with a 1540-nm laser to the untreated control in 17 subjects.[37] After 3 monthly sessions, the areas treated with fractionated laser appeared smoother and more even. Majority of subjects experienced an average improvement of 2 levels on a blinded visual and palpable 0-10 categorical scale for textural scores. No significant improvement in pigmentation was seen. Two subjects had no improvement in texture, which was possibly secondary to the deeper depth of their burn scars, and one subject experienced minor scarring secondary to bulla and crusting.[37] The range of fluencies used was 70–100 mJ/microbeam with lower settings used initially and increased as tolerated. There was no difference in efficacy seen with respect to burn scar age, subject age, or scar location.[37]

There are many studies demonstrating significant clinical improvement of surgical scars, including a case report of near-complete correction of a depressed alar scar following Mohs micrographic surgery for a basal cell carcinoma that was allowed to heal by secondary intention.[38,39] This was achieved with five sessions utilizing the 1550-nm erbium-doped fiber laser fixed at 40 mJ of energy and performing eight passes.[38] Further studies have confirmed the potential for surgical scar revision with nonablative fractional photothermolysis, although longer follow-up periods are necessary to determine lasting effects.[40] A randomized blinded split study comparing the efficacy of nonablative fractionated laser (1550 nm) to pulsed-dye laser (595 nm) on contralateral halves of linear Mohs surgical scars in 15 patients two months post procedure found significantly superior scar pigmentation, thickness, texture, and overall appearance with use of the fractionated laser.[41] Additionally, the ability to improve hypopigmented scarring was unique and not seen in the areas treated with the pulsed-dye laser.[41]

This parallels the findings in one study of seven patients with hypopigmented facial scars which demonstrated improvements of 51–75% in six of the subjects who underwent 2–4 treatments, 4 weeks apart, using the 1550-nm erbium-doped fiber laser with setting of 7–20 mJ and 1,000–2,500 MTZs/cm^2.[42] More recently, fractional resurfacing has been studied in combination with postprocedure topical bimatoprost and either topical tretinoin or pimecrolimus for hypopigmented scarring and was shown to have prolonged improved results, with a mean follow-up of 20.1 months.[43] It has been postulated that this may be secondary to improved melanocyte density over the scar and increased melanogenesis, as well as melanocyte transfer to keratinocytes, but has not been histologically confirmed.[43]

The response of hypertrophic linear scars, 6 months or older in age, to nonablative fractional photothermolysis has been investigated in a prospective controlled trial with subjects randomized to high- or low-density treatment (26 versus 14% coverage; 40 mJ throughout) and results compared to the untreated portion of the scar.[44] Seventeen of the twenty enrolled patients noted a benefit at 3 months, while three subjects treated with high density coverage felt their scar had worsened, and those in the low density arm had just as effective results with fewer side-effects, namely erythema, exfoliation, and pain.[44] Younger scars, those less than 2 years of age, responded better to treatment than those that were greater than 6 years of age, suggesting earlier intervention may be crucial.[44]

These reports highlight the utility of offering nonablative fractional photothermolysis as a means to achieving the best cosmetic result after surgical treatment of skin cancer and other disorders. Figures 8.5A and B show clinical photographs of a postprocedural scar treated successfully with NAFR.

STRIAE DISTENSAE/RUBRA/ALBA

Striae are dermal scars marked by the appearance of atrophic bands secondary to hormonal influences and rapid stretching of the skin. Topical therapies, including tretinoin creams, can be cumbersome and are often ineffective, but nonablative fractional photothermolysis has shown promising results with great patient satisfaction.[45] Because the lesions are located in the superficial dermis, lower energy settings are often used.

The treatment of striae rubra and alba with a 1540-nm erbium glass nonablative fractionated laser was found to be both safe and effective in 51 patients with skin types II – IV.[46] The age of the lesions ranged from 1 year to 40 years and greater than 50% improvement was seen in all, as well as confirmed histologically with neocollagenesis and increased elastic fibers.[46] Better results may be seen in the treatment of striae alba and in those lesions of longer duration, as was demonstrated in a study of twenty-two women who underwent two treatments, 4 weeks apart, using a 1500-nm erbium-doped fiber laser with pulse energy of 30 mJ, density of 6, and eight passes.[47] Increased epidermal and dermal thickness and procollagen type 1 immunoreactivity were seen in post-treatment biopsies.[47] One randomized controlled trial comparing ablative to nonablative fractional therapy on striae distensae in Asian skin showed equally effective results.[48]

BENIGN SKIN NEOPLASMS AND DEPOSITION DISORDERS

Syringomas, Dermatosis Papulosa Nigra, Xanthelasma, Colloid Milium

In general, the treatment of these benign and often recurrent neoplasms is complicated because of their dermal depth and consequent risk of scarring or dyschromia secondary to the high energies needed to target the lesions. Although not first-line therapy due to the nature of the fractionated laser, multiple passes and treatment sessions are often required, but the final results can be impressive.

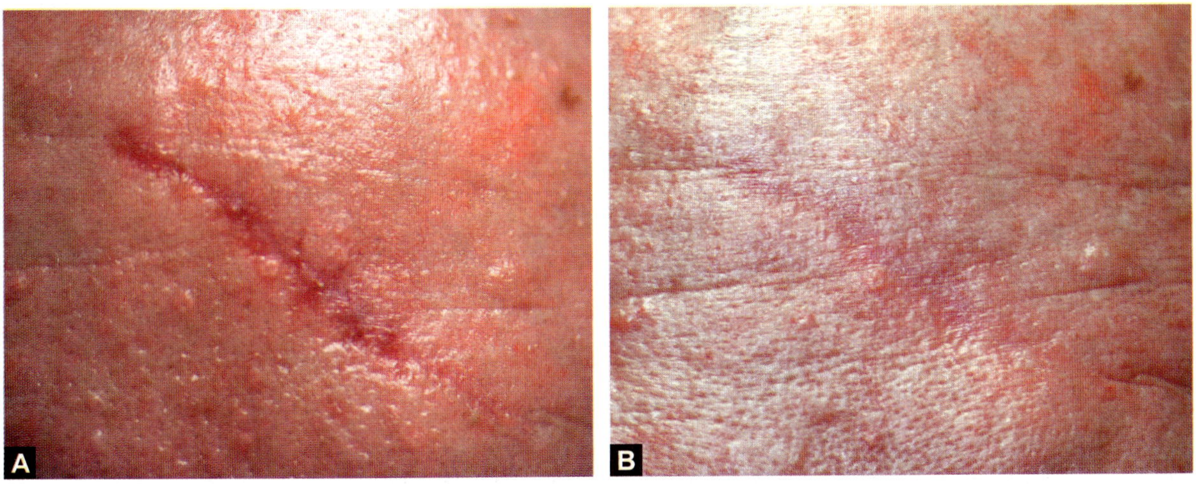

Figs 8.5A and B: Clinical photographs of a postprocedural scar treated successfully with NAFR

There have been reports of syringomas treated successfully with fractional photothermolysis using both ablative and nonablative lasers.[49,50] Treatment of dermatosis papulosa nigra, which are histologically the same as seborrheic keratoses, has been reported using a 1550-nm erbium-doped fiber laser. Three sessions with 8–10 passes of high energy settings (60–70 mJ) with 20% coverage led to near-total improvement (>75% reduction in lesions) in a Pakistani woman with type IV skin.[51] There are no published studies regarding the efficacy of treating sebaceous hyperplasia or cherry angiomas, but given their general characteristics, select small lesions could be the potential targets. Figures 8.6A and B show clinical photographs of dermatosis papulosa nigra treated successfully with NAFR.

Xanthelasma, for which the gold-standard first-line therapy is excision, has also been treated successfully in a 52-year-old Asian woman with a 1550-nm erbium-doped fractionated nonablative laser and 7 sessions using the following parameters: energy fluence starting at 40 mJ and increased incrementally by 5 mJ until a maximum of 70 mJ, and total densities of 250–408 MTZ/cm^2 achieved through eight passes during each treatment.[52] Adult colloid milium, a notoriously difficult to treat condition, has been completely cleared in case reports with 5 sessions using settings of 20 mJ, 125 MTZs/cm^2, and 10 to 12 passes with a 1550-nm erbium-doped fiber laser.[53] Because these case reports are rare in the literature, optimal settings and recurrence rates are not yet available.

PRECANCEROUS LESIONS

Actinic Cheilitis, Actinic Keratoses, Disseminated Superficial Actinic Porokeratoses

Fractionated lasers have been investigated as a potential tool for treating precancerous lesions and in doing so may play a role in decreasing the risk of transformation of these lesions into squamous cell carcinomas. The main benefit is the absence of significant downtime associated with other field modalities such as topical fluorouracil, imiquimod, chemical peels, or photodynamic therapy.

Actinic cheilitis in a 56-year-old Caucasian man was treated with three sessions using a 1927-thulium nonablative fractional laser with fluence of 20 mJ/cm^2, 40% coverage, and four passes. Unlike other treatment modalities, there was no dysesthesia or scarring.[54] Another multicenter study of 15 patients with actinic cheilitis showed 51–75% improvement in 6 patients and 76–100% improvement in 9 patients after 1–2 treatments.[55] The potential for increased recurrence due to skipped areas inherent to a fractionated laser necessitates close clinical follow-up and continued monitoring.

For example, fractional photothermolysis has been shown to decrease the clinical appearance of actinic keratoses in a study of 14 men after 5 sessions with a 1550-nm erbium-doped fiber laser; however, post-treatment histological examination revealed persistent actinic keratoses in almost all specimens.[56] While nonablative fractional photothermolysis as a single modality may not be sufficient in treating

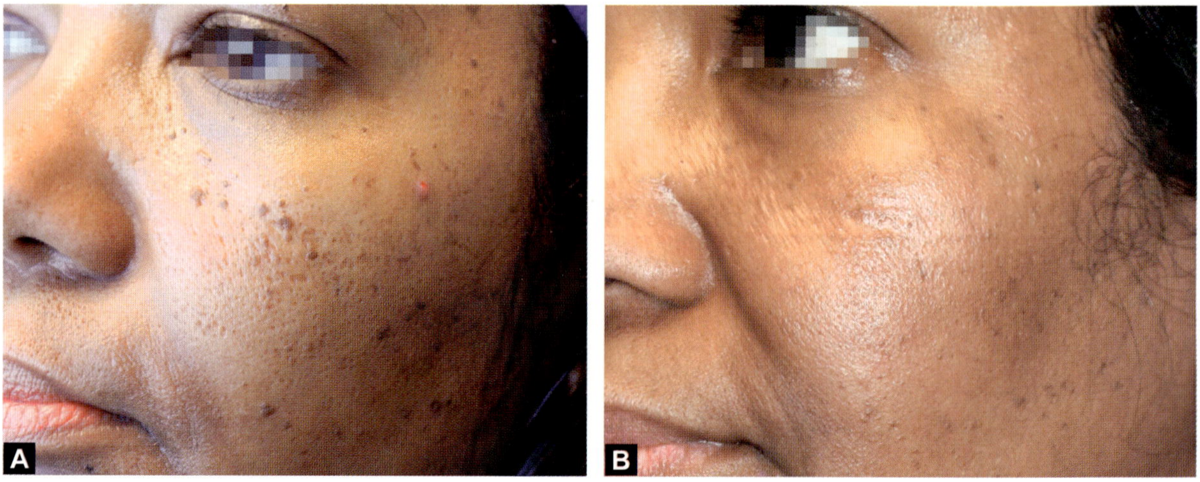

Figs 8.6A and B: Clinical photographs of dermatosis papulosa nigra and acne scarring treated successfully with NAFR in FST VI
Source: Reprinted with permission from Katz T, Goldberg LH, Friedman PM. Dermatosis papulosa nigra treatment with fractional photothermolysis. Dermatol Surg. 2009;35:1840-3

actinic keratoses, there is evidence that photodynamic therapy may be enhanced after treatment with an ablative fractionated laser, presumably secondary to improved photosensitizer uptake.[57]

Two cases of disseminated superficial actinic porokeratoses showed moderate to marked improvement in number of lesions, skin texture, and even relief of associated pruritus after three treatments with 1550-nm erbium-doped fractionated laser.[58]

GRANULOMA ANNULARE

There have been two published case reports of granuloma annulare (GA) being successfully treated with fractional photothermolysis. A 58-year-old woman with generalized GA had complete response of four lesions on her upper arm after two to three treatments with a 1440-nm Nd:YAG laser.[59] The untreated lesions persisted. Eleven treatments with a 1550-nm Er:YAG fractionated laser led to a patient-reported 80–90% improvement in a 60-year-old man with GA using the following parameters: energy 5.8 to 6.8 kJ, setting 70 J/cm^2, and 8 to 14 passes per lesion.[60]

RESIDUAL HEMANGIOMAS

There have been published reports of fractionated lasers used to treat a number of conditions, including residual hemangiomas. After five treatments using two 1550-nm nonablative glass-fiber lasers, a 14-year-old girl with a cosmetically-sensitive involuted facial hemangioma had both improvement in the overall appearance and reduction in volume, allowing her to easily camouflage it with make-up.[61] An 18-year-old woman with redundant skin and fibrofatty tissue of the glabella and temple from a residual hemangioma, which had been previously treated with pulsed-dye laser and CO_2 abrasion, had a remarkable improvement after two sessions with a 1,440-nm erbium-doped fractionated laser.[62] With successful stories such as these, we can anticipate the potential clinical indications will only continue to grow.

POSTPROCEDURE CARE AND COMPLICATIONS

There is minimal downtime after having nonablative fractional photothermolysis. After application of a light moisturizer, patients can re-apply their make-up and resume their normal daily activities. In an early survey of 60 patients, 72% reported limiting their social engagements for an average of about two days post procedure, mainly due to concerns of facial erythema and swelling.[7] Gentle skin care with nonabrasive cleansers, bland emollients and strict photoprotection are important to advocate.

Immediate postprocedure erythema is an expected response and usually lasts from one to three days. Diffuse xerosis that is responsive to moisturizer and mild facial swelling are experienced by the majority of patients as well. The edema is often most prominent in the infraorbital region.[7] Other commonly reported findings include flaking, superficial abrasions, pruritus, and a bronzing or "suntan" appearance. According to an early review, the abrasions were most often to occur on the upper cutaneous lip, lower orbital rim, and forehead, and were presumably attributed to tangential application of the laser or stacking of pulses. Either way, the incidence decreased to nearly zero with increased technical experience, as well as the development of newer modified handpieces.[7,13]

Complications are low risk and usually short-lived with nonablative fractional photothermolysis, but potentially include excessive desquamation, protracted erythema or edema, purpura, erosions, dermatitis, acneiform eruptions and milia, secondary infection with *Staphylococcus*, HSV, or *Candida*, and pigmentary alteration.[63,67] Given the nature of the treatment, the likelihood of scarring is minimal to none, as long as the settings are appropriately selected and the practitioner is skilled. Eruptive keratoacanthomas on the legs after fractional photothermolysis has been reported in two individuals, possibly secondary to follicular disruption.[64]

Side-effects such as prolonged erythema and edema can often be minimized by avoiding multiple passes and remaining cognizant of the potential for unintentional stacking. A split-face comparison of twenty patients who underwent fractional photothermolysis for dermal melasma found that postprocedure erythema and xerosis were significantly reduced after spraying thermal spring water on the affected area multiple times daily after treatment.[65] Immediate postprocedure photomodulation with a 590-nm light-emitting diode has also been shown to decrease the intensity and duration of postfractionated laser erythema, presumably from anti-inflammatory effects.[66]

Significant edema requiring therapy may be treated with pulse steroids (prednisone 40 mg for 3 days).[7] Avoidance of unnecessary antiplatelets agents and anticoagulants in the periprocedural period will minimize purpura.[63] Overall, complications generally increase with treatment of sensitive areas, such as the periorbital regions and neck, and in those with darker skin types or predisposing medical risk factors, such as a history of HSV.[63] The clinician should be aware that punctuate painful erosions are the clinical sign of reactivated HSV.[14]

A retrospective chart review of 961 consecutive treatment sessions with a 1550-nm erbium-doped fiber laser found a short-term complication rate of 7.6%.[67] The most frequent complications were acneiform eruptions (n = 18 or 1.87%), followed closely by HSV outbreaks (n = 17 or 1.77%), and then erosions (n = 13 or 1.35%). Impetigo and purpura each occurred only once.[67] The acneiform eruptions occurred in acne-prone patients and were prevented during further treatments with doxycycline 20 mg twice daily. Prophylaxis with antivirals did not eliminate the risk of secondary infection; 35% of HSV outbreaks occurred despite appropriate prophylactic therapy and approximately 18% occurred in those with no known history of HSV. There were no cases of HSV dissemination or scarring.[67] Emphasizing the use of noncomedogenic and nonocclusive moisturizers and starting antiviral prophylaxis when warranted will help to limit, but likely not eliminate, these untoward side-effects.

Not surprisingly, the incidence of post-inflammatory hyperpigmentation (PIH) after fractional photothermolysis is higher in patients with darker skin phototypes and the pigment changes last on average around 50 days.[67] Even subclinical PIH has been demonstrated histologically with dermal melanophages in the treatment area of a patient with Fitzpatrick skin type VI.[9] In those at risk, the postprocedure use of topical bleaching agents (hydroquinone, kojic acid), as well as retinoic, azelaic, ascorbic, glycolic acids, and full UV spectrum blocking sunscreens to prevent further pigmentation may be helpful.[67]

WHAT LIES AHEAD: THE FUTURE OF FRACTIONAL PHOTOTHERMOLYSIS

The effects of fractional photothermolysis may also be enhanced in combination with other laser modalities. A study of twenty-nine subjects looked at the effects of treatment with a 1550-nm fractionated laser after intense pulsed light therapy, performed immediately afterward or delayed 4 weeks later, and found synergistic improvements in photoaging when the treatments were combined to a single session, with no increased safety concerns or downtime.[68] Similar enhanced results were seen in a study of thirty-six patients in which ten received optimized pulsed light therapy followed by fractional 1540-nm treatment for facial rejuvenation.[69]

The transepidermal channels created during fractional laser treatment have inspired studying the use of this therapy to enhance the delivery of topically applied drugs. Early on this principle was demonstrated with the use of ablative fractional resurfacing to increase the depth and diffusion of MAL (methyl 5-aminolevulinate), a porphyrin precursor used in photodynamic therapy.[70] It has also been shown to augment the delivery of hydrophilic molecules that normally cannot penetrate the skin barrier, such as anti-oxidant vitamin C derivatives.[71] When compared to traditional CO_2 laser pretreatment in the absorption of ascorbic acid 2-glucoside on ex vivo porcine skin, fractional laser therapy achieved similar flux rates for the same fluence level after four passes.[72] Permeability changes did not reach the depth that conventional CO_2 therapy achieved and tissue destruction was less. These findings, however, do not immediately translate into enhanced dermal delivery of the drug and should be interpreted with caution.[73] Ultimately, the clinical significance of deeper penetration, as well as the risks of potential adversity, needs to be further studied.

Also being studied is the dermal delivery of topical or injected live human fibroblasts in ex vivo human abdominoplasty skin after pretreatment with different fractional lasers.[74] While topically-applied cells only penetrated the microchannels created by the Erbium 2940-nm laser, intradermally injected fibroblasts were observed after treatment with all tested fractionated lasers, including the nonablative Thulium 1927-nm laser.[74] Platelet-rich plasma, an autologous human platelet suspension used in skin rejuvenation and wound healing, has been studied in combination with fractional laser in twenty-two Korean women.[75] One month post-treatment, an increased number of fibroblasts, volume of collagen, and length of dermal-epidermal junction was seen. Patient satisfaction was increased as well.[75] We can anticipate additional applications with further advancement of technology and medical science.

In the future, a form of nonablative fractional photothermolysis may even be available for at-home use. Two clinical studies enrolling a total of 124 subjects investigated a new handheld home-use nonablative fractional laser device designed for the reduction of periorbital wrinkles.[76] Approximately 1.5% of the covered skin is targeted per treatment. The device was used daily for 4 weeks during the treatment phase, followed by twice weekly for 4 weeks for maintenance, and was found to be safe, easy to use, and had minimal side-effects, mostly transient erythema and trace edema.[76] Regarding efficacy, 90% of participants had improvement by one or more grades at the end of the active phase, and 79% at the end of the maintenance phase. These evaluations were performed by independent blinded physicians using the Fitzpatrick Wrinkle Scale score.[76]

REFERENCES

1. Berlin AL, Goldberg DJ. Non-Ablative Resurfacing. Chapter in Facial Resurfacing. John Wiley and Sons; 2010.p.20.
2. Manstein D, Herron GS, Sink RK, et al. Fractional photothermolysis: a new concept for cutaneous remodeling using microscopic patterns of thermal injury. Lasers Surg Med. 2004;34:426-38.
3. Wanner M, Tanzi EL, Alister TS. Fractional photothermolysis: treatment of facial and nonfacial cutaneous photodamage with a 1,550-nm erbium-doped fiber laser. Dermatol Surg. 2007;33:23-8.
4. Behroozan DS, Goldberg LH, Glaich AS, et al. Fractional photothermolysis for treatment of poikiloderma of Civatte. Dermatol Surg. 2006;32(2):298-301.
5. Jih MH, Goldberg LH, Kimyai-Asadi A. Fractional photothermolysis for photoaging of hands. Dermatol Surg. 2007;34(1):73-8.
6. Mahmoud BH, Srivastava D, Janiga JJ, et al. Safety and efficacy of erbium-doped yttrium aluminum garnet fractionated laser for treatment of acne scars in type IV to VI skin. Dermatol Surg. 2010;36(5):602-9.
7. Fisher GH, Kim KH, Bernstein LJ, et al. Concurrent use of handheld forced cold air device minimizes patient discomfort during fractional photothermolysis. Dermatol Surg. 2005;41(9 Pt 2):1242-3.
8. Hantash BM, Bedi VP, Sudireddy V, et al. Laser-induced transepidermal elimination of dermal content by fractional photothermolysis. J Biomed Opt. 2006;11(4):041115.
9. Laubach H-J, Tannous Z, Anderson RR, et al. Skin responses to fractional photothermolysis. Laser Surg Med. 2006;38:142-9.
10. Starnes AM, Jou PC, Molitoris JK, et al. Acute effects of fractional laser on photoaged skin. Dermatol Surg. 2012;38:51-7.
11. Wind BS, Meesters AA, Kroon MW, et al. Formation of fibrosis after nonablative and ablative fractional laser therapy. Dermatol Surg. 2012;38:437-42.
12. Walia S, Alster TS. Prolonged clinical and histologic effects from CO_2 laser resurfacing of atrophic acne scars. Dermatol Surg. 1999;25:926-30.
13. Tannous Z. Fractional resurfacing. Clin Dermatol. 2007;25:480-6.
14. Chua SH. Fractionated lasers in the Asian skin (Chapter 10). Textbook of Laser and Light Dermatology in Asian Skin.pp.97-105.
15. Bedi VP, Chan KF, Sink RK, et al. The effects of pulse energy variations on the dimensions of microscopic thermal treatment zones in nonablative fractional resurfacing. Laser Surg Med. 2007;39:145-55.
16. Chan HH, Manstein D, Yu CS, et al. The prevalence and risk factors of post-inflammatory hyperpigmentation after fractional resurfacing in Asians. Lasers Surg Med. 2007;39(5):381-5.
17. Kauvar A, Seckel B, Doherty S. Clinical study of a novel diode-laser-based non-ablative fractional device for treatment of facial wrinkles and dyschromia. Abstract from ASLMS abstracts. Laser Surg Med;44(24), Mar 2012.
18. Jung JY, Cho SB, Chung HJ, et al. Treatment of periorbital wrinkles with 1550- and 1565-nm Er:glass fractional photothermolysis lasers: a simultaneous split-face trial. JEADV. 2011;25:811-8.
19. Sherling M, Friedman PM, Adrian R, et al. Consensus recommendations on the use of an erbium-doped 1550-nm fractionated laser and its applications in dermatologic laser surgery. Dermatol Surg. 2010; 36:461-9.
20. Geronemus RG. Fractional photothermolysis: current and future applications. Laser Surg Med. 2006; 38:169-76.
21. Ruiz-Rodriguez R, Lopez L, Candelas D, et al. Enhanced efficacy of photodynamic therapy after fractional resurfacing: fractional photodynamic rejuvenation. J Drugs Dermatol. 2007;6(8):818-20.
22. Geraghty LN, Biesman B. Clinical evaluation of a single-wavelength fractional laser and a novel multi-wavelength fractional laser in treatment of photodamaged skin. Laser Surg Med. 2009;41:408-16.
23. Saedi N, Petrell K, Durfee M, et al. Evaluating pore size and skin texture after a series of non-ablative fractional 1440 nm laser treatments. Abstract from ASLMS abstracts. Laser Surg Med;44(24), Mar 2012.
24. Dierickx C, Campos V, Pinto C, et al. Deep heating of dermis and non-ablative fractional facial treatment with micro-compression optics. Abstract from ASLMS abstracts. Laser Surg Med;44(24), Mar 2012.

25. Goldberg DJ, Berlin AL, Phelps R. Histologic and ultrastructural analysis of melasma after fractional resurfacing. Laser Surg Med. 2008;40:134-8.
26. Katz TM, Glaich AS, Goldberg LH, et al. Treatment of melasma using fractional photothermolysis: a report of eight cases with long-term follow-up. Dermatol Surg. 2010;36:1273-80.
27. Kroon MW, Wind BS, Beek JF, et al. Nonablative 1550-nm fractional laser therapy versus triple topical therapy for the treatment of melasma: a randomized controlled pilot study. 2011;64:516-23.
28. Behroozan DS, Goldberg LH, Glaich AS, et al. Fractional photothermolysis for treatment of Poikiloderma of Civatte. Dermatol Surg. 2006;32:298-301.
29. Kouba DJ, Fincher EF, Moy RL. Nevus of Ota successfully treated by fractional photothermolysis using a fractionated 1440-nm Nd:YAG laser. Arch Dermatol. 2008;144(2):156-8.
30. Izikson L, Anderson RR. Resolution of blue minocycline pigmentation of the face after fractional photothermolysis. Laser Surg Med. 2008;40:399-401.
31. Katz TM, Goldberg LH, Firoz B, et al. Fractional photothermolysis for the treatment of postinflammatory hyperpigmentation. Dermatol Surg. 2009;35:1844-8.
32. Rokhsar CK, Ciocon DH. Postinflammatory hyperpigmentation after carbon dioxide laser resurfacing. Dermatol Surg. 2009;35:535-7.
33. Ong MWS, Bashir S. Fractional laser resurfacing for acne scars: a review. British Journal of Dermatol [Epub ahead of print]. Accepted 01/21/2012.
34. Hedelund L, Moreau KER, Beyer DM, et al. Fractional nonablative 1540-nm laser resurfacing of atrophic acne scars. A randomized controlled trial with blinded response evaluation. Lasers Med Sci. 2010;25:749-54.
35. Yoo KH, Ahn JY, Kim JY, et al. The use of 1540 nm fractional photothermolysis for the treatment of acne scars in Asian skin: a pilot study. Photodermatol Photoimmunol Photomed. 2009;25(3):138-42.
36. Cho SB, Lee SJ, Cho S, et al. Non-ablative 1550-nm erbium-glass and ablative 10600-nm carbon dioxide fractional lasers for acne scars: a randomized split-face study with blinded response evaluation. JEADV. 2010;24:921-5.
37. Haedersdal M, Moreau KER, Beyer DM, et al. Fractional nonablative 1540 nm laser resurfacing for thermal burn scars: a randomized controlled trial. Laser Surg Med. 2009;41:189-95.
38. Schulz KK, Walling HW. Fractional photothermolysis improves a depressed alar scar following Mohs micrographic surgery. J Drugs Dermatol. 2010;9(1):66-7.
39. Behroozan DS, Goldberg LH, Dai T, et al. Fractional photothermolysis for the treatment of surgical scars: a case report. J Cosmet Laser Ther. 2006;8(1):35-8.
40. Pham AM, Greene RM, Woolery-Lloyd H, et al. 1550-nm nonablative laser resurfacing for facial surgical scars. Arch Facial Plast Surg. 2011;13(3):203-10.
41. Tierney E, Mahmoud BH, Srivastava D, et al. Treatment of surgical scars with nonablative fractional laser versus pulsed dye laser: a randomized controlled trial. Dermatol Surg. 2009;35:1172-80.
42. Glaich AS, Rahman Z, Goldberg LH, et al. Fractional resurfacing for the treatment of hypopigmented scars: a pilot study. Dermatol Surg. 2007;33:289-94.
43. Massaki A, Fabi SG, Fitzpatrick R. Repigmentation of hypopigmented scars using an erbium-doped 1550-nm fractionated laser and topical bimatoprost. Dermatol Surg. 2012;1-7.
44. Lin JY, Warger WC, Izikson L, et al. A prospective randomized controlled trial on the efficacy of fractional photothermolysis on scar remodeling. Laser Surg Med. 2011;43:265-72.
45. Katz TM, Goldberg LH, Friedman PM. Nonablative fractional photothermolysis for the treatment of striae rubra. Dermatol Surg. 2009;35:1430-3.
46. De Angelis F, Kolesnikova L, Renato F, et al. Fractional nonablative 1540-nm laser in treatment of striae distensae in Fitzpatrick skin types II to IV: clinical and histological results. Aesthet Surg J. 2011;31(4): 411-9.
47. Bak H, Kim BJ, Lee WJ, et al. Treatment of striae distensae with fractional photothermolysis. Dermatol Surg. 2009;35:1215-20.
48. Yang YJ, Lee G-Y. Treatment of striae distensae with nonablative fractional laser versus ablative CO_2 fractional laser: a randomized controlled trial. Ann Dermatol. 2011;23(4): 481-9.
49. Akita H, Takasu E, Washimi Y, et al. Syringoma of the face treated with fractional photothermolysis. J Cosmet Laser Ther. 2009;11:216-9.
50. Cho SB, Kim HJ, Noh S, et al. Treatment of syringoma using an ablative 10,600-nm carbon dioxide fractional laser: a prospective analysis of 35 patients. Dermatol Surg. 2011;37(4):433-8.
51. Katz TM, Goldberg LH, Friedman PM. Dermatosis papulosa nigra treatment with fractional photothermolysis. Dermatol Surg. 2009;35:1840-3.
52. Katz TM, Goldberg LH, Friedman PM. Fractional photothermolysis: a new therapeutic modality for xanthelasma. Arch Dermatol. 2009;145(10):1091-4.
53. Marra DE, Pourrabbani S, Fincher EF, et al. Fractional photothermolysis for the treatment of adult colloid milium. Arch Dermatol. 2007;143(5): 572-4.
54. Ghasri P, Admani S, Petelin A, et al. Treatment of actinic cheilitis using a 1,927-nm thulium fractional laser. Dermatol Surg. 2012;38:504-7.
55. Anolik R, Weiss ET, Chapas A, et al. Non-ablative fractional resurfacing with the 1927 nm Thulium

laser is an effective, well-tolerated treatment for actinic cheilitis. Lasers Surg Med. 2011;43 (suppl 23): 927.

56. Katz TM, Goldberg LH, Marquez D, et al. Nonablative fractional photothermolysis for facial actinic keratoses: 6 month follow-up with histologic evaluation. J Am Acad Dermatol. 2011;65:349-56.
57. Togsverd-Bo K, Haak CS, Thaysen-Petersen D, et al. Intensified photodynamic therapy of actinic keratoses with fractional CO_2 laser: a randomized clinical trial. Br J Dermatol;2012 [Epub ahead of print].
58. Chrastil B, Glaich AS, Goldberg LH, et al. Fractional photothermolysis: a novel treatment for disseminated superficial actinic porokeratosis. Arch Dermatol. 2007;143(11):1450-2.
59. Karsai S, Hammes S, Rutten A, et al. Fractional photothermolysis for the treatment of granuloma annulare: a case report. Lasers Surg Med. 2008; 40(5):319-22.
60. Liu A, Hexsel CL, Moy RL, et al. Granuloma annulare successfully treated using fractional photothermolysis with a 1550-nm Erbium-doped yttrium aluminum garnet fractionated laser. Dermatol Surg. 2011;37:712-5.
61. Laubach H-J, Anderson RR, Luger T, et al. Fractional photothermolysis for involuted infantile hemangioma. Arch Dermatol. 2009;145(7): 748-50.
62. Blankenship CM, Alster TS. Fractional photothermolysis of residual hemangioma. Dermatol Surg. 2008;34:1112-4.
63. Metelitsa AI, Alster TS. Fractionated laser skin resurfacing treatment complications: a review. Dermatol Surg. 2010;36:299-306.
64. Mamelak AJ, Goldberg LH, Marquez D, et al. Eruptive keratoacanthomas on the legs after fractional photothermolysis: report of two cases. Dermatol Surg. 2009;35:513-8.
65. Barolet D, Lussier I, Mery S, et al. Beneficial effects of spraying low mineral content thermal spring water after fractional photothermolysis in patients with dermal melasma. J Cosmet Dermatol. 2009;8(2):114-8.
66. Alster TS, Wanitphakdeedecha R. Improvement of postfractional laser erythema with light-emitting diode photomodulation. Dermatol Surg. 2009; 35(5):813-5.
67. Graber EM, Tanzi EL, Alster TS. Side effects and complications of fractional laser photothermolysis: experience with 961 treatments. Dermatol Surg. 2008;34: 301-7.
68. Kearney C, Brew D. Single-session combination treatment with intense pulsed light and nonablative fractional photothermolysis: a split-face study. Dermatol Surg. 2012 May 10. [Epub ahead of print].
69. Dover J, Saedi N, Mickle C, et al. A new combined treatment for facial rejuvenation using an optimized pulse light source followed by a fractional laser. Abstract from ASLMS abstracts. Laser Surg Med; 44(24), Mar 2012.
70. Haedersdal M, Sakamoto FH, Farinelli WA, et al. Fractional CO_2 laser-assisted drug delivery. Laser Surg Med. 2010;42:113-22.
71. Hsiao C-Y, Huang C-H, Hu S, et al. Skin pretreatment with lasers promotes the transdermal delivery of vitamin C derivatives. Lasers Med Surg. 2011; 26:369-76.
72. Hsiao C-Y, Huang C-H, Hu S, et al. Fractional carbon dioxide laser treatment to enhance skin permeation of ascorbic acid 2-glucoside with minimal skin disruption. Dermatol Surg. 2012;38:1284-93.
73. Alexiades-Armenakas M. Fractional laser resurfacing to enhance skin permeation. Commentary in Dermatol Surg. 2012;38:1294-5.
74. McDaniel D, Steel C, Mazur C. Dermal delivery of topically applied fluorescently labeled human skin fibroblasts following various fractional laser treatments. ASLMS 2012 Annual Conference. Late Breaking Abstract 6.
75. Shin M-K, Lee J-H, Lee S-J, et al. Platelet-rich plasma combined with fractional laser therapy for skin rejuvenation. Dermatol Surg. 2012;38:623-30.
76. Leyden J, Stephens TJ, Herndon JH. Multicenter clinical trial of a home-use nonablative fractional laser device for wrinkle reduction. J Am Acad Dermatol. 2012;67(5):975-84.

CHAPTER 9

Ablative Fractional Resurfacing

Sara Risner-Rumohr, Parisa Ravanfar, Paul M Friedman

INTRODUCTION TO ABLATIVE LASER RESURFACING

The traditional ablative resurfacing laser—the confluent carbon dioxide (CO_2) laser, has been used since the 1990s by dermatologists for the treatment of facial rhytides.[1,2] The erbium-doped yttrium aluminum garnet (Er:YAG) laser began to be used in the late 1990s showing efficacy in treating superficial rhytides and atrophic scars comparable to CO_2 resurfacing.[3-5] The traditional confluent ablative resurfacing laser devices are discussed in more detail in Chapter 7.

INTRODUCTION TO FRACTIONAL LASER RESURFACING

Fractional resurfacing technology was the response to the limitations seen with the traditional confluent ablative laser resurfacing devices. Manstein et al. in 2004 published the concept of fractional photothermolysis with the prototype nonablative fractional resurfacing photothermolysis device (NAFR), a 1.5-µm wavelength laser system (Reliant MTZ SR prototype, Reliant Technologies, Palo Alto, CA).[6] Many nonablative lasers preceded this novel fractional laser advancement, which included pulsed-dye lasers and Q-switched Nd:YAG lasers. These lasers were observed to improve the clinical appearance of rhytides and had corresponding histological changes in the dermal collagen.[7-9] This motivated the search for nonablative wavelengths that would target water and thus deliver thermal-effects to the dermis where the majority of the ultraviolet-induced photodamage occurs at depths of 100–400 µm.[10] By utilizing longer wavelengths (infrared lasers) in which the water absorption coefficient is lower than in the visible light spectrum, thus enabling the lasers to penetrate deeper into the dermis to promote collagen repair and skin tightening. In addition, the longer wavelength lasers would not have the epidermal effects of the 585–595-nm pulse-dye or the 1064-nm Q-switched Nd:YAG lasers.[10-12] Three infrared nonablative laser systems,1320-nm Nd:YAG, 1450-nm diode and 1540-nm Er:Glass were developed. (Trade named examples include: CoolTouch II®: 1320-nm Nd:YAG, SmoothBeam®: 1450-nm diode, Aramis, 1540 Er:glass).[13,14] These advances led to the development of infrared fractional lasers, NAFR devices such as the 1550-nm erbium-doped laser (e.g. Fraxel SR®, Solta Medical).

The concept of fractional photothermolysis must first be understood in order to discuss the clinical applications. It is a novel way to deliver thermal coagulative injury to the dermis without confluent epidermal damage. This is achieved by creating noncontiguous microscopic columns (called microscopic thermal zones or MTZs) to produce a grid of tiny thermal wounds that facilitate enhanced tissue contraction surrounded by columns of normal tissue which results in reduced recovery time and less adverse effects[6] (Fig. 9.1). With ablative fractional resurfacing (AFR) the conversion of radiant energy to heat at the point of absorption instantly raises the temperature of tissue water to more

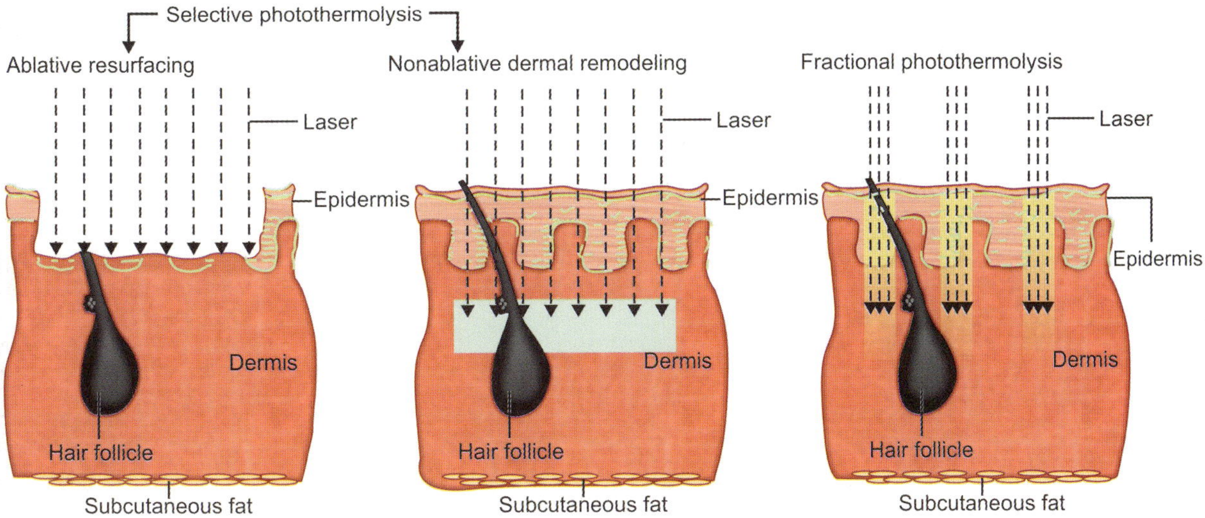

Fig. 9.1: Diagram of AFR vs confluent ablation

Source: Reprinted with permission from Hantash, BM and Mahmood, MB. Fractional photothermolysis: a novel aesthetic laser surgery modality. Dermatologic Surgery. 2007;33:525-34.

than 100°C, leading to tissue water vaporization. The threshold for vaporization of human skin is 5 J/cm^2 with the CO_2 laser. The original study by Manstein et al. reported an overall clinical improvement in periorbital rhytides and skin texture of 19% with this prototype NAFR device.[6] (Note: Kindly refer to Chapter 8—Nonablative Fractional Resurfacing, for a more in-depth review of the NAFR and other nonablative technologies as their specific indications, benefits and risks vary greatly from the ablative fractional resurfacing lasers and will not be covered in this chapter).

INTRODUCTION TO ABLATIVE FRACTIONAL LASER RESURFACING

Hantash et al. first published the use of an ablative fractional resurfacing (AFR) device that produced MTZs at specified depths and densities. The AFR devices result in confluent columns of thermal injury involving both ablation and coagulation that extends from the stratum corneum to the deeper reticular dermal layers in a noncontiguous pattern.[15] This study also demonstrated the histologic effects of AFR with persistent collagen remodeling for at least 3 months post procedure. This may explain the observed enhanced tissue contraction and tightening outcomes of AFR devices over the NAFR devices.[15-18] In the literature, it has been suggested that the improvement in skin laxity and texture seen with AFR devices could be further optimized with longer pulse durations (1000–1500 μs) leading to greater depth of penetration, however longer pulse durations can lead to increasing the MTZ width causing more collateral thermal injury leading to more scarring complications.[19] Longer pulse duration for targeting skin laxity delivers higher densities of MTZs to maximize the surface area treated. A higher density of MTZs treated leads to more effective treatment of dyschromia and skin texture abnormalities, although higher densities can lead to increased post-procedural erythema and edema and increased risk for postinflammatory hyperpigmentation.[19] Studies have also shown long-term sustainability of the clinical outcomes after AFR resurfacing.[20] One study observed that 10 patients treated with a fractional CO_2 laser maintained 74% of their overall improvement in facial rhytides and photodamage at 1- and 2-year follow-up compared to 3-month follow-up.[20]

Today, there are many AFR devices on the market, both Er:YAG and CO_2 lasers and a few Er:YSGG lasers (See Table 9.1 for examples). There are very few published comparative studies or standardized treatment protocols for the clinical use of AFR devices. Most of the AFR devices are continuous lasers equipped with fractionated scanners or stamping devices that provide a regular pixilated pattern of MTZs. One exception is the Fraxel Re:pair® laser (Solta Medical) that uses a Intelligent Optical Tracking System (IOTS), that automatically adjusts to the speed of the practitioner to provide a random pattern of injury that in theory reduces the possibility of bulk heating with multiple passes that

Table 9.1: Various device models and device modifications

Company	*Device*	*Laser*	*Wavelength (nm)*	*Mode*	*Energy Output (Joule or Work)*	*Pulse Length*	*Spot Size (mm)*	*MTZ Density/Scanned Area*
Alma Lasers, Buffalo Grove, IL	Harmony^{XL} Platform, Pixel 2940	Fraction al ER: YAG	2940 nm	Scanner	300– 2,500 mJ/p	Short, medium, long, 1–2 ms pulse durations	250 μm spot	11mm × 11mm scanner area with depth of 300 μm. Typically, 2–4 passes of 20–60 μm ablation and 30–50 μm of thermal effect with a MTZ of 150 μm
Alma Lasers, Buffalo Grove, IL	Harmony^{XL} Platform, Pixel Omnifit or Pixel CO_2	Fraction al CO_2 system	10,600 nm	Scanner	70 W	CW Superpulse	11mm^2	
Cutera, Brisbane, CA	Xeo Platform, Pearl Fractional	Fraction al Er: YSGG	2790 nm	Scanner	60–320 mJ per microspot	600 μs	300 μm spot size	10 mm × 14 mm scanned area, 8–12% density of MTZs
DEKA, Eclipse Med, Dallas, TX	SmartXide Dermal Optical Thermoly-sis (DOT) 30 W/50 W	Scanned fraction al CO_2	10,600 nm	Scanner	150 W/250 W max	200 μs–80 ms. Ablative pulse width <150 μs. Thermal pulse width: 0.2–2.0 ms	350 μm spot size	15 mm × 15 mm scanner area, 200–1500 μm depth, 25% coverage density of MTZs
Eclipse Aesthe-tics	Equinox	CO_2 fraction al laser, RF excited tube	10,600 nm		1–300 mJ	0.05–10 ms		
Ellman Inter-national, Inc., Elluminé Frac-tional CO_2 Laser System	CO_2 fractional laser, Flexible fiber	Scanned CO_2 fraction al laser	10,600 nm	Scanner	Up to 105 mJ	2–7 ms, adjustable		
Focus Medical, Ltd	Natura-Lase CO_2	Frac-tional CO_2	10,600 nm		50 W	Up to 10 ms		
Hironic Co., Ltd	MIXEL	Frac-tional CO_2	10,600 nm		60 mJ	Up to 5,000 μs		
Ilooda Co., Ltd.	Fraxis	Frac-tional CO_2	10,600 nm		Up to 30 W	0.1–5 ms		

Contd...

Contd...

Industra Technologies	2940 Dual Mode, Er: YAG Laser	Er: YAG	2940 nm		Up to 60 mJ/MTZ	300 μs–5 ms		
Lasering USA	Slim Evolution II, MiXto SX Pro	Scanned fractional CO_2	10,600 nm	Scanner	0.5–30 W	2.5–16 ms	300 μm/ 180 μm spots size	20 nm × 20 nm scanned area, ablation depth 200 μm, thermal depth additional 300 μm settings typically of 8–25 watts power, 20–40% density
Lumenis Inc., Santa Clara, CA	UltraPulse Active Fx	Scanned fractional CO_2	10,600 nm	Scanner	1–225 mJ	<1 ms	1.3 mm	9 mm × 9mm/10 mm × 10 mm scanned area, 10–300 μm depth, up to 3200 μm with stacked pulses
Lumenis Inc., Santa Clara, CA	UltraPulse DeepFx	Scanned fractional CO_2	10,600 nm	Scanner	2.5–50 mJ	<2 ms	0.12 mm	
Lumenis Inc., Santa Clara, CA	UltraPulse Total Fx	Scanned fractional CO_2	10,600 nm	Scanner	1–170 mJ (superficial), 1–30 mJ (deep)	<2 ms	1.3 mm and 0.12 mm spot size delivery systems	
Lumenis Inc., Santa Clara, CA	AcuPulse Multi Mode	Scanned fractional CO_2	10,600 nm	Scanner		<2 ms	1.3 mm and 0.12 mm with one hand, piece	
Lutronic, Princeton Junction, NJ	eCO_2, Dynamic stamping	Fractional CO_2	10,600 nm	Scanner	2–240 mJ	Variable	100 μm/ 300 μm/ 120 μm spot size	14 mm × 14 mm scanned area, typical depth of 2500 μm
Palomar	Palomar Icon	2940 fractional	2940 nm	Stamping delivery	2–5.5 mJ/0.1 mm	0.25–5 ms	100 μm spot size	10 mm × 10 mm/ 6 mm × 6 mm scanned area, depth of 200 μm
Sandstone Medical Technologies	UltraFine-FS fractional scanner	Scanner adapts to most CO_2 lasers	10,600 nm	Scanner	Up to 40 W for Matrix Ls-40 with fractional scanner	Adjustable to 100 ms		
Sandstone Medical Technologies	Cortex Resurfacing Work Station	CO_2/ Er: YAG laser	10,600 mm/ 2940 nm		Up to 40 W/up to 1J	Adjustable to 100 ms		

Contd...

Contd...

Sciton	ProFractional-XC	Er: YAG	2940 nm		Up to 400 J/cm	Variable		
Sciton	ProFractional-XC	Er: YAG	2940 nm		Up to 400 J/cm	Variable	430 μm spot size	Ablation depth 25–100 μm depth and treatment density of 5.5%, 11% or 22% with or without depth- specific coagulation
Solta Medical, Hayward, CA	Fraxel re:pair	Fractional CO_2, Intelligent optical tracking system (IOTS) continuous motion delivery system	10,600 nm		Up to 70 mJ/MTZ	0.15–3 ms pulse duration	<140 μm spot size	
Syneron & Candela, Quadralase Candela Corporation, Wayland, MA	eLaser Sublative Rejuvenation CO_2, RE	Fractional CO_2	10,600 nm		Up to 60 W	30–60 mJ, 60–90 mJ, 50–80 mJ, 60–70 mJ, 1–10 mJ		

can occur with a scanner or stamping device. One split-face study compared a rolling scanner AFR device (UltraPulse Encore Deep FX®) to a scanned stamping device (Fraxel Re:pair® laser, Solta Medical) for the treatment of photoaged skin, rhytides, skin textural abnormalities, and dyschromia and found both devices were effective and safe, but with the stamping device associated with longer operative times and more intraoperative pain.[21] This study demonstrated that with the use of manufacturer settings for the two devices, the stamping device led to deeper ablative depth with similar density of MTZs (500 μm compared to 200 μm for the rolling scanner) but did not result in improved clinical outcomes. The authors argue that there is likely a threshold for the depth of ablative injury beyond which further penetration is not clinically significant in the treatment of photoaging with fractional CO_2 resurfacing. They propose that as long as the injury zone targets the papillary dermis, where the majority of histological photoaging occurs, the AFR devices will result in clinical improvement of photoaging.[21] All available devices have operator-adjusted settings such as pulse duration, spot size, energy and MTZ density. Most AFR devices have small spot sizes (<200 μm) which allow deeper penetration, although some also offer larger spot sizes (>300 μm) that are used when shallower penetration is desired for fine superficial rhytides (e.g. Lumenis Encore® with the Active FX® and Total FX®). The depth of penetration with the AFR devices with small spot sizes can be further augmented based on energy settings and pulse stacking. By increasing the energy settings, deeper penetration is achieved but this also increases the width of the MTZs leading to collateral thermal injury.[15]

A more recent AFR technology advancement has been the development of the fractionated Er:YSGG devices. The Er:YSGG AFR devices emit energy at 2790-nm wavelength which like the confluent Er:YSGG lasers takes advantage of a water absorption coefficient between CO_2 and Er:YAG. Studies have demonstrated that the new AFR device is safe and effective for the treatment of photodamage and perioral rhytides.[22,23] Few studies have compared the efficacy between available AFR devices. One randomized double-blind split-face study compared one treatment with a fractional CO_2 laser to treatment with a fractional Er:YAG laser for periorbital rhytides. No appreciable difference in profilometric wrinkle depth reduction (approximately 20%) or patient satisfaction between the two AFR devices was observed.[24]

The safety profile of AFR devices offer an advantage compared to traditional confluent ablative laser devices with lower incidences of prolonged erythema, postinflammatory pigmentary changes and scarring.[6,25-27] The improved safety profile is the result of the pixilated pattern of MTZs where the thermally damaged tissue is surrounded by normal tissue that promotes more rapid re-epithelialization. This leads to a shorter recovery time with less post-procedural complications. The recovery period is significantly shorter with re-epithelialization complete after full-face AFR in 3–6 days compared to the 2–3 weeks observed with traditional ablative CO_2 laser devices.[29] It is important that the AFR devices not be considered without risk, there have been reports of most of the common complications as seen with traditional ablative lasers, including scarring.[19,25,26,28] The superiority of AFR resurfacing over traditional ablative laser resurfacing has been well established in the literature and is based on a better safety profile and recovery time, rather than on clinical outcomes.

The NAFR devices also have favorable safety profiles, but the AFR devices are suspected to result in higher clinical efficacy over the NAFR devices. However, to date, there are limited published comparative prospective studies between NAFR and AFR devices evaluating the presumed superiority of AFR devices in skin tightening and textural outcomes. Weiss in 2008 presented a small (10 subject) prospective split-face study comparing an AFR device (Fractional CO_2 laser, UltraPulse Encore,Lumenis®) to the nonablative fractional erbium-doped laser (Fraxel SR®)with a median improvement of periocular rhytides of 75% for AFR device compared to median improvement of 25% seen with the NAFR erbium device.[16] Tierney in 2011 published a review of the literature and a small prospective single-blinded study of the treatment of lower eyelid rhytides and laxity with an AFR device (SmartXide DOT laser).[30] The study showed that with two to three treatments there was a mean improvement of 62.6%, 65.3% and 62.1% in 25 subject patients of periorbital skin texture, laxity and rhytides, respectively. The overall cosmetic outcome mean was 65.7%,[30] which is much higher than the older studies of NAFR devices resulting in a 19% clinical improvement in periorbital rhytides.[6] Newer generations of NAFR device systems have been shown to have improved skin tightening outcomes compared to the prototypical NAFR devices, one study reported a 25% improvement in skin tightening in the periorbital area using a nonablative 1550-nm erbium-doped device (Fraxel SR) which is higher than the 19% overall improvement noted with the prototype NAFR device.[31] These few studies have demonstrated AFR devices' relative superiority over NAFR devices.[30]

One disadvantage of AFR resurfacing devices is based on the pattern of MTZs restricting full epidermal coverage and thus limited ability to improve skin texture, tone and pigmentation. One small prospective study demonstrated that the combination of a confluent Er:YSGG and fractional Er:YSGG laser device in the same treatment resulted in a clinically significant mean improvement in photodamaged skin up to a 6-month follow-up with good tolerability.[32] This novel combination treatment results in complete ablation of the superficial epidermis, with coagulation of the deeper epidermis and fractional coagulation in the deeper dermis. More randomized controlled, prospective studies are needed to compare available ablative resurfacing tools and to develop treatment protocols specific to various treatment goals to assist dermatologists in optimizing their clinical outcomes.

RHYTIDES

All available resurfacing devices, both traditional confluent and fractional lasers have been designed for the primary treatment of facial rhytides. Most published studies on AFR have primary study outcomes based on improvement of facial rhytides and have established AFR efficacy as nearly analogous

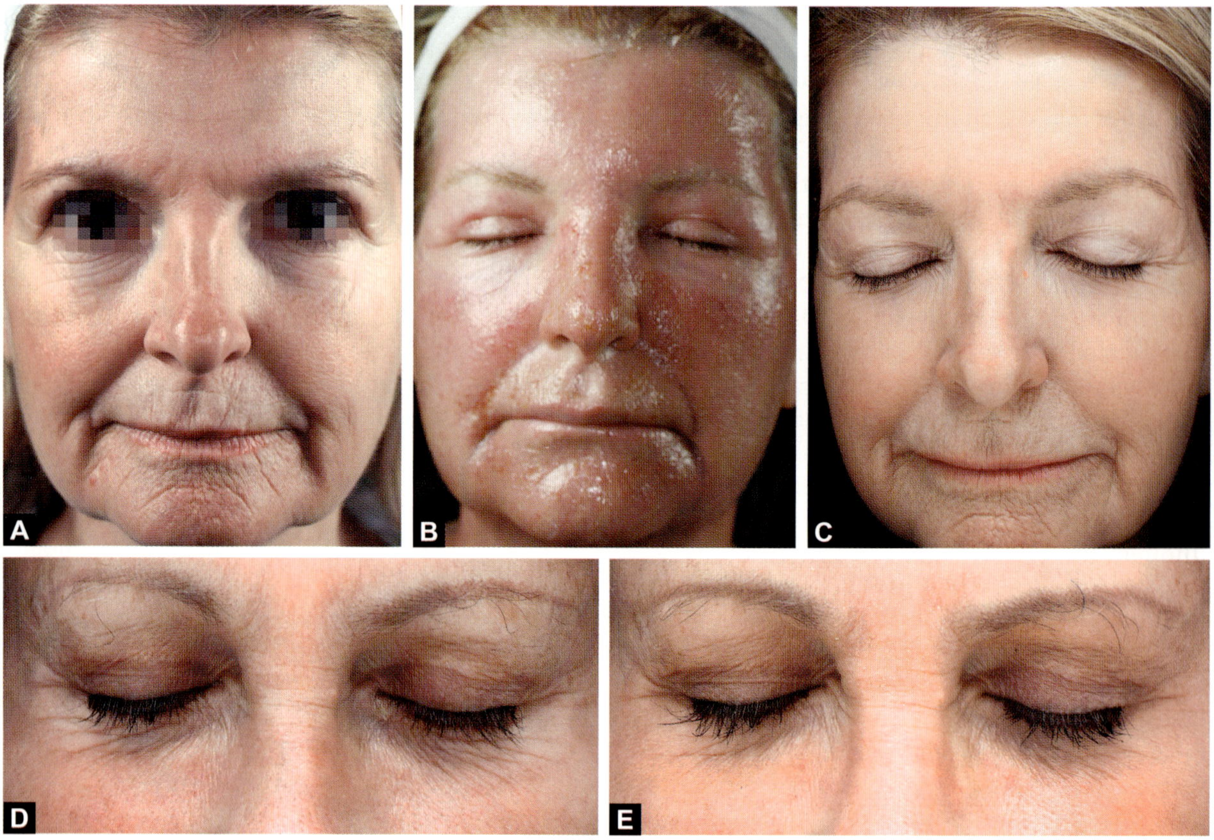

Figs 9.2A to E: Clinical photographs of rhytides treatment with AFR

to those results achieved by traditional confluent resurfacing with improved safety profiles and less downtime.[27,33] The fractional resurfacing laser devices with specific settings that confer deeper dermal penetration and wider thermal injury zones are more effective in the treatment of rhytides. Early studies demonstrated improved AFR efficacy for fine facial rhytides compared to deep rhytides, although deeper rhytides are responsive to AFP.[32,34] Non-movement associated rhytides in the periorbital and perioral areas respond to ablative laser resurfacing with predictable clinical outcomes (Figs 9.2A to E). This is compared to movement-associated rhytides in the glabellar and forehead area that tend to yield less favorable results. Few novel studies have combined ablative laser resurfacing with botulinum toxin for the treatment of movement-associated rhytides with encouraging results.[35] A split-faced study confirmed AFR surpasses the prototype NAFP devices in clinical outcomes for photoaging and periocular rhytides.[16]

PHOTOREJUVENATION

Pigmentation Changes (Lentigines, Dyschromia, Skin-tone Irregularities) and Epidermal Dyspigmentation

With the wide variety of therapeutic modalities available to dermatologists, most consider a combined approach optimal for the treatment of dyschromia and photoaging. These modalities often include nonablative and ablative lasers in conjunction with chemical peels, topical agents such as retinoids and bleaching agents and a wide array of cosmeceuticals. Most epidermal pigmentation such as photoaging-associated dyschromia and solar lentigines, lentigo simplex and *café-au-lait* macules (CALMs) can be removed with single pass of traditional confluent ablative resurfacing devices.[36-38] It has been demonstrated that both epidermal and dermal pigment can be effectively extruded through the MTZs after an AFR treatment.[19] There are many studies confirming the efficacy of AFR lasers for the treatment of photoaging such as dyschromia and poikiloderma.[27,34,39,40] There are few comparative studies between traditional ablative and ablative fractional laser modalities and between AFR devices for the treatment of epidermal dyspigmentation. One split-face study compared a CO_2 AFR device with an Er:YAG AFR device in the treatment of photodamage and resulted in improved skin texture and color on the side treated with CO_2 AFR device.[41] Other studies comparing AFR CO_2 to AFR Er:YAG devices resulted in no difference in efficacy or complications between the two AFR technologies, both demonstrated clinical improvement in photodamage.[42] However, AFR devices are typically considered clinically inferior for the treatment of skin-tone irregularities and dyschromia compared to confluent ablative resurfacing based on the pattern of MTZs. This is thought to be a result of the pattern of MTZs, as they limit full epidermal coverage and thus limit the ability to improve full-face skin-tone irregularities and dyschromia.

However, contrary to this theory; some studies have also documented the superiority of AFR over traditional resurfacing for photoaging.[43] Furthermore, some practitioners argue the superiority of AFR devices over traditional confluent ablative lasers for the treatment of photoaging because of the versatility of the AFR devices in treating both facial dyschromia along with other common areas such as chest, back and extremities that are high risk for scarring and hypopigmentation with traditional ablative lasers.[34] Ablative fractional resurfacing devices with higher density modes are best suited to treat dyschromia. Melasma is a dyspigmentation disorder with pigment deposits in the dermis and epidermis. It is often very difficult condition to treat with laser resurfacing and has a high risk of complications: especially rebound hyperpigmentation. In general, ablative resurfacing is not recommended for the treatment of melasma. NAFR laser resurfacing on the other hand has been shown to be an effective treatment of melasma as well as other dermal dyspigmentation such as minocyclin-induced pigmentation and Nevus of Ota.[44-46]

Textural Changes (Skin Laxity, Pore-size and Solar Elastosis-related Textural Changes)

In addition to treating dyschromia and rhytides, AFR devices have been used successfully in treating skin textural abnormalities, skin laxity and pore-size with less risk than full-face traditional ablative laser resurfacing. Traditional confluent ablative resurfacing lasers are still considered the gold standard laser for textural abnormalities. Although some researchers have theorized that AFR devices may even confer greater efficacy than traditional confluent ablative lasers because of the ability of the AFR devices to penetrate deeper in the dermis with the pixilated pattern of MTZs.[17,18] It often requires multiple passes of traditional ablative resurfacing laser to penetrate deep enough to promote skin-tightening effects. One study suggested that AFR devices with settings of longer pulse durations lead to improved skin-tightening outcomes.[19] Few studies have compared AFR devices, one study confirmed the superiority of CO_2 AFR device over Er:YAG AFR device for the treatment of photoaging and skin textural abnormalities.[41] One study by La Towsky et al. compared four AFR devices: Fraxel Re:pair (Solta Medical Inc, Hayward, CA), Active and Deep FX (Total FX; Lumenis, Santa Clara, CA), Quadralase (Candela, Wayland, MA), and Pearl Fractional (Fx; Cutera, Brisbane, CA).[47] All four AFR devices improved rhytides, lentigines, texture and pore size with no statistical differences between the devices for outcomes, intraoperative pain or side-effects. Pore-size responded less than textural photodamage across all the tested devices, with median overall improvement at 6 months between 26% and 50%, and 1 to 25% for pore-size.[47]

SCARS

There is a long tradition of treating atrophic acne scars and other atrophic scars with traditional confluent ablative laser resurfacing. The Food and Drug Administration approved the use of AFR devices for the treatment of acne scars in 2006, with successful clinical outcomes. Multiple small studies and case reports have evaluated AFR devices with satisfactory outcomes for acne scarring.[48-50] In addition, AFR devices may allow treatment for extrafacial acne scarring, which has not been safe with traditional ablative resurfacing technologies.[48] Early indications are that AFR devices may enhance results for acne scarring treatment more than NAFR.[34] Figures 9.3A and B show clinical photographs of atrophic acne scars treated by AFR. A study compared fractional ablative and nonablative laser resurfacing for acne scars and suggested that AFR has an overall higher improvement range (26–83%) compared to NAFR (26–50%).[51] However, more side-effects were noted with AFR resurfacing compared to NAFR resurfacing such as postinflammatory hyperpigmentation,

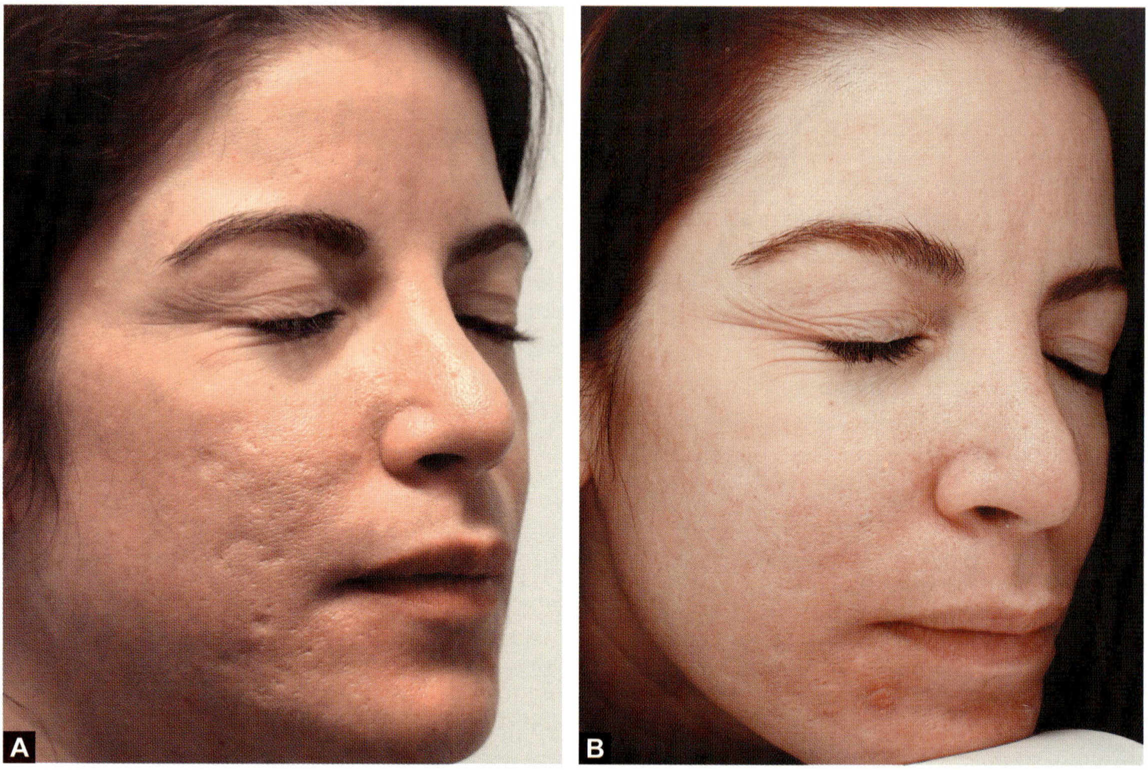

Figs 9.3A and B: Clinical photographs of acne scar treatment with AFR with 2-year follow up

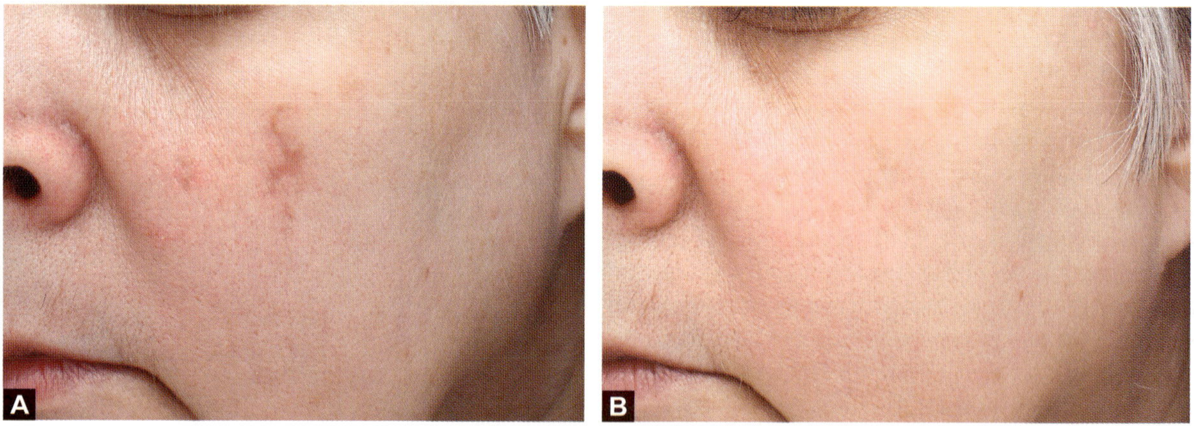

Figs 9.4A and B: Clinical photographs of postprocedural, atrophic scar treatment with AFR

prolonged erythema and higher intraprocedural pain.[51] A retrospective study evaluated NAFR and AFR devices in the treatment of acne scars in ethnic skin with Fitzpatrick phototypes III–V. Over 50% improvement in acne scars was demonstrated for AFR and NAFR device groups demonstrating the effectiveness of both modalities in treating acne scars in darker skin types. Both the AFR and NAFR devices had few adverse outcomes, and no statistical difference in PIH was noted, concluding that both laser modalities have good safety profiles in treating acne scars in darker skin types.[52]

Non-acne scars have also been successfully treated with ablative laser resurfacing such as post-varicella scars, traumatic or post-procedural scars, burn scars, contractures and striae distensae.[53-56] Figures 9.4A and B show clinical photographs of postprocedural scar treated successfully with AFR. Systemic scleroderma-related scarring, perioral rhytides and morphea-induced contractures have

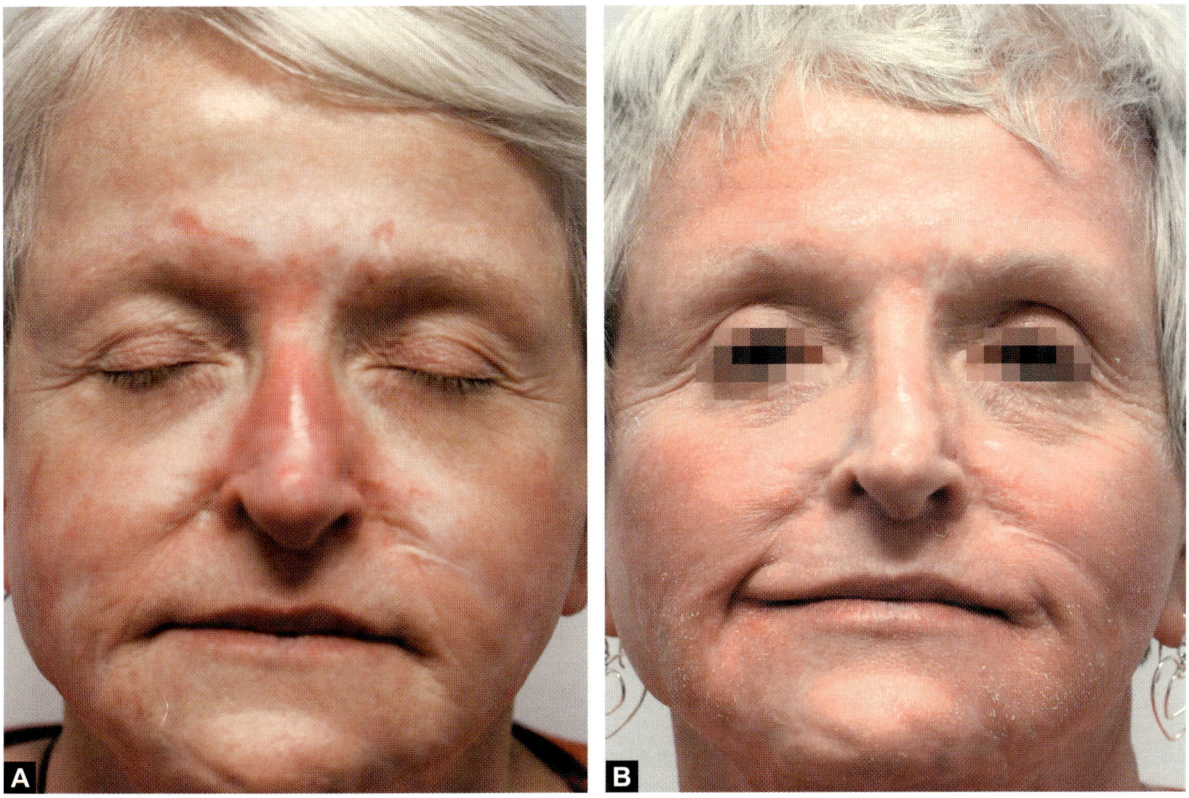

Figs 9.5A and B: Clinical photographs of burn scars treatment with AFR

all been successfully treated with ablative resurfacing although caution should be taken as resurfacing can also exacerbate scleroderma.[57] Waibel and Beer in 2009 reported the first case report of a successful outcome from a fractional ablative laser resurfacing treatment for a severe third-degree burn scar (Lumenis Encore, one pass of Deep FX at 12.5 mJ/cm^2 and one pass of Active FX at 80 mJ/cm^2).[58] Figures 9.5A and B show clinical photographs of burn scars treated successfully with AFR. Waibel et al. reported a study of a 2940 Er:YAG AFR laser used as an effective treatment for third-degree burn scars.[59] The study demonstrated histological confirmation of the removal of scar tissue with the resurfacing vaporization and promotion of normal wound healing with decrease of dystrophic collagen fibers in the clinically improved treatment areas.[59] The treatment of burn scars with an erbium-doped, 1550-nm nonablative fractional laser was also reported in a small prospective study.[60] Although there is limited literature on the use of AFR devices for burn scars evaluating the clinical and histological outcomes, it has been argued much like with the treatment of deep facial rhytides, possible advantages of AFR compared to traditional ablative lasers and NAFR lasers secondary to the fractional photothermolysis inducing unique thermal damage patterns of superficial ablation and depth of penetration with MTZs.[61] One proposed mechanism for the advantage of AFR devices for burn scars is the ability of AFR devices to stimulate heat shock proteins that promote wound healing by promoting keratinocyte migration, proliferation and differentiation. It has been proven that fractional photothermolysis thermal damage results in increased expression of heat shock proteins.[61] Hantash in 2007 argued one step further that the increased expression of heat shock proteins can activate transient amplifying epidermal stem cells located in the basal layer which replace the damaged epidermal tissue.[15]

KERATOSES AND OTHER EPIDERMAL LESIONS

The removal of epidermal lesions such as seborrheic keratoses, dermatosis papulosa nigra and pre-malignant actinic keratoses (AKs) can easily be addressed by ablative laser resurfacing. It has also been hypothesized that by addressing photoaging as the primary goal of therapy, ablative laser resurfacing may in fact not only treat currently present keratoses but may also decrease the formation of future AKs. Traditional ablative laser resurfacing has been shown to be effective in the treatment of diffuse actinic keratoses and actinic cheilitis by targeting the entire epidermis with surface ablation.[36,62,63] There are limited comparative studies between confluent and fractional ablative laser modalities. More research is needed to evaluate treatment outcomes for premalignant and malignant epidermal neoplasms such as histological clearance; local recurrence and cosmetic outcomes to develop standardized treatment protocols. One study combined the use of a fractional CO_2 laser device with photodynamic therapy (PDT) with methyl aminolaevulinate (MAL) to PDT-MAL alone for the treatment of AKs. The AFR plus PDT-MAL was significantly more effective for the treatment of AKs and secondary outcome of improved photoaging compared to PDT-MAL alone.[63]

Other benign epidermal lesions such as seborrheic keratoses, dermatosis papulosa nigra, epidermal nevi and refractory viral warts have been reported to be successfully treated with ablative laser resurfacing, yet there are limited publications comparing fractional and confluent ablative resurfacing for benign epidermal lesions.[36,65-69]

OTHER INDICATIONS

Over the years, traditional confluent ablative laser resurfacing has been a powerful destructive modality utilized in the treatment of various refractory dermatoses. Often, treatment courses required aggressive settings and a series of treatment sessions leading to a high risk of scarring and pigmentary alterations and limiting the modalities used in treating chronic dermatoses such as recalcitrant Darier disease, Hailey-Hailey disease and hidradenitis suppurativa.[70,71] In addition, sebaceous hyperplasia, rhinophyma and various dermal lesions such as melanocytic nevi, trichoepitheliomas and syringomas, xanthelasma, neurofibromas, plexiform neurofibromas, angiofibromas and pearly penile papules have all been reported to have been successfully treated with ablative laser resurfacing.[72-80] Figures 9.6A and B show clinical photographs of rhinophyma treated successfully with AFR. At this time there are limited studies evaluating the use of AFR devices for these indications.[81] One novel study demonstrated the benefit of using an AFR device in combination with electrosurgical debulking and pulsed-dye laser for the treatment of angiofibromas in the setting of tuberous sclerosis.[82]

CONTRAINDICATIONS

There are very few true contraindications for ablative laser resurfacing, relative contraindications should be considered during the patient selection and consenting process. A careful history should be taken with attention to a history of keloids and hypertrophic scars or to a history of conditions that are triggered by the Koebner phenomenon such as vitiligo, psoriasis and lichen planus. Avoiding the most common locations for scarring locations such as chest, neck and facial locations of the upper lip, mandible and the periorbital area or modifying the treatment settings

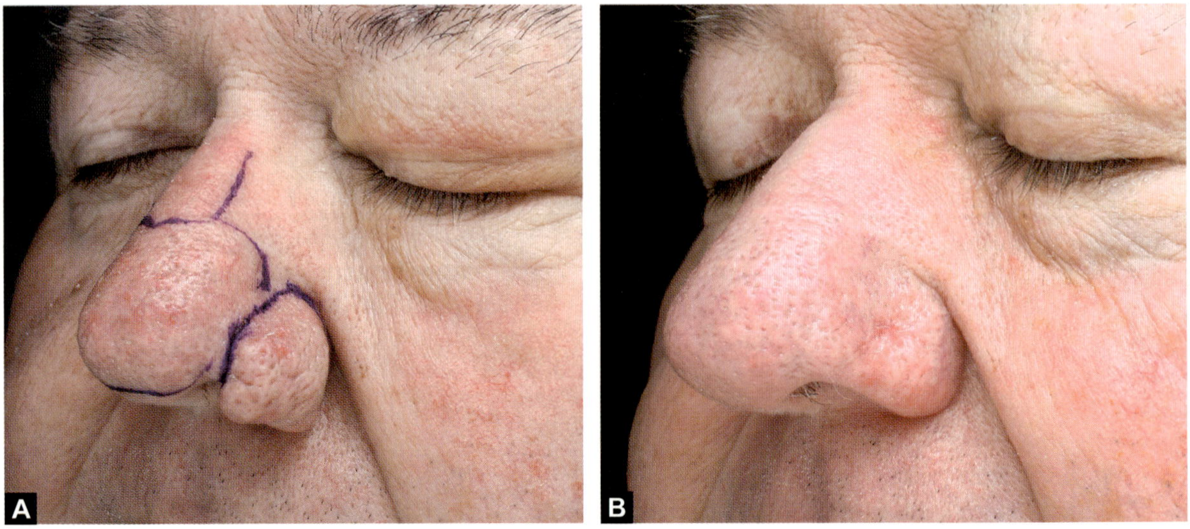

Figs 9.6A and B: Clinical photographs of rhinophyma treated successfully with AFR

in these areas should be considered.[83] Confluent ablative resurfacing is discussed separately in Chapter 7. In addition, a history of oral isotretinoin therapy within the last 6 months is a relative contraindication to any elective surgical procedure with potential impaired wound healing from the retinoid therapy. Darker skinned patients should be counseled on the higher risk of pigment alterations. Pregnancy and exogenous hormone therapies also confer an increased risk of hyperpigmentation and the safety of AFR resurfacing has not been tested in pregnant patients. Therefore, AFR resurfacing, like many elective dermatologic procedures, should be avoided in pregnant patients.

NOVEL APPLICATIONS AND POSSIBILITIES

Combining laser modalities for optimizing the treatment of rhytides and photodamage is an area of ongoing interest. There are published reports of improved outcomes with combining ablative fractional laser resurfacing with other nonablative technologies such as radiofrequency, intense-focused ultrasound, intense pulsed light and nonablative fractional photothermolysis resurfacing. In addition, many creative novel applications utilizing AFR devices to facilitate the introduction of therapeutic agents are being actively researched.

One example is the combination of AFR with PDT-MAL for the treatment of keratosis.[64] Few studies have explored AFR devices in combination with topical applications of wound healing modifiers for the treatment of scars. Lee et al. in 2011 reported a small split-face study comparing a fractional CO_2 laser with saline control to combination of fractional CO_2 laser with platelet-rich plasma (PRP), a wound healing modifier with clinical outcomes of erythema, edema and clinical improvement of acne scars.[84] The authors' conclusions were that the treatment with PRP after ablative CO_2 fractional resurfacing enhances recovery of laser-damaged skin and synergistically improves the clinical appearance of acne scarring.[84] A small split-face study evaluating fractional laser resurfacing with normal saline injection (CO_2 or Er:YAG) versus fractional laser resurfacing in combination with PRP and harvested adult mesenchymal stem cell reinjection intradermally and subcutaneously for the treatment of acne scars. The combination therapy resulted in improved efficacy but had no effect on recovery time.[85] Massaki et al. published a small open study evaluating the combination treatment using an NAFR device in combination with bimatoprost and either topical retinoids or topical calcineurin inhibitors for postprocedural hypopigmented scars.[86] This study resulted in greater than 50% improvement with prolonged results up to mean on 20 months.[86] This is an exciting area of research, as AFR devices uniquely create microchannels for the topical agents to penetrate deeper, thus combination therapy has been theorized to improve absorption and clinical outcomes.

The possibilities are limitless such as the introduction of corticosteroids, wound healing modulators like PRP or stem-cells with AFR for the treatment of scars and contractures.[87,88] Other combination therapies have been proposed such as the introduction of dermal fillers such as poly-L-lactic acid with AFR for facial rejuvenation or the introduction of botulinum toxin with AFR for the treatment of movement-associated rhytides.[89]

CONCLUSION

As a laser-resurfacing practitioner, it is important to engage in careful patient selection and to provide realistic expectations and outcome counseling. Ablative fractional laser resurfacing is an area of continued growth and development in order to maximize clinical outcomes while minimizing complications. There are limited published protocols available and all the AFR devices allow the practitioner great flexibility to personalize the settings. Therefore, a basic understanding of laser physics and the pattern of injury delivered by the ablative resurfacing devices is imperative to provide safer, more effective personalized treatments.

SUMMARY

Indications

The primary indication for ablative fractional laser resurfacing is for the treatment of photodamaged skin; promoting skin tightening, skin textural, pigmentary improvement and reduction in facial rhytides. It is also used for a wide variety of dermatologic indications. Table 9.2 summarizes the indications for ablative fractional resurfacing lasers.

Advantages

Ablative fractional laser resurfacing can lead to long-lasting, clinical outcomes with an improved

Table 9.2: Indications for ablative fractional resurfacing lasers and confluent ablative resurfacing lasers

Published Efficacy for Ablative Fractional Resurfacing Lasers	*Published Efficacy for Confluent Ablative Resurfacing Lasers*
Epidermal dyspigmentation: photoaging, dyschromia, Poilkiloderma of Civatte[9,20,21,23,37-39,40-42,47]	Adnexal tumors
Epidermal tone irregularity: skin laxity/photoaging[17,20,41,47,56]	Dermal lesions: sebaceous hyperplasia, neurofibromas, angiofibromas, rhinophyma, xanthelasma, congenital melanocytic nevi[72-80]
	Dermal dermatoses: Hailey-Hailey, Darier's, hidradenitis suprativa[70,71]
Rhytides[16,20,22 24,29,30,34,43,56]	Epidermal dyspigmentation/photodamage[1,9]
Scars[48,49,51,52,54-56,58,59,61]	Epidermal tone irregularity, skin laxity/photodamage[1,2,3,4,59]
Striae distensae[53,56]	Epidermal lesions: keratoses, actinic cheilitis, superficial basal cell carcinoma, squamous cell carcinoma in situ, verrucae, lentigos, epidermal nevi, *café-au-late* macules, disseminated superficial actinic porokeratosis[36,62,63,68,69]
Angiofibromas[78,81]	Rhytides[1-5,32,33]
Epidermal lesions: keratoses[64]	Scars[50]
	Striae distensae

Table 9.3: Complications and perioperative management of ablative fractional resurfacing lasers[19,25,26,28,29]

Complication or Perioperative Consideration	*Perioperative Management*
Acne, milia	Avoiding occlusive dressings and petrolatum-based products. Treat with topical benzoyl peroxide, retinoids, alpha- or beta-hydroxyacids or oral tetracycline-based antibiotics
Bleeding, purpura	Avoiding antiplatelets and blood thinners, arnica
Edema, Inflammation	Head elevation, arnica
Contact dermatitis	Avoiding products with perfumes, dyes, lanolin and other common allergens. Treat with avoidance, topical steroids and oral antihistamines
Infection	Avoid any concurrently infected areas. Appropriate patient selection with complete history of risk factors: history of refractory infections, immunosuppression, comorbidities with high risk of poor wound healing and infection such as poorly controlled diabetes, smoking, Cushing disease, scleroderma, systemic steroid use. Appropriate prophylactic antimicrobials and antivirals, and treatment antimicrobials as indicated
Postinflammatory hyperpigmentation	Appropriate patient selection and laser settings. Treat with sun protection, bleaching creams, chemical peels and other laser modalities
Isotretinoin use	Delay treatment for 6 months
Pruritus, dermatographism	Cool compresses, oral antihistamines
Pain	Local anesthetics, regional nerve blocks, tumescent anesthesia, epidermal cooling techniques, oral pain medication, oral sedatives, occlusive dressings
Persistent erythema	Coverage make-up
Pregnancy	Delay treatment
Relative hypopigmentation	Fanning, other laser modalities
Risk for Koebner Phenomenon	Appropriate patient selection with complete history of risk factors: history of lichen planus, psoriasis, vitiligo
Scarring, keloids	Appropriate patient selection and laser settings, Treat with silicone dressings, sun protection, other laser modalities

safety profile over traditional confluent ablative laser resurfacing. There is a wide range of available resurfacing devices; all allow great flexibility to personalize the settings.

Disadvantages

Ablative fractional laser resurfacing can produce a significant wound, necessitating longer recovery time, potential adverse outcomes, and both short-term and long-term complications. Table 9.3 highlights the major complications and perioperative management of ablative fractional resurfacing lasers. A basic understanding of the laser physics and the patterns of injury delivered by the ablative fractional resurfacing devices are imperative to provide safer, more effective, personalized treatments.

REFERENCES

1. Fitzpatrick RE, Goldman MP, Satur NM, et al. Pulsed carbon dioxide laser resurfacing of photoaged facial skin. Arch Dermatol. 1996;132:395-402.
2. Alster TS, Garg S. Treatment of facial rhytides with a high energy pulsed carbon dioxide laser. Plast Reconstr Surg. 1996;98:791-4.
3. Hughes PS. Skin contraction following Erbium:YAG laser resurfacing. Dermatol Surg. 1998;24:109-11.
4. Alster TS. Clinical and histologic evaluation of six Erbium:YAG lasers for cutaneous resurfacing. Laser Surg Med. 1999;24;87-92.
5. Zachary CB. Modulating the Er:YAG laser. Lasers Surg Med. 2000; 26(2):223-6.
6. Manstein D, Heron GS, Sink RK, et al. Fractional photothermolysis: a new concept for cutaneous remodeling using microscopic patterns of thermal injury. Lasers Surg Med. 2004;34:426-38.
7. Berlin AL, Hussain M, Goldberg DJ. Cutaneous photoaging treated with a combined 595/1064 nm laser. J Cosmet Laser Ther. 2007;9(4):214-7.
8. Bernstein EF. The new-generation, high-energy, 595-nm, long pulse-duration pulsed-dye laser improves the appearance of photodamaged skin. Lasers Surg Med. 2007;39(2):157-63.
9. Papadavid E, Katsambas A. Lasers for facial rejuvenation: a review. Int J Dermatol. 2003;42(6):480-7.
10. Hardaway CA, Ross EV. Non-ablative laser skin remodeling. Dermatol Clin. 2002;20:97-111.
11. Goldberg DJ. New collagen formation after dermal remodeling with an intense pulsed light source. J Cut Laser Ther. 2000;2(2):59-61.
12. Goldberg DJ, Silapunt S. Histologic evaluation of a Q-switched laser in the nonablative treatment of wrinkles. Dermatol Surg. 2001;27(8):744-6.
13. Goldberg DJ. Non-ablative subsurface remodeling: clinical and histologic evaluation of a 1320-nm Nd:YAG laser. J Cut Laser Ther. 1999;1(3):153-7.
14. Goldberg DJ, Rogachefsky AS, Silaput S. Non-ablative laser treatment of facial rhytides: a comparison of 1450-nm diode laser treatment with dynamic cooling as opposed to treatment with dynamic cooling alone. Lasers Surg Med. 2002;30(2):79-81.
15. Hantash BM, Bedi VP, Kapadia B, et al. In vivo histological evaluation of a novel ablative fractional resurfacing device. Lasers Surg Med. 2007;39: 96-107.
16. Weiss R, Weiss M, Beasley K. Prospective split-face trial of a fixed spacing array computed scanned fractional laser versus hand scanned 1550nm fractional for rhytides. Presented at the American Society for Laser Medicine and Surgery Conference; April 4, 2008; Kissimmee, FL.
17. Rahman Z, MacFalls H, Jiang K, et al. Fractional deep dermal ablation induces tissue tightening. Lasers Surg Med. 2009;41:78-86.
18. Berlin AL, Hussain M, Phelps R, et al. A prospective study of fractional scanned nonsequential carbon dioxide laser resurfacing: a clinical and histopathologic evaluation. Dermatol Surg. 2009;35:222-8.
19. Avram MM, Tope WD, Yu T, et al. Hypertrophic scarring of neck following ablative fractional carbon dioxide laser resurfacing. Lasers Surg Med. 2009:41(3):185-8.
20. Ortiz AE, Tremaine AM, Zachary CB. Long-term efficacy of fractional resurfacing device. Lasers Surg Med. 2010;42(2):168-70.
21. Ciocon DH, Engelman DE, Hussain M, et al. A split-face comparison of two ablative fractional carbon dioxide lasers for the treatment of photodamaged facial skin.Dermatol Surg. 2011:1524.
22. Goldberg D, Ciocon D, Engelman D, et al. Treatment of perioral rhytides with the new fractional ablative ER: YSGG (2790-nm) laser. Presented at the American Society of Laser Medicine and Surgery Conference. April 2010, Phoenix, AZ.
23. Ross EV, Swann M, Soon S, et al. Full-face treatments with the 2790-nm Erbium: YSGG laser system. J Drugs Dermatol. 2009;8(2):248-52.
24. Karsai S, Czamecka A, Junger M, et al. Ablative fractional lasers (CO_2 and Er:YAG): a randomized controlled double-blind split-face trial of treatment of peri-orbital rhytides. Lasers Surg Med. 2010; 42(2):160-7.
25. Biesman N. Fractional ablative skin resurfacing: complications. Lasers Surg Med. 2009;41:177-8.
26. Fife D, Fitzpatrick ER, Zachary CB. Complications of fractional laser resurfacing: four cases. Lasers Surg Med. 2009;41:179-84.
27. Tierney EP, Kouba DJ, Hanke CW. Fractional photothermolysis: review of treatment indications and efficacy. Dermatol Surg. 2009;35:1445-61.

28. Garber EM, Tanzi EL, Alster TS. Side effects and complications of fractional laser photothermolysis: experience with 961 treatments. Dermatol Surg. 2008;34:301-5.
29. Hunzeker CM, Weiss ET, Geronemus RG. Fractionated CO_2 laser resurfacing: our experience with more than 2000 treatments. Aesthet Surg. 2009;29(4):317-22.
30. Tierney EP, Hanke CW, Watkins L. Treatment of lower eyelid rhytides and laxity with ablative fractionated carbon-dioxide laser resurfacing: Case series and review of the literature. J Am Acad Dermatol. 2011;64(4):730-40.
31. Sukal SA, Chapas AM, Bernstein LJ, et al. Eyelid tightening and improved eyelid aperture through nonablative fractional resurfacing. Dermatol Surg. 2008;34:1454-8.
32. Munavalli G. Single pass resurfacing for improvement of lower eyelid rhytides. Abstract presented at American Society for Laser Medicine and Surgery Conference, April 2008, Kissimmee, FL.
33. Brightman L, Chapas A, Hunzeker C, et al. Blepharoplasty-like results with periorbital fractional CO_2 laser. Lasers Surg Med. 2009;21(Suppl):77.
34. Geronemus R. Fractional photothermolysis: current and future applications. Lasers Surg Med. 2006; 38:169-76.
35. West TB, Alster TS. Effect of botulinum toxin type A on movement-associated rhytides following CO_2 resurfacing. Derm Surg. 1999;25:259-61.
36. Fitzpatrick RE, Goldman MP, Ruiz-Esparza J. Clinical advantage of the CO_2 laser superpulsed mode. Treatment of verruca vulgaris, seborrheic keratoses, lentigines, and actinic cheilitis. J Derm Surg Oncol. 1994;20:449-56.
37. Alora MB, Arndt KA. Treatment of café-au-lait macule with erbium:YAG laser. J A, Acad Dermatol. 2001;45:566-8.
38. Polder KD, Landau JM, Vergilis-Kalner IJ, et al. Laser eradication of pigmented lesions: a review. Dermatol Surg. 2011;37(5):572-95.
39. Lapidoth M, YAGima Odo ME, Odo LM. Novel use of erbium:YAG (2,940-nm) laser for fractional ablative photo-thermolysis in the treatment of photodamaged facial skin: a pilot study. Dermatol Surg. 2008;34:1048-53.
40. Tierney EP, Hanke CW. Treatment of Poikiloderma of Civatte and ablative fractional laser resurfacing: prospective study and review of the literature. JDD. 2009;8(6):527-34.
41. Lomeo G, Cassuto D, Scrimali L, et al. Er:YAG versus CO_2 ablative fractional resurfacing: a split face study. Abstract presented at American Society for Laser Medicine and Surgery Conference, April 2008, Kissimmee, FL.
42. Al-Dujaili Z, Hussain M, Goldberg D. Ablative fractional laser resurfacing: split face comparison between CO_2 and Er:YAG lasers. Presented at the American Society for Laser Medicine and Surgery Conference; 2011.
43. Ross V, Swann M, Barnette D. Use of a micro-fractional 2940 nm laser in the treatment of wrinkles and dyspigmentation. Abstract presented at American Society for Laser Medicine and Surgery Conference, April 2008, Kissimmee, FL.
44. Katz TM, Glaich AS, Goldberg LH, et al. Treatment of melasma using fractional photothermolysis: a report of eight cases with long-term follow-up. Dermatol Surg. 2010;36(8):1273-80.
45. Tannous ZS, Astner S. Utilizing fractional resurfacing in the treatment of therapy-resistant melasma. J Cosmet Laser Ther. 2005;5(1):39-43.
46. Polder KD, Bruce S. Treatment of melasma using a novel 1,927-nm fractional thulium fiber laser: a pilot study. Dermatol Surg. 2012: 38(2):199-206.
47. LaTowsky BC, Abbasi N, Dover J, et al. A randomized, controlled trial of four ablative fractionated lasers for photoaging: a quadrant study. Dermatol Surg. 2012;38(9):1477-89.
48. Ortiz A, Elkeeb L, Truitt A, et al. Evaluation of a novel fractional resurfacing device for the treatment of acne scarring. Abstract presented at American Society for Laser Medicine and Surgery Conference, April 2008, Kissimmee, FL.
49. Chapas AM, Brightman L, Sukal S, et al. Successful treatment of acneiform scarring fractional resurfacing. Lasers Surg Med. 2008;40:381-6.
50. Kim S. Clinical trial of a pinpoint irradiation technique with the CO_2 laser for the treatment of atrophic acne scars. J Cosmet Laser Ther. 2008; 29:1-4.
51. Ong MW, Bashir SJ. Fractional laser resurfacing for acne scars: a review. Br J Dermatol. 2012;166;6:1160-9.
52. Alaijan AM, Alsuwaidan SN. Acne scars in ethnic skin treated with non-ablative fractional 1,550 nm and ablative fractional CO_2 lasers: comparative retrospective analysis with recommended guidelines. Lasers Surg Med. 2011:43(8):787-91.
53. Yang YJ, Lee GY. Treatment of striae distensae with nonablative fractional versus ablative CO_2 fractional laser: a randomized controlled trial. Ann Dermatol. 2011;23(4):481-9.
54. Cervelli V, Gentile P, Spallone D, et al. Ultrapulsed fractional CO_2 laser for the treatment of post-traumatic, and pathological scars. J Drugs Dermatol. 2010;9(11):1328-31.
55. Waibel JS, Beer KR. Fractional laser resurfacing for thermal burns. J Drugs Dermatol. 2008;7(1):12-4.
56. Alexiades-Armanaka M, Saranoff D, Gotkin R, et al. Multi-center clinical study and review of fractional ablative CO_2 laser resurfacing for the treatment of rhytides, photoaging, scars and striae. JDD. 2011;10(4):352-62.

57. Apfelberg DB, Varga J, Greenbaum SS. Carbon dioxide laser resurfacing of peri-oral rhytides in scleroderma patients. Dermatol Surg. 1998; 24(5):517-9.
58. Waibel JS, Beer KR. Ablative fractional laser resurfacing for the treatment of a third-degree burn. J Drugs Dermatol. 2009;8(3):294-7.
59. Waibel J, Graber E, Davis S, et al. Effects of erbium fractional resurfacing on third degree burn scars. Presented at the American Society for Laser Medicine and Surgery Conference; 2011.
60. Waibel J, Wulkan AJ, Lupo M, et al. Treatment of burn scars with the 1550-nm nonablative fractional Erbium laser. Lasers Surg Med; 2012.
61. Tanzi EL, Alster TS. Laser treatment of scars. Skin Therapy Lett. 2004;9(1):4-7.
62. Callen JP, Bickers DR, Moy RA. Actinic keratoses. J Am Acad Dermatol. 1997;36:650-3.
63. Laws RA, Wilde JL, Grabski WJ. Comparison of electrodessication with CO_2 laser for the treatment of actinic cheilitis. Dermatol Surg. 2000; 26(4):349-53.
64. Togsverd-Bo K, Haak CS, Thaysen-Petersen D, et al. Intensified photodynamic therapy of actinic keratoses with fractional CO_2 laser: a randomized clinical trial. Br J Dermatol. 2012;166(6):1262-9.
65. Lauchli S, Kempf W, Dragieva G, et al. CO_2 laser treatment of warts in immunosuppressed patients. Dermatology. 2003;206:148-52.
66. Katz TK, Goldberg LH, Friedman PM. Dermatosis papulosa nigra treatment with fractional photothermolysis. Dermatol Surg. 2009;35:1840-3.
67. Polder KD, Landau JM, Vergilis-Kalner IJ, et al. Laser eradication of pigmented lesions: a review. Dermatol Surg. 2011;37(5):572-95.
68. Geronemus RG, Kauvar AN, McDaniel DH. Treatment of recalcitrant verrucae with both the ultrapulse CO_2 and PLDL pulsed dye lasers. Plast Reconstr. 1998;101:2010.
69. Boyce S, Alster TS. CO_2 laser treatment of epidermal nevi: long-term success. Dermatol Surg. 2002;28: 611-4.
70. Beier C, Kaufmann R. Efficacy of erbium:YAG laser ablation in Darier disease and Hailey-Hailey disease. Arch Dermatol. 1999;135(4):423-7.
71. Madan V, Hindle E, Hussain W, et al. Outcomes of treatment of nine cases of recalcitrant severe hidradenitis suppurativa with carbon dioxide laser. Br J Dermatol. 2008;159(6):1309-14.
72. Nerad JA, Anderson RL. CO_2 laser treatment of eyelid syringomas. Ophthal Plast Reconstr Surg. 1988;4:91-4.
73. Alster TS, West TB.Ultrapulse CO_2 laser ablation of xanthelasma. J Am Acad Dermatol. 1996;34:848-9.
74. Magid M, Garden JM. Pearly penile papules: treatment with carbon dioxide laser. J Dermatol Surg Oncol. 1989;15(5):552-4.
75. Goon PK, Dalal M, Peart FC. The gold standard for decortication of rhinophyma: Combined erbium:YAG/ CO_2 laser. Aesthetic Plast Surg. 2004; 28:456-60.
76. Greenbauns SS, Krull EA, Watrick K. Comparison of laser and electrosurgery in the treatment of rhinophyma. J Am Acad Dermatol. 1998;18:363-8.
77. Madan V, Ferguson JE, August PJ. Carbon dioxide laser treatment of rhinophyma: a review of 124 patients. Br J Dermatol. 2009;16(4):814-8.
78. Verma KK, Ovung EM, Sirka CS. Extensive facial angiofibromas in tuberous sclerosis treated with carbon dioxide laserbrasion. Dermatol Surg. 2001; 67:326-8.
79. Ostertag JU, Theunissen CC, Neumann HA. Hypertrophic scars after therapy with CO_2 laser for the treatment of multiple cutaneous neurofibromas. Dermatol Surg. 2002;28:296-8.
80. Horner BM, El-Muttradi NS, Mayo BJ. Treatment of congenital melanocytic nevis with laser. Ann Plast Surg. 2005;55:276-80.
81. Singh S, Peterson JD, Friedman PM. Management of mild to moderate rhinophyma using ablative fractional photothermolysis. Dermatol Surg. 2013;39(7):1110-3.
82. Weiss ET, Geronemus RG. New technique using combined pulsed dye laser and fractional resurfacing for treating facial angiofibromas in tuberous sclerosis. Lasers Surg Med. 2010;42(5):357-60.
83. Nanni CA, Alster TS. Complications of carbon dioxide laser resurfacing: an evaluation of 500 patients. Dermatol Surg. 1998;24:315-20.
84. Lee JW, Kim BJ, Kim MN, et al. The efficacy of autologous platelet rich plasma combined with ablative carbon dioxide fractional resurfacing for acne scars: a simultaneous split-face trial. Dermatol Surg. 2011;37(7):931-8.
85. Bowen R. Cell assisted laser resurfacing for treatment of acne scars. Presented at the American Society for Laser Medicine and Surgery Conference; 2011.
86. Massaki ABMN, Fabi SG, Fitzpatrick R. Repigmentation of hypopigmented scars using an erbium-doped 1,550-nm fractionated laser and topical bimatoprost. Dermatol Surg. 2012;38:995-1001.
87. Waibel JS, Wulkan AJ, Shumaker PR. Treatment of hypertrophic scars using laser and laser assisted corticosteroid delivery. Lasers Surg Med. 2013;45(3):135-40.
88. Bloom BS, Brauer JA, Geronemus RG. Ablative fractional resurfacing in topical drug delivery: an update and outlook. Dermatol Surg. 2013;39(6):839-48.
89. Waibel J, Wulkan A, Kent K. Treatment of atrophic scars using laser and laser assisted poly-l-lactic acid. Lasers Surg Med. 2013;45(S25):15.

CHAPTER 10

Photodynamic Therapy

Jennifer Peterson, Ane Massaki, Mitchel P Goldman

INTRODUCTION

Aminolevulinic acid (ALA) was the first photosensitizer prodrug to be US Food and Drug Administration (FDA) approved for use in topical photodynamic therapy (PDT). Since its approval over a decade ago, many aspects of ALA-PDT have been examined. Studies investigating the treatment of nonhyperkeratotic actinic keratoses (AKs) with ALA-PDT have led to advances in treatment. Incubation times of ALA have decreased, multiple light sources have been used to elicit the reaction, and cosmetic benefits of treatment have been discovered. In the discussion that follows, background on ALA-PDT is provided. In addition, clinical studies regarding the treatment of AKs, nonmelanoma skin cancer (NMSC), acne and photorejuvenation are summarized. Finally, a practical guide for treatment is provided for the reader to optimize treatment while avoiding common pitfalls of treatment.

HISTORY

In 1990, Kennedy and colleagues[1] introduced the first topical porphyrin derivative, known as 5- δ-ALA, which is a natural precursor of protoporphyrin IX (PpIX) in the heme pathway. Therefore, ALA is the prodrug photosensitizing agent with the ability to penetrate the stratum corneum of the skin and be absorbed by actinically damaged skin cells as well as pilosebaceous units whereas PpIX is the photosensitizer. Exogenous ALA-forming PpIX is rapidly cleared from the body, reducing the potential for phototoxicity to days instead of several months.

Later, lipophilic ALA ester derivatives, including methyl aminolevulinate (MAL), were developed, showing stronger porphyrin fluorescence and better tumor selectivity, most likely because of better penetration through cellular membranes compared with the hydrophilic ALA.[2]

MECHANISM OF PHOTODYNAMIC THERAPY

Photodynamic Therapy Mechanism of Action

Porphyrins exhibit a maximum absorption in the Soret band (360–400 nm) followed by 4 smaller peaks between 500 nm and 635 nm (Q bands)[3] (Fig. 10.1).

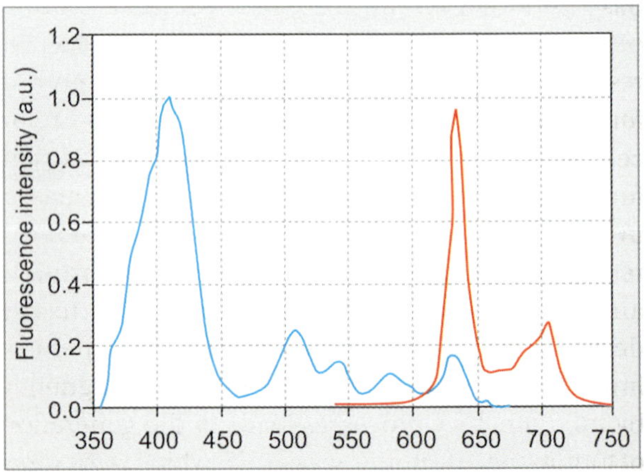

Fig. 10.1: Porphyrin absorption curve displays maximum absorption in the Soret band (360–400 nm) followed by four smaller peaks between 500 nm and 635 nm (Q bands)

PDT involves the activation of a photosensitizer by light in the presence of an oxygen-rich environment. Topical PDT involves the application of ALA or MAL to the skin for varying periods of time. This leads to the conversion of ALA to PpIX, an endogenous photoactivating agent. PpIX accumulates in rapidly proliferating cells of premalignant and malignant lesions,[4] as well as in melanin, blood vessels and sebaceous glands.[5] Upon activation by a light source and in the presence of oxygen, the sensitizer (PpIX) is oxidized, a process called "photobleaching".[6] During this process, free radical oxygen singlets are generated, leading to selective destruction of tumor cells by apoptosis without collateral damage to surrounding tissues.[7,8] Selective destruction of malignant cells is due in part to their reduced ferrochelatase activity, leading to excessive accumulation of intracellular PpIX.[9] Recent in vitro research suggests that any remaining malignant cells following PDT have reduced survival.[10]

Although the precise mechanisms (at a cellular level) underlying the efficacy of topical PDT in the treatment of NMSC are not fully known, both apoptosis[11,12] and necrosis[13,14] have been described, with their respective importance being related to intracellular localization of the photosensitizer and illumination parameters. In addition to direct damage of neoplastic cells, vascular injury plays an important role for the tumor destruction,[15-17] particularly with systemic photosensitizers. Oxygen radicals produced during the photodynamic process decrease the barrier function of endothelial cells, exposing the vascular basement membrane that leads to the activation of platelets and polymorphonuclear leukocytes,[18,19] resulting in arteriolar vessel constriction, thrombus formation, blood flow stasis causing indirect tumor cell kill.[15,16] In addition, the impairment of vascular functions activates acute phase proteins (proteinases, peroxidases, complement factors and cytokines) resulting in massive accumulation of neutrophils and macrophages[20,21] that will contribute to the destruction of tumor tissue. The establishment of immune response against the treated malignancy by inflammatory processes leads to the generation of tumor-specific immune cells,[22,23] which represents a unique feature of PDT and a major advantage over conventional anticancer therapy.[22]

Topical Photosensitizers: Aminolevulinic Acid and Methyl Aminolevulinate

δ-5-aminolevulinic acid is a hydrophilic, low-molecular weight molecule within the heme biosynthesis pathway.[4,24] As mentioned above, ALA is considered a prodrug.[25] In vivo, it is converted to PpIX, a photosensitizer in the PDT reaction. In the United States, ALA is available as a 20% topical solution manufactured under the name Levulan Kerastick (DUSA Pharmaceuticals, Inc, Wilmington, MA). FDA approved since 1999, Levulan is approved for the treatment of nonhyperkeratotic AKs on the face and scalp in conjunction with a blue light source, such as the Blu-U (DUSA Pharmaceuticals, Inc, Wilmington, MA).[26] It is supplied as a cardboard tube housing two sealed glass ampules, one containing 354 mg of δ-ALA hydrochloride powder and the other 1.5 ml of solvent.[9] These separate components are mixed within the cardboard sleeve just prior to use.

Esters of ALA (methyl ester methyl aminolevulinate or MAL) are lipophilic derivatives of the parent molecule. Their chemical structure provides increased lipophilicity, allowing superior penetration through cellular lipid bilayers compared to ALA.[5,27] MAL is available as a 16.8% cream in a 2 g tube and is produced under the name of Metvixia™ (Galderma Laboratories, Ft. Worth, TX). The cream vehicle contains peanut and almond oils and should, therefore, not be used in patients with a history of allergic reaction to either of these nuts. Since 2004, Metvixia™ and the CureLight Broadband (Model CureLight 01) were FDA approved for the treatment of nonhyperkeratotic AKs of the face and scalp in immunocompetent patients. More recently in June 2008, Metvixia™ can be used in conjunction with the Aktilite CL128 lamp (Galderma Laboratories, Ft. Worth, TX) as well. MAL may offer better tumor selectivity[2,27-29] and less pain[2,30,31] during PDT with less patient discomfort[31] compared to ALA.

Light Irradiation

No standardized guidelines for the "optimal irradiance, wavelength and total dose characteristics for PDT" exist according to the British Dermatology group and the American Society of Photodynamic Therapy Board.[25,32,33] However, certain laser and light sources are predictably chosen for PDT activation. Their wavelengths correspond closely with the four absorption peaks along the porphyrin curve. The Soret band (400–410 nm), with a maximal absorption at 405–409 nm, is the highest peak along this curve for photoactivating PpIX. Smaller peaks designated as the "Q bands" exist at approximately 505–510 nm, 540–545 nm, 580–584 nm and 630–635 nm.[4,5,24] There are advantages and disadvantages to exploiting the wavebands in either the Soret band or Q band for PDT. The Soret band peak is 10–20 fold larger than the Q bands, and blue light sources are often used to activate PpIX within this portion of the porphyrin curve, targeting lesions up to 2 mm in depth.[2] Longer wavelengths found within the Q bands produce a red light that penetrates more deeply (5 mm into the skin), but necessitates higher energy requirements.[4,24]

Light Sources

Light sources utilized in PDT can be categorized in a variety of ways, including incoherent versus coherent sources, or by color (and wavelengths) emitted. Incoherent light is emitted as noncollimated light and is provided through broadband lamps, light emitting diodes (LEDs) and intense pulsed light (IPL) systems. Incoherent light sources are easy to use, affordable, easily obtained and portable due to their compact size.[34] The earliest uses in PDT were filtered slide projectors that emitted white light.[4] Metal halogen lamps such as the Curelight (Photocure, Oslo, Norway, 570–680 nm) are often employed in PDT as they provide an effective light source in a time, power and cost-effective manner.[4,35] The only widely available fluorescent lamp used in conjunction with PDT is the Blu-U (DUSA Pharmaceuticals, Inc, Wilmington, MA) with a peak emittance at 417 ± 5 nm. LEDs provide a narrower spectrum of light irradiation, usually in a 20–50 nm bandwidth via a compact, solid but powerful semiconductor.[4,36] LEDs are simple to operate and are typically small in size, emitting light from the ultraviolet (UV) to infrared (IR) portion of the electromagnetic spectrum. However, the diminutive size of most LED panels necessitates multiple rounds of light illumination to treat larger areas. IPL is yet another source of incoherent light, emitting a radiation spectrum from approximately 500 nm to 1,200 nm.[36] Cutoff filters allow customization of the delivered wavelengths. This light source is particularly useful in photorejuvenation, targeting pigment, blood vessels and even collagen.

Lasers provide precise doses of light radiation. As a collimated light source, lasers deliver energy to target tissues at specific wavelengths chosen to mimic absorption peaks along the porphyrin curve. Lasers used in PDT include the tunable argon dye laser (blue-green light, 450–530 nm),[28] the copper vapor laser-pumped dye laser (510–578 nm), long-pulse pulsed dye lasers (585–595 nm), the Nd:YAG KTP dye laser (532 nm), the gold vapor laser (628 nm) and solid-state diode lasers (630 nm).[35] Although laser sources allow the physician to delivery light with exact specifications in terms of wavelength and fluence, the fluence rate should be kept in the range of 150–200 mW/cm^2 to avoid hyperthermic effects on tissue.[2,4] In fact, there is evidence to support cumulative light doses of greater than 40 J/cm^2 can deplete all available oxygen sources during the oxidation reaction, making higher doses of energy during PDT unnecessary.[6]

CLINICAL APPLICATIONS IN GENERAL DERMATOLOGY

Actinic Keratoses

Background

Actinic keratoses are a premalignant skin condition, comprising 14% of all dermatology office visits.[37,38] The concern for untreated AKs is their rate of transformation to cutaneous squamous cell carcinoma (SCC). The reported conversion rate of AK to SCC varies widely, estimated as 0.025–16% per lesion per year.[39-43] A small percentage of SCC metastasizes[44] and this is more likely in higher-risk areas, such as mucous membranes (e.g. lips).[45] It has been suggested that the AK/SCC continuum be graded as "cutaneous intraepithelial neoplasia", in a manner analogous to cervical malignancy. Both lesions express tumor markers including the tumor suppressor gene *p53*[46] and over 90% of biopsied SCCs have adjacent AKs within the examined histopathologic field.[47]

Treatment Options for Actinic Keratoses

Given the premalignant potential of AKs, and the metastatic potential of SCC, early treatment is paramount to preventing disease progression. Treatment options for AKs depend on a variety of factors including severity of involvement, duration or persistence of lesions, patient tolerability or desire for cosmesis, affordability/insurance coverage and physician comfort with available treatment modalities.[38,43]

While solitary or few lesions may be approached with local, surgical treatments such as cryotherapy, curettage, excision or dermabrasion, field treatment may be more appropriate when numerous lesions are identified. In addition, field therapy will simultaneously treat subclinical AKs. Chemical peels, laser resurfacing, 5-fluorouracil (5-FU), topical diclofenac, topical retinoids and topical immunomodulators (imiquimod) are all reasonable treatment options in addition to PDT.

A comparison of PDT to other field treatment options for AKs yields comparable clearance rates.[48,49] In fact, a comparison of 100% clearance rates from phase III clinical trials reported complete AK clearance with ALA-PDT of 72%, comparable to 5-FU (72%), and superior to imiquimod (49%) and diclofenac (48%).[50] A direct comparison study by Kurwa and coworkers[51] found comparable lesion area reduction rates between ALA-PDT (73%) and 5-FU (70%).

Advantages/Disadvantages of Aminolevulinic Acid-Photodynamic Therapy for Actinic Keratoses

Clearance rates of AKs following PDT has ranged from 68% to 98%.[52,53] Assuming near equivalent or even superior clearance rates of PDT compared to other field treatment options, PDT has several advantages in the treatment of AKs. Improvement of photodamage, superior cosmesis and better patient satisfaction were documented in two studies by Szeimies et al. and Goldman and Atkin.[49,53] Other procedures used for the clearance of AKs, such as cryotherapy or chemical peels, can result in hypopigmentation or even scarring.[49,54] PDT, perhaps surprisingly to some, is a cost-effective means of treating AKs. Gold found ALA-PDT with a blue light source to be the least expensive treatment option for AKs compared to 5-FU, imiquimod and diclofenac. In fact, ALA-PDT was approximately one-half the cost of a similar course of imiquimod for field AK treatment.[50]

Disadvantages of PDT are largely related to minor and expected adverse events following the procedure. Minor pain and erythema may occur during or following the procedure. Mild crusting and edema may occur, lasting up to one week. However, other treatment modalities for AKs have similar if not longer recovery periods. There are financial costs associated with the procedure. If PDT is performed for AK treatment and photorejuvenation, there is an associated out-of-pocket cost to the patient. The physician must also make an initial investment in the laser and light devices, although many of the light sources have multiple applications beyond PDT.

Treatment Results of Aminolevulinic Acid-Photodynamic Therapy for Actinic Keratoses

A variety of light sources have been investigated for use in PDT for the treatment of AKs. As the PDT reaction is activated from an emission spectra ranging from 400 nm to 800 nm,[55] the authors have organized clinical studies according to the light source utilized. Table 10.1 provides a summary of peer-reviewed articles on the use of ALA-PDT and MAL-PDT in AK treatment.

Table 10.1: Published clinical studies on aminolevulinic acid and methyl aminolevulinate-photodynamic therapy for actinic keratoses

Reference	*ALA Preparation*	*Location of AKs*	*Incubation Period (Hours)*	*No. of Lesions Treated (No. of Patients)*	*Light Source (Wavelength in nm)*	*Response Rate*	*Follow-up (Months)*
Kennedy[1] (1990	20% emulsion	Not specified	3–6	10	Tungsten (> 600)	90% CR	18
Wolf[8] (1993)	20% emulsion	Face and scalp	4–8	9	Tungsten, unfiltered	100% CR	3–12
Calzavara-Pinton[4] (1995)	20% cream	Face	6–8	50 (from pool of 85 patients with AKs, BCCs, SCCs, Bowen's)	Argon dye laser (630)	100% CR	24–36

Contd...

Contd...

Morton[56] (1995)	20% emulsion	Face and scalp	4	4	Xenon (630)	100% CR	12
Fijan[57] (1995)	20% emulsion	Not specified	20, occluded	43 (9)	Halogen (570–690)	81% CR	3–20
Szeimies[58] (1996)	10% emulsion	Head, hands, arms	6, occluded	36 (10)	Waldmann red lamp (580–740)	71% CR head	1
Fink-Puches[59] (1997)	20% emulsion	Head, neck, forearms, dorsal hands	4, occluded	251 (28)	Halogen slide projector (300–800) with cutoff filters at 515, 530, 570, 610	71% CR	36
Fritsch[60] (1997)	10% ointment	Face and scalp	6, occluded	(6)	Green lamp (543–548) vs red Waldmann lamp (570–750)	100% CR for both green and red light	15
Jeffes et al.[61] (1997)	0–30% emulsion	Face, scalp, trunk, extremities	3, occluded	240 (40)	Argon dye laser (630)	91% CR face and scalp; 45% CR trunk and extremities	2
Karrer et al.[62] (1999)	20% emulsion	Scalp, face	6, occluded	200 (24)	Red light lamp (580–740) or PDL (585)	84% CR (red light); 79% CR (PDL)	1
Kurwa et al.[51] (1999)	20% emulsion	Hands	4, occluded	(14)	Metal halide lamp (580–740)	73% lesion area reduction; comparable to 5-FU	6
Itoh[63] (2000)	20% emulsion, 2 or more sessions	Face, neck, extremities	4, occluded	53 (10)	Red lamp (peak 630, range 600–700), excimer dye laser (630)	82% CR face and neck; 56% CR extremities	12
Dijkstra[55] (2001)	20% gel, 2 sessions	Unspecified	8, occluded	4	Violet lamp (400–450)	50% CR	3–12
Jeffes[48] (2001)	20% solution	Face, scalp	14–18	70 (36)	Blue light (417)	85% CR	4
Markham[37] (2001)	% concentration unspecified, cream	Scalp	4, occluded	(4)	Red light (580–740)	75% CR	6
Varma[64] (2001)	20% ointment	Not specified	4, occluded	127 (88 patients with mixed diagnoses)	Waldmann red lamp (580–740)	77% CR after 1st, 99% after 2nd, RR of 28%	6

Contd...

Contd...

Ruiz-Rodriguez[65] (2002)	20% emulsion	Face, scalp	4, occluded	38	IPL (590–1200)	76% CR 1 session; 91% CR 2 sessions	3
Alexiades-Armenakas[54] (2003)	20% solution	Head, extremities, trunk	3 with occlusion; 14–18 without occlusion	3622 (36)	Long-pulsed PDL (595)	90–100% CR	8
Clark[35] (2003)	20% ointment	Not specified	4	23	Metal halide (590–730); Halogen lamp (570–680), diode laser (630)	91% CR	11
Goldman[53] (2003)	20% solution	Face, long-incubation PDT	15–20	(32)	Blue light (417)	94% CR of AKs; improved skin texture, pigmentation	3–6
Smith[66] (2003)	20% solution, 2 sessions	Face, scalp	1	(35)	Blue light (417) or PDL (595)	80% CR for blue light; 60% CR for PDL	1
Dragieva[67] (2004)	20% emulsion; transplant patients	Face, scalp	5, occluded	32 (20)	Red light (580–740)	94% CR at 4 weeks; 72% at 48 weeks	12
Piacquadio[68] (2004)	20% solution, 1–2 sessions	Face, scalp	14–18	1402 (243)	Blue (417)	91% CR 1 session; 83% CR 2 sessions	3
Touma[9] (2004)	20% solution	Face	1–3	(17)	Blue lamp (417)	87–94% CR	5
Gilbert[69] (2005)	20% solution, 5-FU daily × 5 days pre-PDT	Face	0.5–0.75	(15)	IPL (560–1,200)	90% CR with combination therapy	12
Kim[70] (2005)	20% emulsion	Face	4, occluded	12 (7)	IPL (555–950)	50%	3
Tschen[71] (2006)	20% solution, (1–2 treatment sessions)	Face, scalp	14–18	968 (110)	Blue (417)	72–76% CR 1 session; 86% 2 sessions	12
Nakano[33] (2009)	20% cream (3 treatment sessions)	Face	4, occluded	(30)	Excimer dye laser (630 nm)	100% CR in lesions < 10 mm; 70% CR in lesions > 10 mm diameter	12

Contd...

Contd...

MAL	*Study*	*Location*	*Incubation Period (Hours)*	*No. of Lesions Treated (No. of Patients)*	*Light Source (Wavelength in nm)*	*Response Rate*	*Follow-up (Months)*
Szeimies[49] (2002)	1× MAL-PDT vs 2× freeze-thaw cryotherapy	Face, scalp, other	3, occluded	699 AK (367 treated by MAL-PDT) in 193 patients	Noncoherent red light (570–670 nm), total light dose of 75 J/cm^2 and a light intensity of 70–200 mW/cm^2	MAL-PDT—69% and cryo-therapy—75%	3
Freeman[72] (2003)	2× MAL-PDT vs 2× placebo-PDT vs 1 freeze cycle cryotherapy	Face and scalp	3, occluded	763 AK in 200 patients (295 treated by MAL-PDT)	Red light (570–670 nm) and a total light dose of 75 J/cm^2, light intensity of 50–250 mW/cm^2	MAL-PDT—91%, placebo-PDT 30% and cryotherapy 68%	3
Pariser[73] (2003)	2× MAL-PDT vs 2× placebo-PDT	Face and scalp	3, occluded	502 AK (260 treated with MAL-PDT) in 80 patients	Noncoherent red light (wavelength 570–670 nm, light dose of 75 J/cm^2, light intensity of 50–200 mW/cm^2	MAL-PDT—89%, placebo-PDT 38%	3
Dragieva[74] (2004)	MAL-PDT in transplant patients, 2× MAL-PDT vs 2× placebo-PDT	Face, scalp, neck and extremities	3, occluded	34 lesional areas comprising 129 AK (17 areas with 62 AK treated with MAL-PDT) in 17 OTR patients	Noncoherent light source (600–730 nm), light dose of 75 J/cm^2, light intensity of 80 mW/cm^2	94% CR at 4 weeks; 72% at 48 weeks	MAL-PDT in trans-plant patients, 2× MAL-PDT vs 2× placebo-PDT
Tarstedt[75] (2005)	Compari-son: 1× MAL-PDT repeated if necessary at 3 months vs 2× MAL-PDT	Face and scalp	3, occluded	400 AK in 211 patients	Red LED light source (634 ± 3 nm, 37 J/cm^2, 50 mW/cm^2)	1× MAL-PDT repeated if necessary-92% (81% after first treatment) vs 2× MAL-PDT—87%	3 after last treatment

Contd...

Contd...

Morton[76] (2006)	1× MAL-PDT vs cryotherapy (2 freeze cycle), repeat at 12 week, if required	Face and scalp	3, occluded	1,505 AK in 119 patients	Red LED light source (634 ± 3 nm, 37 J/cm², 50 mW/cm²)	MAL-PDT—89% (84% after one treatment) vs	3 after last treatment
Perrett[77] (2007)	MAL-PDT in transplant patients, 2× MAL-PDT vs topical 5-FU twice daily for 3 weeks	Head, trunk and extremities	3, occluded	18 lesional areas were treated (10 carcinoma in situ and 8 AK) in 8 OTR patients	Noncoherent red light source (633 ± 15 nm light dose of 75 J/cm², light intensity of 80 mW/cm²	8 of 9 lesional areas (89%) cleared with MAL-PDT vs 1 of 9 lesional areas (11%) cleared with 5-FU	6
Kauffman[78] (2008)	1× MAL-PDT vs 2× freeze-thaw cryo-therapy, repeat at 12 week, if required	Extremities (98%), trunk and neck	3, occluded	1,343 AK in 121 patients (691 treated with MAL-PDT)	Red LED light source (634 ± 3 nm, 37 J/cm², 50 mW/cm²)	MAL-PDT—78% vs	6
Palm[79] (2011)	MAL blue light vs red light	Face, scalp, chest, and back	1	(18)	PDL (7 mm, 10–12 J/cm², 40 ms) ± IPL, + Blue light (407 nm, 10 J/cm², 16 min, 40 sec) vs Red LED light (630 nm, 37 J/cm², 8 min, 49 sec)	No difference in improvement in AKs, wrinkles,	1

5-FU: 5-fluorouracil; AKs: Actinic keratoses; ALA: 5-aminolevulinic acid; BCCs: Basal cell carcinomas; CR: Complete response; IPL: Intense pulsed light; LED: Light emitting diodes; MAL: Methyl aminolevulinate; OTR: Solid organ transplant recipients; PDL: Pulsed-dye laser; PDT: Photodynamic therapy; RR: Relative risk; SCCs: Squamous cell carcinomas; SGH: Sebaceous gland hyperplasia

Blue Light

Perhaps the most popular emission spectrum utilized in the United States, blue light was the first FDA-approved form of light for activating ALA (Fig. 10.2). As a result, numerous published studies exist on the use of blue light in ALA-PDT not only for the treatment of AKs, but also for other skin conditions responsive to this treatment modality. As the relatively shorter wavelength of blue light only penetrates 1–2 mm, but is potent in its photochemical effect, blue light is often selected for the treatment of superficial lesions such as nonhyperkeratotic AK lesions.[80]

In 2001, Jeffes et al.[48] reported the usage of ALA-PDT with a 14–18 hour incubation using blue light (417 nm) to AKs of the face and scalp in 36 patients. Light exposure duration was 16 minutes and 40 seconds, now considered standard of treatment. At

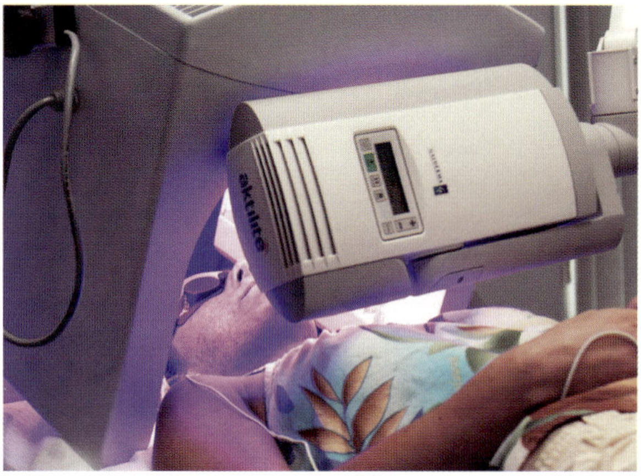

Fig. 10.2: Noncoherent blue lamp is a common choice for photoactivating 5-aminolevulinic acid in the United States. The Blu-U (DUSA Pharmaceuticals, Inc, Wilmington, MA) emits light at a bandwidth of approximately 417 ± 5 nm. Red light (Aktilite; Galderma Laboratories, Ft. Worth, TX) emits light at a bandwidth of approximately 630 ± 40 nm and is US Food and Drug Administration approved for activation of Metvixia. During our illumination, we simultaneously deliver blue and red light. The patient is placed directly under the blue light with the red light placed at the outlet of the blue light

8 weeks following a single treatment, 88% of lesions cleared. A similarly designed study with 64 patients[81] displayed 75% or more clearance of AK lesions following one treatment. However, 14% of patients required reduced power density during blue light irradiation due to intolerable side effects including stinging and burning.

Piacquadio and coworkers[68] followed in 2004, with a similarly designed protocol in 243 patients with nonhyperkeratotic AKs. Complete clearance at 12 weeks following one PDT session was 70%. A second treatment resulted in a complete clearance rate of 88%. Facial lesions responded more favorably than scalp lesions, with complete response rates of 78% and 50% respectively, at week 12 following treatment. In terms of patient feedback, 94% of patients rated their cosmetic outcome following PDT as good or excellent. A recurrence rate analysis for this treatment cohort between 8 weeks and 12 weeks posttreatment was 5%.[81]

Multiple studies have demonstrated a reduction in AKs in addition to photorejuvenative effects on the treated areas of the skin.[53,81] In 2004, Touma et al.[9] reported on the efficacy of short-contact ALA-PDT. Not only did this allow for PDT to be conducted in a single clinic visit rather than over 2 days, but side effects related to the longer 14–18 hour incubations were reduced. A clearance rate of 93%, 84% and 90% were achieved in the 1-, 2- and 3-hour incubation groups respectively. Clearance rates were maintained through 5 months of follow-up. In addition, the subjects in this study also showed a modest, but significant improvement in photoaging.

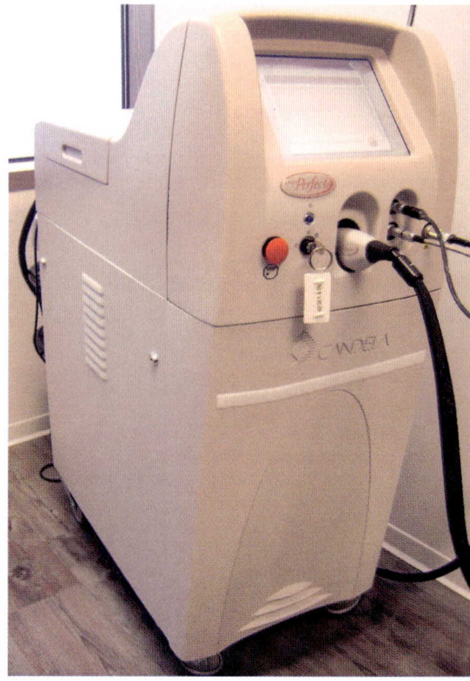

Fig. 10.3: Pulsed-dye lasers may be used as a light source for aminolevulinic acid-photodynamic therapy to target individual lesions including actinic keratoses, sebaceous hyperplasia and solar lentigines. Image of Vbeam Perfecta (595 nm) laser

Green Light

One study by Fritsch and coworkers[60] used a green light source for the treatment of AKs with ALA-PDT concluded green light (543–548 nm) was less painful than red light in the treatment of facial AKs during PDT.

Yellow-Orange Light: Pulsed-Dye Laser

Long-pulsed pulsed-dye lasers (585–595 nm) (Fig. 10.3) target the chromophore oxyhemoglobin, allowing selective destruction of blood vessels. As AKs often appear as erythematous scaly plaques, the inflammatory nature of these lesions can be targeted with this vascular laser. Alexiades-Armenakas and coworkers[54] were the first to report on its use in ALA-PDT. Thirty-six patients and a total of 3,622 lesions (face and scalp = 2,620, extremities = 949 and trunk = 53) were treated. ALA was applied with either a 3 hour, unoccluded incubation versus a 14- to 18-hour incubation. No difference in clearance was observed between the two incubation time groups. Clearance rates were highest for head lesions at 100%. According to this large cohort study, it appeared that PDL (pulsed-dye laser) at subpurpuric doses allows an efficient and less painful means of accomplishing PDT.

In 2003, Smith and coworkers[66] found AK clearance rates were similar with topical 5-FU and ALA-PDL (79% vs 80%), but clearance rates of PDT using a blue light source were lower (60%). Additionally, improvements in global photodamage, hyperpigmentation and tactile roughness were also observed.

Red Light Sources

The longer wavelength of red light allows deeper tissue penetration, up to 5 mm. Red light is used frequently during PDT with MAL (see Fig. 10.2). Red light may also be used for photoactivation of PpIX during ALA-PDT. Several laser and light sources emit wavelengths in the red light spectrum, usually targeted around 630 nm. These include the argon pumped dye laser, excimer laser, metal halide lamps and red LED lamps.

Several studies have reported clearance rates of facial AKs between 71% and 99%. Kurwa et al.[51] used a metal halide lamp for ALA-PDT to treat the dorsal hands, resulting in a 79.5% decrease in AKs lesions. Itoh and coworkers[63] treated Japanese patients with AKs on the face, neck and extremities. With two or more treatments, clearance rates at 12 months were higher for lesions on the head and neck (81.8%) compared to the extremities (55.6%). One possible explanation for an increased resistance of AK of the extremities would be the lack of pilosebaceous units in these areas, which are important to a better absorption of prodrug and so, to a better response. No serious adverse effects were reported in these patients with darker skin types. These studies mirror the results of other reports of decreased AK clearance rates in nonfacial and nonscalp sites. Research by Varma et al.[64] found complete clearance rates for AKs after one and two treatments were 77% and 99% respectively. However, the recurrence rate at 12 months was 28%. Moseley and coworkers[82] demonstrated a 92% AK clearance rate after two treatments, with 100% clearance after three ALA-PDT sessions.

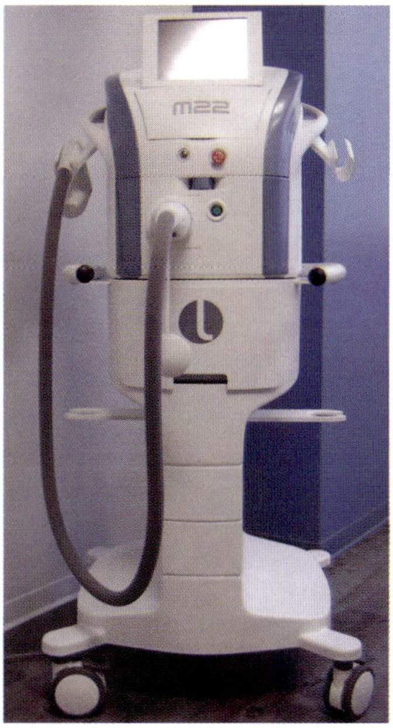

Fig. 10.4: Intense pulsed light devices are particularly effective in aminolevulinic acid-photodynamic therapy for photorejuvenation. Cooled conductive gel and forced air cooling units minimize discomfort during treatment. Image of Lumenis M22 System Intense pulsed light

Intense Pulsed Light

Intense pulsed light devices (Fig. 10.4) emit noncollimated, noncoherent light with wavelengths in the range of 515–1,200 nm, which corresponds to the visible light and near-infrared spectrum.[36] Various filters can be used to block certain wavelengths below the cut-off point of the desired filter. A small study by Kim et al.[70] documented the use of ALA-IPL for the treatment of AKs exclusively. Twelve facial AK lesions in seven patients treated with a single session of ALA-PDT showed a 50% clearance rate at 12 weeks follow-up. This clearance rate is markedly lower than reported averages, but it is difficult to formulate sound conclusions based on the small sample size. Further studies evaluating the simultaneous improvement of AKs and photorejuvenation are discussed below.

Treatment Results of Methyl Aminolevulinate-Photodynamic Therapy for Actinic Keratoses

Three randomized comparison/control studies of MAL-PDT using the same protocol (MAL 3h, 570–670 nm, 75 J/cm^2, 50–250 mW/cm^2) cleared 69% of predominantly thin and moderate thickness AKs of the face or scalp after a single treatment,[49] increasing to 89–91% when two treatments 7 days apart were performed.[72,73] In comparison, cryotherapy cleared 68% and 75%[49,72] in two of these studies, with placebo responses of 30–38%.[72,73] Superior cosmetic response was observed in the MAL-PDT group in both studies that compared PDT with cryotherapy.[49,72]

Similar studies[76] have also found MAL-PDT with a red LED light source (634 ± 3 nm, 37 J/cm^2, 50 mW/cm^2) resulted in a significantly higher cure rate than cryotherapy (87% vs 76%), significantly superior cosmesis and overall subject preference (efficacy and skin discomfort).

Using the same LED at MAL dosing parameters as above, Tarstedt et al.[75] found a single treatment with MAL-PDT, repeated after 3 months in cases in which lesions remained, was equally as effective (93% with single MAL-PDT vs 89% with double treatment) as using two treatments, 7 days apart for thin AKs. However, for thicker AKs, they found that clearance rates were greater after double treatment (84% vs 70% with single treatment). After this study, most countries in Europe revised their MAL-PDT license in AK and started to recommend an initial single treatment for thin AK, with repeat after 3 months if necessary.

Finally, multiple AKs, particularly those that develop within the context of the field of cancerization,[83] frequently challenge the authors' clinical routine. In these patients, PDT appears to be very effective, with a patient complete response rates varying from 82% to 68%[72,73,84] and generally well tolerated. A recent randomized study by Serra-Guillen[85] compared tolerance and satisfaction in the treatment of AK of the face and scalp between 5% imiquimod cream and MAL-PDT. Among 58 patients included, there were a significantly greater percentage of patients very satisfied with the MAL-PDT treatment than in the imiquimod group (93% in MAL-PDT vs 62% in imiquimod). Although the percentage of patients with good tolerance to the MAL-PDT was higher (38% for PDT vs 21% for imiquimod), these differences were not statistically significant.

Palm and Goldman performed a randomized, split-area study on 18 patients with AKs and photodamage using MAL-PDT with 60 minute incubation. All patients received illumination with pulsed-dye lasers and/or intense pulsed light, followed by split face treatment of either blue or red light. No differences were found at 1 month follow-up in the improvement of AKs, wrinkles, pigmentation or erythema between red or blue light for PDT activation. Additionally, no difference in the incidence or severity of adverse events occurred between red and blue light treated areas.[79]

Combination Therapy for Actinic Keratosis Treatment

Several small case studies have demonstrated a possible synergistic effect of ALA-PDT with other treatment options for AKs. Gilbert[69] investigated 15 patients with multiple AKs treated with a 5-day course of nightly 5-FU cream to the face followed by short-contact PDT activated by an IPL light source. A clearance rate of 90% was observed at 1 year follow-up. Martin[86] performed a split-area study with three patients treated with ALA-PDT alone versus sequential therapy with 5-FU (7–10 days) and short-contact ALA-PDT (1 hour ALA incubation followed by blue light 417–432 nm illumination). Six months after the initial visit, the combined regimen showed enhanced efficacy in treating AK, suggesting synergistic effects of 5-FU and ALA-PDT. Shaffelburg[87] conducted a split-face study of 24 patients with multiple AKs, in which ALA-PDT was performed on the entire face. One half of the face was also randomized to receive additional subsequent treatment with a 12-week regimen of imiquimod. Clearance rates at 12 months were superior on the combination treatment side, with 89.9% complete lesion clearance compared to 74.5% on the ALA-PDT treatment side alone.

Treatment Protocol

Skin Preparation

Optimal results following ALA-PDT can be achieved with proper preparation prior to the procedure itself. The stratum corneum is a major barrier to the penetration of 5-ALA.[38,81] Hyperkeratotic lesions must be treated with light curettage prior to 5-ALA application. Otherwise, ALA is preferentially absorbed by the hyperkeratotic scale rather than the lesion intended for treatment.[37] Some physicians use occlusion to improve delivery of 5-ALA through thicker lesions. Tegaderm™, opaque Mepore®, or Glad Press-N-Seal® may be used for these purposes.

Methods of proper skin preparation to reduce stratum corneum thickness also include light chemical peels, tape stripping, microdermabrasion,

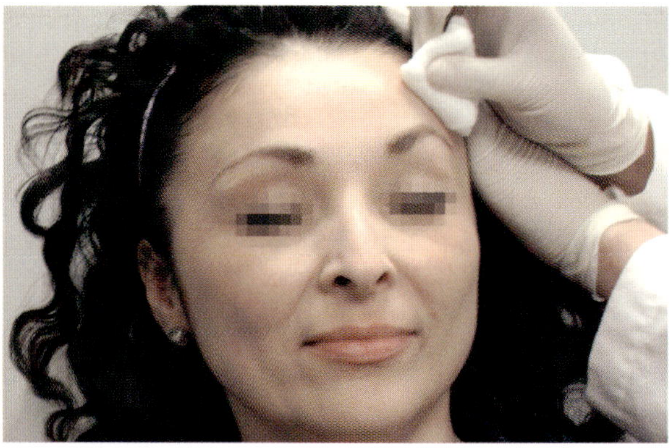

Fig. 10.5: Acetone-soaked gauze following microdermabrasion enhances 5-aminolevulinic acid delivery. Firm pressure should be used during scrubbing to remove excess skin lipids and keratinocytes

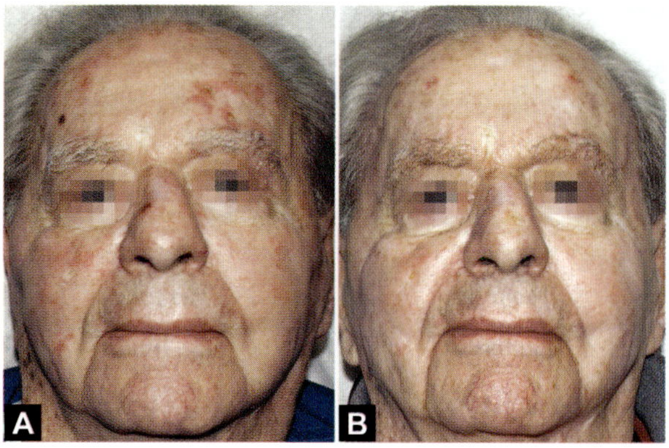

Figs 10.6A and B: Significant reduction in the number of actinic keratosis following a single aminolevulinic acid-photodynamic therapy treatment utilizing sequential activation with pulsed-dye laser, intense pulsed dye laser to nonhair bearing areas and simultaneous illumination with blue and red lights

oscillating sonic cleansing brushes (Clarisonic, Redmond, WA) and degreasing of the skin with acetone.[32,88-90] All of the above measures can improve the absorption of ALA by the skin.[21] The authors routinely use a vibrating microdermabrasion system (Vibraderm, Great Plains, TX) with subsequent acetone degreasing to prepare the skin for 5-ALA application (Fig. 10.5).

Finally, patients with a history of herpes simplex virus are prophylaxed with oral antivirals. One week prior to PDT, patients are asked to discontinue the usage of topical retinoids, alpha hydroxy acids and beta hydroxy acids, and avoid chemical peels for one month prior.

Incubation Time

5-ALA is FDA approved for use with a 14–18-hour incubation and subsequent photoactivation with blue light.[26] However, longer incubation times often results in an increased severity of adverse effects following ALA-PDT (Figs 10.6A and B),[48] and furthermore, shorter incubation times (1–3 hours) have demonstrated similar efficacy in AK clearance.[9,66] The authors routinely use a 60-minute incubation time in the treatment of AKs or for photorejuvenation. When treating thicker, larger or more invasive lesions, the authors extend the incubation time to 3 hours and occlude the treated area with Glad Press'n Seal®. Additionally, on the extremities the authors incubate using a simultaneous application of heating pads, set on low setting, to encourage the conversion of PpIX. Current FDA approval for MAL-PDT involves applying a 16.8% cream (approximately 1 gm, 1 mm thick) with the usage of nitrile gloves. MAL should then be occluded for 3 hours followed by illumination with a narrow spectrum red light lamp.

Light Sources

Blue, red, green and broadband light sources may be used to activate PpIX during ALA-PDT for AKs or photorejuvenation. There are some evidences blue light may be more effective for superficial AKs due to the shorter wavelength and increased potency during PDT of blue light.[6] Red light has a deeper depth of penetration but is often used with MAL rather than ALA. Broadband light sources including IPL have the advantage of improving signs of photodamage. It is our practice, both in the treatment of AKs and photorejuvenation, to use multiple light sources during ALA-PDT. With a typical treatment, the authors treat individual lesions first with subpurpuric doses of a PDL, followed by full-face treatment by an IPL and lastly, illumination with a blue and/or red light source. It should be noted that the IPL also results in hair reduction, so judicious use should be exercised in hair-bearing areas such as the scalp and beard area.

Patient Comfort and Photoprotection and Follow-Up

The authors do not routinely use topical or intralesional anesthesia prior to ALA-PDT. With one hour incubation time, the authors' clinical experience is the procedure is well-tolerated by the overwhelming majority of patients. The authors use forced air cooling and refrigerated conductive gel during the

IPL portion of photoactivation and a cooling fan with aerosolized water during blue light exposure. For longer incubation periods, the use of oral analgesics, topical lidocaine preparations and ice packs in conjunction with PDT may increase patient comfort.[53] Borelli and colleagues[30] recently examined the effects of subcutaneous infiltration anesthesia (SIA) on pain in PDT. They compared the pain related to ALA-PDT in 16 patients who received oral analgesics (1 g paracetamol, 20 mg codeine) and SIA on one side of the face, containing a mixture of ropivacaine, prilocaine and epinephrine. Significantly less pain was reported by 94% of the patients with SIA. However, SIA should not contain vasoconstrictors, such as epinephrine, as their use could reduce the oxygen supply in the skin and thus compromise the effectiveness of PDT.

Immediately following treatment, the authors apply an Aloe vera based gel or a cooled, bland, gentle skin cream to the treated skin to calm erythema and irritation. A sunblock (physical blocker) containing zinc oxide and titanium dioxide is applied to the treated skin. To avoid phototoxicity during daylight hours, the authors' patients are scheduled for treatment in the late afternoon, so they may depart the clinic during twilight hours. Patients are given a protective visor if the face was treated, and patients are asked to wear sunglasses and protective clothing during their ride to home.

The authors instruct patients to avoid sunlight and bright indoor light sources for 36 hours following treatment. The authors request patients return to clinic at 1 week and 2 months following PDT for routine follow-up. They perform subsequent rounds of ALA-PDT at 1–2 month intervals. They counsel patients to anticipate 2 ALA-PDT sessions for the treatment of AKs. These recommendations are consistent with consensus guidelines from the American Society of Photodynamic Therapy.[25]

Clinical Technique

Summarized below is the authors' treatment protocol for ALA-PDT.[5] This is supplied as an example but is by no means the only way to successfully perform PDT. This may be used as a general guideline and practitioners must decide for themselves the most effective and efficient use of ALA-PDT in their office.

Aminolevulinic Acid-Photodynamic Therapy for Actinic Keratoses

- Cleanse the patient's skin with mild soap and water (Cetaphil cleanser or Neutrogena foaming facial wash).
- Perform microdermabrasion with the Vibraderm over the treated area.
  - If a microdermabrasion system is unavailable, consider using a oscillating skin brush (Clarisonic Pro, Clarisonic, Redmond, WA) on high setting for 2 minutes while cleansing the skin
- Scrub the skin vigorously using a 4 inches × 4 inches acetone-soaked gauze.
- Break the two glass ampules in the Levulan Kerastick as per the package insert.[26] Shake the stick for about two minutes.
- Apply the ALA solution to the treatment area. This is best accomplished by painting the Levulan on using the application stick. At least two coats of the solution are recommended and the entire contents of the Kerastick should be used. It is important to get close to the eyes; otherwise it will be apparent that the periorbital skin was not treated.
- Allow the Levulan to incubate for 60 minutes on the skin. The patient should remain indoors and away from sunlight during the incubation period.
- Remove the Levulan prior to any light treatment by requesting the patient to wash his/her face with a gentle soap and water.
- Activate the Levulan with the appropriate light source(s):
  - Illumination is begun with the PDL to individual lesions (if PDL unavailable, proceed to IPL)
    - 595 nm with a 7 mm spot size, 40 ms pulse width and 10–12 J/cm^2 (Cynergy, Cynosure Inc, Westford, MA) with forced cold air cooling (Zimmer, LaserMed, LLC, Shelton, CT).
    - 595 nm with a 7 mm spot size, 40 ms pulse width, dynamic cooling 30/30 and 10–12 J/cm^2 or Vbeam Perfecta, Candela).
  - Next, the intense pulsed light source is utilized in nonhair bearing areas.

- For skin types I–III the authors use the 560 nm cut-off filter and the 590 nm filter for skin types IV (Lumenis One or the Lumenis M22, Lumenis Ltd., Yokneam, Israel).
  a. If predominant hyperpigmentation (solar lentigines or postinflammatory hyperpigmentation): double pulse technique, 3.0 msec pulse duration for both pulses.
  b. If combination of hyperpigmentation (solar lentigines or postinflammatory hyperpigmentation) and erythema: double pulse technique, 3.5 msec pulse duration for both pulses.
  c. Predominance of fine telangiectasias: double pulse technique, 4 msec pulse duration for both pulses.
- 10–30 ms delay is set between pulses in skin types I–III and 30–40 ms in skin type IV
- Fluence range of 17–22 J/cm^2, with decreased doses is recommended for nonfacial locations
- Other IPL devices can also be used successfully, though treatment settings must be adjusted appropriately to each device.

– Finally, simultaneous illumination with blue and red light (see Fig. 10.2)
  - Blue light source (Blu-U, DUSA Pharmaceuticals Inc., Wilmington, MA) positioned 25 to 50 mm from the skin, 16 minutes 40 seconds, light dose 10 J/cm^2.
  - Red light source (Aktilite CL128, Galderma, Ft. Worth, TX) positioned 50–80 mm from the skin, 8 minutes 49 seconds, 37 J/cm^2.

- Mineral based sunscreen is applied and patient is discharged home.
- Instruct the patient on strict photoprotection for the following 36 hours. The patient is to remain indoors, out of direct sunlight.
- Patients are given Avene Thermal Spring Water spray to apply to their skin 4–6 times a day.
- Repeat the treatment in 4–8 weeks. If there was little reaction, increase the incubation time, reevaluate your skin preparation technique, or consider combination therapy.

Clinical examples of AKs treated with a multi-laser PDT approach are presented in Figures 10.7 and 10.8.

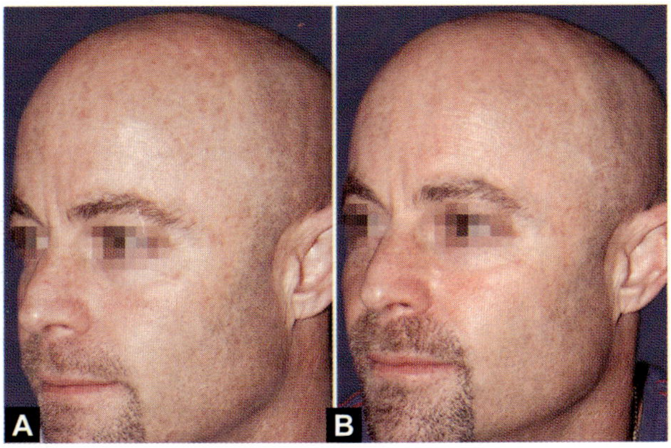

Figs 10.7A and B: Before and one month following a single multilaser aminolevulinic acid-photodynamic therapy to the face of a middle-aged male with reduction in actinic keratosis along with improvement in signs of photoaging including solar lentigines and erythema

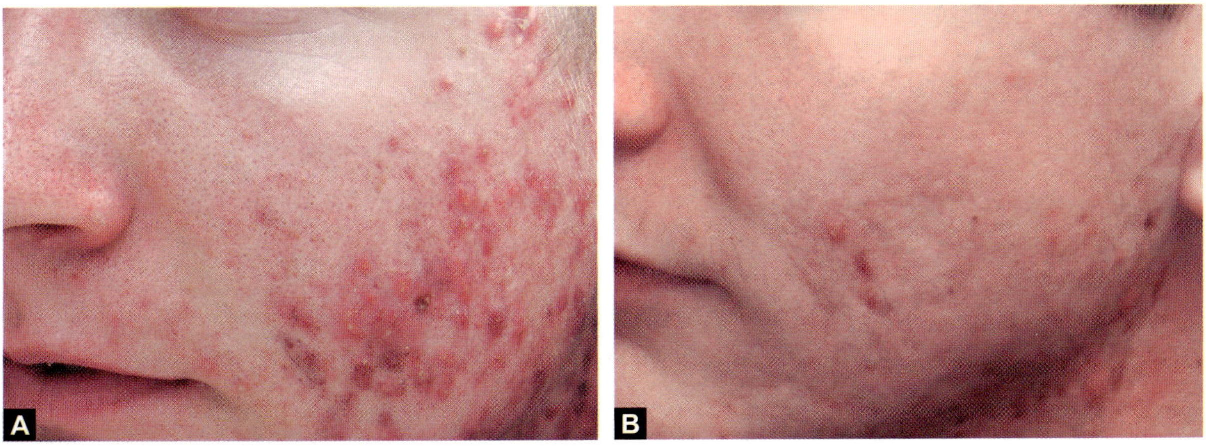

Figs 10.8A and B: Young adult male with cystic and scarring acne before and 15 months after his third aminolevulinic acid-photodynamic therapy treatment showing a dramatic decrease in the severity of cystic acne. The patient also displayed a decrease in the depth and erythema of the acne scars

Nonmelanoma Skin Cancer

Basal cell carcinoma (BCC) is the most common malignant skin tumor in the Caucasian population and is classified together with SCC as NMSC. It is estimated that NMSC affects at least 1–2% of the population annually,[40,44] with 0.9–1.2 million new cases of NMSC diagnosed each year in United States; of these 80% are BCC and 16% are SCC.[40] Risk factors to NMSC include exposure to ultraviolet radiation, light complexion, male gender, increasing age, immunosuppression, precancerous skin lesion and ionizing radiation.[44,91]

Treatment of NMSC usually is based on clinical type, tumor size, location and other important factors should be considered such as maintaining close to normal skin appearance, downtime, treatment compliance, therapeutic risks related to comorbidities and medications (anticoagulants, immunosuppressive therapy). Apart from surgical excision, which is the standard treatment for cutaneous SCC, other treatment options exist including curettage and electrocautery, cryotherapy, radiotherapy, cytotoxic agents, and immune response modifiers.

Photodynamic therapy with MAL is an innovative treatment modality that has been approved in Europe for the treatment of superficial BCC (sBCC), nodular BCC (nBCC), AKs, and Bowen's disease.[92] Herein, we revise the evidence for the efficacy and safety of PDT in the treatment NMSC.

Bowen's Disease/Squamous Cell Carcinoma

Bowen's disease (BD) also known as squamous cell carcinoma in situ (SCCIS), is particularly common in elderly patients, frequently occurring on the lower part of the legs[73] and is associated with a small risk of progression (about 3%) to an invasive SCC.[75] This condition has been widely proposed as an indication for topical PDT with several studies confirming the efficacy of ALA-PDT. Topical ALA-PDT clears, on average, 86–93% of lesions of BD following one or two treatments[93] (Table 10.2). Three small randomized trials using nonlicensed ALA formulations and identical protocols demonstrated that PDT was equivalent in efficacy to cryotherapy,[94] superior to 5-FU[95] and significantly more effective when delivered narrowband red light instead of green light,[96] possibly related to deeper tissue penetration.

Table 10.2: Published clinical studies on aminolevulinic acid and methyl aminolevulinate-photodynamic therapy for squamous cell carcinoma in situ

Reference	*ALA Preparation*	*Location of SCCIS*	*Incubation Period (Hours)*	*No. of Lesions Treated (No. of Patients)*	*Light Source (Wavelength in nm)*	*Response Rate*	*Follow-up (Months)*
Morton[94] (1996)	20% emulsion		4	20	Desktop lamp—300 W xenon short arc (125 J/cm^2 at a fluence rate of 70 mW/cm^2)	100% CR	12
Salim[95] (2003)	20% emulsion	Legs	4	33 (20)	Red light (630 ± 15 nm, 100 J/cm^2)	88% CR	12
Morton[96] (2000)	20% emulsion	Legs	4	61	Red (630 ± 15 nm, 125 J/cm^2) or Green (540 ± 15 nm, 62.5 J/cm^2) light	88% CR—Red light; 48% Green light	12
Leman[97] (2002)	20% emulsion	Unspecified	4	107 (68)	Filtered red light (Xenon source, 630 ± 15 nm, 100–125 J/cm^2)	83%	64

Contd...

Contd...

Reference	*MAL Preparation*	*Location of SCCIS*	*Incubation Period (Hours)*	*No. of Lesions Treated (No. of Patients)*	*Light Source (Wavelength in nm)*	*Response Rate*	*Follow-up (Months)*
Morton[98] (2001)	20% emulsion	Face, trunk and limbs	4–6	40	Filtered red light (Xenon source, 630 ± 15 nm, 100–125 J/cm^2)	78%	12
Morton[99] (2006)	16.8% cream	Unspecified	3	124	Broadband red light (570–670 nm, 75 J/cm^2)	80%	12
Morton[100] (2004)	16.8% cream	Unspecified	3	124 (96)	Broadband red light (570–670 nm, total light dose 75 J/cm^2)	85%	12

ALA: 5-aminolevulinic acid; CR: Complete response; MAL: Methyl aminolevulinate; SCCIS: Squamous cell carcinoma in situ

More recently, a large multicenter study has been completed comparing MAL-PDT with cryotherapy or topical 5-FU.[99] In this randomized placebo-controlled study, 225 patients with 275 histologically confirmed SCCIS, with 111 lesions treated with two MAL-PDT treatments, 7 days apart, with a repeat cycle after 3 months, if necessary. Cryotherapy was performed as a single freeze-thaw cycle to achieve an ice field that persisted for at least 20 seconds and 5-FU was topically applied daily for 3 weeks. Both treatment modalities were also repeated if required. After 3 months, MAL-PDT achieved clearance of 93% in comparison with 86% and 83% for cryotherapy and topical 5-FU respectively. The remission rate after 12 months was 80% with MAL-PDT versus 67% with cryotherapy ($P = 0.047$) and 69% ($P = 0.19$) with 5-FU. Recurrence rates for 24 months have been presented with an 18% rate with MAL-PDT comparable with 23% for cryotherapy and 21% for 5-FU. Cosmetic outcome at 3 months was good or excellent for 94% of patients from the PDT group in comparison with 66% for the cryotherapy and 76% for 5-FU.

Data concerning long-term clearance are limited but in one retrospective study of 617 patients, Thestrup-Pedersen and colleagues[101] found relapse rates (> 5 years) of 34% for cryotherapy, 19% for curettage, 14% for 5-FU, 6% for radiotherapy and 5% for surgery. With a 64-month recurrence rate of 17% in BD noted by Leman et al.[97] following ALA-PDT, PDT, comparing with more established therapies, seems to have an acceptable long-term efficacy.

While there is high efficacy of topical PDT for in situ SCC, studies have shown the depth of therapeutic effect is the limiting factor for PDT in invasive SCC with poorer response rates and increased recurrence rates. Although topical PDT has shown efficacy, in view of its metastatic potential, topical PDT cannot be currently recommended for the treatment of invasive SCC.[102,103]

Superficial Basal Cell Carcinoma

Basal cell carcinomas are locally aggressive tumors that very rarely metastasize and can be divided in three major groups: superficial, nodular and infiltrating morpheaform lesions. Superficial BCC (sBCC) usually differs from the other subtypes as it tends to appear at a younger age, frequently occurs on the trunk, limbs and neck, and often is multiple.[104] A large number of treatment modalities exist, including surgical techniques (excisional surgery, curettage and electrocautery, Mohs micrographic surgery, cryosurgery), immune response modifiers, cytotoxic agents and PDT. Table 10.3 shows the main clinical studies of topical ALA and MAL-PDT in sBCC.

Table 10.3: Published clinical studies on aminolevulinic acid-photodynamic therapy and methyl aminolevulinate-photodynamic therapy for superficial basal cell carcinoma

Reference	*ALA Preparation*	*Location of sBCC*	*Incubation Period (Hours)*	*No. of Lesions Treated (No. of Patients)*	*Light Source (Wavelength in nm)*	*Response Rate*	*Follow-up (Months)*
Kennedy[1] (1990)	20% emulsion	Not specified	3	80 lesions	Slide projector with a cutoff filter at 600 nm	90% CR	2–3
Calzavara-Pinton[105] (1995)	20% emulsion ALA-PDT repeated *eod* until clinical dis-appearance	Head, trunk and limbs	6–8 occluded	23 lesions	Argon dye laser (630)	91% CR	24–36
Fijan[57] (1995)	1× ALA-PDT in combination with des-ferrioxamine (no lesion preparation specified), repeated after 3–6 months if required	Face, scalp, trunk and extremities	Not specified	34 (32)	Halogen lamp with a red filter	88% CR after 1 treatment, 97% after 2 treatments	20
Wennberg[106] (1996)	20% emulsion 1× ALA-PDT	Not specified	3 occluded	190 (37)	Filtered xenon lamp (620–670 nm)	92% CR	6
Fink-Puches[107] (1998)	20% emulsion 1× ALA-PDT	Face, scalp, neck, trunk (65 lesions) and lower extremity	4 occluded	95 (47)	UV-A or full-spectrum visible light, > 515, > 570, or > 610 nm)	Initial response (2–4 weeks): 86% CR, recurrence rate of 44% after median of 19 months	Median of 19 months
Haller[108] (2000)	20% cream Routine 2× ALA-PDT, 7 days apart	Face, trunk and limbs	3–4 occluded	26 (6)	Red light (630 ± 15 nm)	1–2 month lesion CR: 100%; 1 lesions recurred at 16 months	Median of 27 months

Contd...

Contd...

Soler[109] (2000)	ALA-PDT 15 minutes of pretreatment with 99% DMSO before topical 20% ALA with DMSO (2%) and ethylenediaminetetra-acetic acid (2%)	Face, scalp, trunk and extremities	3 occluded	245 (83)	Broadband lamp with continuous spectrum (570–740 nm) or a red-light laser (630 nm)	Red light: 86% CR vs Broadband lamp: 82% CR	6
Wang[110] (2001)	20% cream 1× ALA-PDT × Cryotherapy 2× freeze-thaw cryotherapy, repeat at 12 week, if required	Head and neck, trunk and limbs	6 occluded	39 sBCC (22 treated with ALA-PDT); 49 nBCC (25 treated with ALA-PDT)	Frequency doubled Nd:YAG laser pumping a dye laser (635 nm, 60 J/cm^2, 80 ± 20 mW/cm^2)	12 month histologically recurrences: 38% for ALA-PDT vs 7% for cryotherapy; Excellent or good cosmetic outcome (sBCC + nBCC) in 93% treated with ALA-PDT vs 54% with cryotherapy	12
MAL	*Study*	*Location*	*Incubation Period (Hours)*	*No. of Lesions Treated (No. of Patients)*	*Light Source (Wavelength in nm)*	*Response Rate*	*Follow-up (Months)*
Soler[111] (2001)	1× MAL-PDT (lesion preparation)	Face, scalp, trunk and extremities	Mean 4 occluded	131 sBCC	Broadband halogen light (570–670 nm) mean light dose of 50–200 J/ cm^2, light intensity of 100–180 mW/cm^2	91% CR after 3 months, 9% relapse at 35 months	24–48

Contd...

Contd...

Horn[112] (2003)	MAL-PDT "difficult to treat" BCC (European trial); 2× MAL-PDT retreated after 3 months if necessary (lesion preparation)	Face, scalp, neck, trunk and extremities	3, occluded	49 sBCC	Red light (570–670 nm), dose of 75 J/cm^2, light intensity of 50–200 mW/cm^2	85% CR after 3 months (histological control); 22% recurrence at 24 months	24
Vinciullo[113] (2005)	MAL-PDT "difficult to treat" BCC (Australian trial); 2× MAL-PDT retreated after 3 months if necessary (lesion preparation)	Face, scalp, neck, trunk and extremities	3, occluded	92 sBCC	Red light (570–670 nm), dose of 75 J/cm^2, light intensity of 50–200 mW/cm^2	93% CR at 3 months, 82% at 24 months	24
Surrenti[114] (2007)	2× MAL-PDT (7 days apart) with additional monthly MAL-PDT sessions up to a maximum 8 where necessary (lesion preparation)	Face, neck, trunk and extremities	3, occluded	94 (69)	Red LED light source (634 ± 3 nm, 37 J/cm^2, 50 mW/cm^2)	89% CR 1 month after 2 sessions, 2.4% recurrence at 12 months; no additional clinical benefit beyond 2 MAL-PDT sessions	12
Basset-Seguin[115] (2008)	1× MAL-PDT vs double freeze-thaw cryotherapy retreated with 2× MAL-PDT (7 days apart) or double freeze-thaw cryotherapy after 3 months if necessary (lesion preparation)	Face, scalp, neck, trunk and extremities	3, occluded	219 (114 treated with MAL-PDT)	Red light (570–670 nm), dose of 75 J/cm^2, mean light intensity of 150 mW/cm^2	MAL-PDT—97% at 3 months vs cryo-therapy—95%	60

Contd...

Contd...

Szeimies[116] (2008)	2× MAL-PDT (7 days apart), retreated after 3 months if necessary vs surgery	Face, scalp, neck, trunk and extremities	3, occluded	246 (128 treated with MAL-PDT)	Red LED light source (634 ± 3 nm, 37 J/cm², 50 mW/cm²)	MAL-PDT-92% at 3 months vs cryo-therapy—99%; 9.3% recurrence with MAL-PDT vs none with surgery at 12 months	12
Fantini[117] (2010)	1 or 2× MAL-PDT (7 days apart), a third PDT session after 3 months if required (lesion preparation)	Head, neck, trunk and limbs	3, occluded	116	Red LED light source (634 ± 3 nm, 37 J/cm², 50 mW/cm²)	CR: 82%	Mean of 23.5

ALA: 5-aminolevulinic acid; CR: Complete response; DMSO: Dimethyl sulfoxide; MAL: Methyl aminolevulinate; nBCC: Nodular basal cell carcinoma; sBCC: Superficial basal cell carcinoma

In 1990, Kennedy et al.[1] were the first to report a 79% complete response rate at 3 months for 300 cases of sBCC treated with ALA-PDT (3–6 hours application of 20% ALA followed by filtered red light, 600+ nm). In 2001, Morton and colleagues[98] treated 98 large or multiple sBCC with ALA-PDT and noted an 89% clearance rate after one or more treatments. Another study by Clark et al.[35] treated up to four times with ALA applied for 6 hours followed by irradiation with red lamps (570–720 nm) or a 630 nm diode laser with a light dose of 125 J/cm² and found a 97% clearance for sBCC. The number of treatments increased with lesion diameter and the recurrence rate was 4.8% with a median follow-up of 55 weeks.

A comparison study by Wang et al.[110] with ALA-PDT (6-hour application of ALA, 635 nm dye laser; 60 J/cm²) and cryotherapy for the treatment of sBCC and nBCC noted no significant difference in efficacy between the two groups. However, ALA-PDT was associated with fewer adverse events, faster healing times and better cosmetic results. It should be noted that lesions were followed clinically and biopsied at 3 months; they were retreated on clinical grounds or for histopathological tumor and biopsied again at 12 months. They found that despite only 5% of the ALA-PDT treated sBCC were clinical failures at 12 months, an additional 20% of the treatment sites that were clinically clear had residual BCC on biopsy.

Several trials in Europe, USA and Australia have been performed to investigate the efficacy and safety of MAL-PDT for the treatment of both sBCC and nBCC. Initial efficacy is consistently high, with clearance rates at 3 months after MAL-PDT ranging from 80% (in difficult to treat cases, recurrent or large lesions, or H-zone lesions)[112,118] to 97% in primary sBCC. Long-term, nearly two-thirds of all recurrent BCC lesions appear in the first 3 years after treatment.[119,120]

Szeimies and colleagues[116] compared MAL-PDT (one cycle of two treatment sessions, 7 days apart, re-treatment after 3 months with a second cycle if required) and surgery in sBCC. Three months after last treatment, the efficacy of MAL-PDT was similar to that of surgery: 92.2% showed complete clearance at 3 months with MAL-PDT vs 99.2% with surgery. However, at 12 months, 9.3% of lesions recurred with MAL-PDT compared with none with surgery. Cosmetic outcome was superior for MAL-PDT at all time points, with 94.1% lesions treated with MAL-PDT had an excellent or good cosmetic result compared with 59.8% with surgery.

In difficult-to-treat populations, i.e. large lesions, in the H-zone, or in patients at high risk of surgical complications, Vinciullo et al.[113] treated 95 patients with 148 BCC lesions (superficial, nodular or mixed superficial and nodular) with MAL-PDT (3-hour occlusion, 570–670 nm, 75 J/cm^2, 50–200 mW/cm^2) and achieved an estimated lesion complete response rate of 90% at 3 months, 84% at 12 months and 78% at 24 months. Overall cosmetic outcome was rated as excellent or good in 79% and 84% of the patients at 12 and 24 months respectively. Therefore, MAL-PDT does show good efficacy and is an attractive option when surgery would be inappropriate or the patient wants to maintain normal skin appearance.

Nodular Basal Cell Carcinoma

Clinical results for nBCC using 5-ALA-PDT varied more markedly than those obtained for sBCC, with clearance rates ranging from 64% to 92%.[121] This difference might be due to inadequate penetration of ALA into the deeper portions of the skin and the malignancy.[122] To enhance effectiveness, several modalities including debulking the lesion before PDT exist. Thissen and colleagues[123] reported a clearance rate of 92% (22 of 24 tumors) after a single cycle of ALA-PDT (noncoherent red light, 100 mW/cm^2, 120 J/cm^2) with debulking curettage performed 3 weeks earlier.

Five phase III studies in which a total of 220 nBCC were treated[112,113,124-127] with MAL-PDT has demonstrated significant efficacy with 3-month complete response rates of 73–94%. It should be noted that histologically controlled studies have confirmed the reliability of efficacy data (73% and 79%). A comparison study of MAL-PDT vs surgery for nBCC[127,128] has provided a 3-month response rate noninferior to surgery (91% compared with 98% for surgery) and a 60-month recurrence rate of 14% compared with 4% with surgery. However, estimated sustained lesion complete response were 76% for MAL-PDT compared with 96% for surgery.

Although thickness of nBCC has not specifically been assessed in other trials, a retrospective study of MAL-PDT for nBCC found recurrence rates of 7% and 14% for thin (< 2 mm) and thick (> 2 mm) nBCC respectively at a median 35-month of follow-up, suggesting that thin nBCC might be particularly responsive to MAL-PDT.[111]

Since the penetration of MAL is higher than of ALA and a standardized protocol involving lesion preparation, light source (red light) and dose has been developed for nBCC in the countries where MAL-PDT is approved for this particular condition, current evidence supports the use of MAL rather than ALA for PDT of nBCC.[129] Table 10.4 shows the main clinical trials of topical ALA and MAL-PDT in nBCC.

Table 10.4: Published clinical studies on aminolevulinic acid-photodynamic therapy and methyl aminolevulinate-photodynamic therapy for nodular basal cell carcinoma

Reference	*ALA Preparation*	*Location of nBCC*	*Incubation Period (Hours)*	*No. of Lesions Treated (No. of Patients)*	*Light Source (Wavelength in nm)*	*Response Rate*	*Follow-up (Months)*
Fijan[57] (1995)	1× ALA-PDT in combination with desferrio-xamine (no lesion preparation specified), repeated after 3–6 months if required	Face, scalp, trunk and extremities	Not specified	22 (32)	Halogen lamp with a red filter	32% CR after 1 treatment, 59% after 2 treatments	3–20

Contd...

Contd...

Calzavara-Pinton[105] (1995)	Various cutaneous malig-nancies. ALA 20% emulsion; ALA-PDT repeated *eod* until clinical dis-appearance	Head, trunk and limbs	6–8	30	Argon dye laser (630)	1-month lesion CR (histologi-cally controlled): 61%; 33% recurrence after median of 29 months	24–36
Thissen[123] (2000)	1× ALA-PDT using 20% ALA cream and DMSO (lesion preparation)	Not specified	6 occluded	24 (23)	Red light (630–635 nm, 120 J/cm^2, 100 mW/cm^2)	3–6 months lesion CR: 92%; 5% recurrence after median of 17 months	17
Wang[110] (2001)	20% ALA cream; 1× ALA-PDT × cryotherapy 2× freeze-thaw cryo-therapy, repeat at 12 weeks, if required	Head and neck, trunk and limbs	6 occluded	49 nBCC (25 treated with ALA-PDT); 39 sBCC (22 treated with ALA-PDT)	Frequency doubled Nd:YAG laser pumping a dye laser (635 nm, 60 J/cm^2, 80 ± 20 mW/cm^2)	12-month histologi-cally recurrences: 13% for ALA-PDT vs 21% for cryotherapy	12
Christen-sen[130] (2009)	1 or 2× ALA-PDT (7 days apart) using 20% ALA cream and DMSO (lesion preparation)	Face, scalp, trunk and extremities	3 occluded	36 nBCC; 24 sBCC	Broadband halogen light source (550–700 nm, 150–230 mW/cm^2)	3 month CR (sBCC + nBCC): 91%, 17% of nBCC recurred after 72 months	72
MAL	*Study*	*Location*	*Incubation Period (Hours)*	*No. of Lesions Treated (No. of Patients)*	*Light Source (Wavelength in nm)*	*Response Rate*	*Follow-up (Months)*
Soler[111] (2001)	1× MAL-PDT (lesion preparation)	Face, scalp, trunk and extremities	Mean 4 occluded	82 thin nBCC (< 2 mm thickness), 86 thick nBCC (> 2 mm)	Broadband halogen light (570–670 nm) light dose of 50-200 J/cm^2, light intensity of 100–180 mW/cm^2	Thin nBCC: 93% CR and thick nBCC: 86% CR after 3 months, 7% of thin nBCC and 14% of thick nBCC relapsed at 35 months	24–48

Contd...

Contd...

Horn[112] (2003)	MAL-PDT "difficult to treat" BCC (European trial); 2× MAL-PDT retreated after 3 months if necessary (lesion preparation)	Face, scalp, neck, trunk and extremities	3, occluded	52 nBCC	Red light (570–670 nm), dose of 75 J/cm^2, light intensity of 50–200 mW/cm^2	75% CR after 3 months (histological control); 14% recurrence at 24 months	24
Rhodes[127] (2004)	2× MAL-PDT (7 days apart) vs surgery (lesion preparation), retreatment after 3 months if required	Face, scalp, neck, trunk and extremities	3, occluded	105 nBCC (53 treated with MAL-PDT)	Red light (570–670 nm), dose of 75 J/cm^2, light intensity of 50–200 mW/cm^2	MAL-PDT: 91% CR vs surgery: 98% 3 months after last treatment, NR or recurrence after 24 months: 19% in the MAL-PDT vs 4% in the surgery group	24
Vinciullo[113] (2005)	MAL-PDT "difficult to treat" BCC (Australian trial); 2× MAL-PDT retreated after 3 months if necessary (lesion preparation)	Face, scalp, neck, trunk and extremities	3, occluded	36 nBCC	Red light (570–670 nm), dose of 75 J/cm^2, light intensity of 50–200 mW/cm^2	82% CR at 3 months, 67% at 24 months	24
Kuijpers[124] (2006)	2× MAL-PDT × 2× ALA-PDT (20% cream) 7 days apart (lesion preparation)	Face, neck, trunk and extremities	3, occluded	43 (22 treated with ALA-PDT and 21 with MAL-PDT)	Broadband halogen light (600–730 nm), dose of 75 J/cm^2, light intensity of 100 mW/cm^2	CR at 2 months (histologically controlled): 72, 7% with ALA-PDT vs 71, 4% with MAL-PDT	8

Contd...

Contd...

Rhodes[128] (2007)	2× MAL-PDT 7 days apart (repeated if necessary, lesion preparation) × Surgery	Face, scalp, neck, trunk and extremities	3, occluded	105 (53 treated with MAL-PDT)	Red light (570–670 nm), dose of 75 J/cm^2, light intensity of 50–200 mW/cm^2	Sustained CR at 5 years: MAL-PDT 76% vs Surgery 96%; recurrence at 5 years: 14% in the MAL-PDT vs 4% in the surgery group	60
Surrenti[114] (2007)	2× MAL-PDT (7 days apart) with additional monthly MAL-PDT sessions up to a maximum 8 where necessary (lesion preparation)	Face, neck, trunk and extremities	3, occluded	24	Red LED light source (634 ± 3 nm, 37 J/cm^2, 50 mW/cm^2)	52.2% CR one month after 2 sessions, no additional clinical benefit beyond 2 MAL-PDT sessions	12
Foley[131] (2009)	2× MAL-PDT (7 days apart) retreated after 3 months if required (lesion preparation) × Placebo-PDT for nBCC < 5 mm in depth	Face, scalp, neck, trunk and extremities	3, occluded	150 (75 lesions treated with MAL-PDT)	Red light (570–670 nm), dose of 75 J/cm^2, light intensity of 50–200 mW/cm^2	histo-logically verified CR: 73% with MAL-PDT vs 27% with the Placebo-PDT	6
Fantini[117] (2010)	1 or 2× MAL-PDT (7 days apart), a third PDT session after 3 months if required (lesion preparation)	Head, neck, trunk and limbs	3, occluded	78	Red LED light source (634 ± 3 nm, 37 J/cm^2, 50 mW/cm^2)	CR: 33% (tumor thickness superior of 0.5 mm and the presence of ulceration were predictors of negative outcome)	Mean of 23.5

CR: Complete response; DMSO: Dimethyl sulfoxide; LED: Light emitting diodes; MAL: Methyl aminolevulinate; nBCC: Nodular basal cell carcinoma; PDT: Photodynamic therapy; NR: Noncomplete response

More recently, photodynamic diagnosis using MAL (13 hour incubation) in conjunction with a Wood lamp examination has been reported as an adjunctive to accentuate tumor margins before Mohs micrographic surgery (MMS). A high degree of consistency between post-Mohs micrographic surgery defect and fluorescent examination size was seen in this study. Therefore, this technique has the potential for increasing the efficiency of MMS by decreasing the number of stages.[132] Another study by Lee and colleagues,[133] using 20% ALA ointment 6 hours before MMS for NMSC, failed to find any efficacy of photodynamic diagnosis though the authors concluded that many variables such as tumor thickness, type of photosensitizer, incubation time might affect the fluorescence, therefore future large-scale studies are still needed.

Unique Patient Populations

Solid organ transplant recipients (OTR) suffer from a 10–250 fold increase in AKs due to their ongoing immunosuppressive therapy. In addition, the precancerous and cancerous lesions developing in the OTR population are often more aggressive,[134] requiring frequent and ongoing cancer surveillance. PDT, a safe and effective treatment option for precancerous and malignant lesions, offered a new treatment modality for controlling AKs and NMSCs in the OTR population. Although initial response rates of AKs following PDT were comparable in the OTR patient population compared to normal controls,67 longer-term follow-up demonstrated statistically significant decreases in clearance rates in the OTR population. In addition, SCC of the dorsal hands and forearms were not prevented in OTRs in a 2-year follow-up study, although there was a trend toward decreased keratotic regions in the areas treated.[135] PDT may still be a viable treatment option in this population, but it may require adjustments to typical treatment protocols including increased frequency of PDT sessions[67] and use of longer wavelengths (red light) for deeper skin penetration.[135]

In summary, PDT is still considered a promising antitumor strategy that has a range of application alone or combined with other approved or experimental therapeutic, thereby improving the therapeutic efficacy. This will represent a main focus of clinical research in modern oncology.

Aminolevulinic Acid-Photodynamic Therapy for Squamous Cell Carcinoma in Situ and Superficial Basal Cell Carcinomas

The treatment is performed as previously described with the following specific change: Levulan is allowed to incubate for 180 minutes on the skin with occlusion utilizing Tegaderm™, opaque Mepore®, or Glad Press'n Seal®.

Acne Vulgaris

Acne results from the obstruction and inflammation of the sebaceous glands and affects 80% of the human population. The pathogenic mechanisms of acne are multifactorial and complex and include epithelial hyperproliferation, follicular plugging with formation of comedones, increased sebum production by sebaceous glands, inflammation and the presence and proliferation of *Propionibacterium acnes* within the follicle.[136] Acne typically begins in adolescence with hormonal changes and more often affects males, but in 30% of women can persist during the entire fertile period.[137] There are several different presentations of acne ranging from comedonal, papular, pustular and cystic acne. In many cases, a combination of these presentations of acne can be present on an individual simultaneously.

First-line therapy for acne vulgaris is conventional prescription topical and/or oral medications. However, many patients have contraindications, partial response or significant adverse effects. Oral isotretinoin is currently most effective treatment that is known to reduce 80% to 90% of the acne lesions after 4 months of treatment;[138,139] however, despite its undeniable effectiveness isotretinoin is not a curative drug. Relapse within 2 years may be seen up to half of the patients that will require two or more courses of treatment.[140,141] Besides, its use is associated with many side effects, some of which can be very serious. The most important issue is its teratogenicity, but common adverse events include: dry skin/lips, epistaxis, ophthalmological symptoms and headaches. Laboratory abnormalities have been described, warranting adequate monitoring of liver functions and serum lipids.[142] In addition, bone mineralization abnormalities,[143] inflammatory bowel disease and depression[144] have been reported. PDT, and light-based treatments can offer alternative treatments for acne with their own advantages and disadvantages.

Photodynamic therapy may promote acne improvement via antibacterial activity against *P. acnes*, selective damage to sebaceous glands, reduction of follicular obstruction and hyperkeratosis, and via immunological host responses.[145,146] Visible light is able to activate natural endogenous porphyrins produced by *P. acnes*, generating ROS that destroy the bacteria.[146] Therefore, it is expected that topical application of ALA, producing additional porphyrins, makes the combination more effective than light alone.[147] A variety of light sources for the treatment of acne with PDT have been studied, including noncoherent red and blue light, PDL, IPL and a combination of these.

Hongcharu and colleagues[145] first described the efficacy of topical ALA followed by light exposure (20% ALA 3 hours, 550–700 nm, 150 J/cm^2) for acne on the back of 22 subjects. Histological exams demonstrated vacuolization of sebocytes and keratinocytes followed by sustained atrophic glands, granulomatous reaction and perifollicular fibrosis up to 3 weeks after irradiation. Significant improvement in inflammatory acne was observed for 10 weeks after a single treatment and for at least 20 weeks after four treatments. Both sebum excretion and bacterial porphyrin fluorescence were decreased with sustained reduction of sebum output for at least 20 weeks of follow-up.

Itoh and colleagues[148] using low-fluence red light (600–700 nm, 17 mW/cm^2, total dose of 13 J/cm^2) and 20% topical ALA under occlusion for 4 hours reported improvement of acne lesions in 13/13 patients treated with one session. Recurrence of lesions started after 3–6 months, suggesting that one session may not be enough for sustained results.

Since then, several open studies report a clinical benefit of ALA-PDT in facial acne with application times varying from 0.25 hour to 4 hours and a variety of light sources, including blue light, red light, IPL and PDL. Unfortunately, reports of these studies are difficult to compare because of protocol variations with small number of patients, short follow-up periods and variable light dosimetry. Table 10.5 provides a summary of peer-reviewed articles on the use of ALA-PDT and MAL-PDT in acne treatment.

Table 10.5: Published clinical studies on aminolevulinic acid and methyl aminolevulinate-photodynamic therapy for acne vulgaris

Reference	*Photosensitizer/ Duration/ Study Design*	*Location/ Pretreatment*	*No. of Sessions*	*No. of Patients*	*Light Source (Emission λ, nm)*	*Response*	*Follow-up (Weeks)*
Hongcharu[145] (2000)	20% ALA, 3 hours occlusion/3 test sites and 1 control site on back per patient (ALA only, ALA-PDT, red light only, control); two randomized groups: 1 vs 4 sessions (1 week apart)	Back/70% isopropyl alcohol	1 vs 4	22	Broad-spectrum (550–700 nm, 150 J/cm^2)	Only ALA-PDT showed significant reduction in inflammatory lesions, Four sessions better than one	20

Contd...

Contd...

Itoh[148] (2001)	20% ALA, 4 hours occlusion	Face/Not mentioned	1	13	Broad-spectrum (600–700 nm, 17 mW/cm², 13 J/cm²)	100% with some improvement, new lesions after 3–6 months	24
Goldman[149] (2003)	20% ALA, 15 minutes/ Blue light only vs ALA-PDT	Face/2% Salicylic acid cleanser	2 sessions of blue light alone weekly, 2 sessions of ALA-PDT at 2 week intervals	22 (12 blue light vs 10 ALA-PDT)	Blue light (417 nm)	68% decrease of papules in the ALA-PDT vs 40% decrease in the blue light alone	2 weeks after last treatment
Pollock[146] (2004)	20% ALA, 3 hours occlusion/3 test sites and 1 control site on back per patient (ALA only, ALA-PDT, red light only, control)	Back/Not mentioned	3, one week apart	10	Diode laser (635 nm, 25 mW/cm², 15 J/cm²)	Significant reduction of mean acne lesions count (69%) in the ALA-PDT site only	3 weeks after last treatment
Gold[150] (2004)	20% ALA, 1 hour	Face/ Cetaphil cleanser	4 (1 week apart)	15	IPL (430–1,100 nm, 3–9 J/cm²)	3 patients did not respond, 12 patients had 71.8% reduction in acne lesions	12
Taub[151] (2004)	20% ALA, 15–30 minutes	Face, Back and chest/ Acetone scrub and alcohol scrub	2–4 (4–8 weeks apart)	18	Blue light (417 nm) or IPL(400–980 nm, 18–25 J/cm² + radio-frequency)	5 patients did not improve, 11 had at least 50% improvement	Average follow-up time of 4 months
Hong[152] (2005)	20% ALA, 4 hours under occlusion/ split-face ALA-PDT vs controls	Face/Not mentioned	1	8	Halogen lamp red light (630 ± 63 nm, 30 mW/cm², 18 J/cm²)	41.9% (treated) vs 15.4% (control) reduction of inflamed lesions at 6 months	6 months

Contd...

Contd...

Santos[153] (2005)	20% ALA, 3 hours/split-face: IPL alone vs IPL + ALA	Face/Not mentioned	2 (2 weeks apart)	13	IPL cutoff filter, 560 nm, 26–34 J/cm^2	Improvement significantly higher in ALA-PDT side: 10/13 had good or excellent results vs IPL only: 3/13 had good results at 8 weeks	8 weeks
Rojana-matin[154] (2006)	20% ALA, 30 minutes under occlusion/ Split-face IPL + placebo vs IPL + ALA	Face/Soap and water	3 (3–4 weeks apart)	14	IPL cutoff filter 560–590 nm, 25–30 J/cm^2	IPL + ALA: 87.7% vs IPL + placebo: 66.8% reduction of inflammatory lesions	12 weeks
Alexiades-Armenakas[155] (2006)	20% ALA, 45 minutes/ ALA topical + LP PDL or blue light vs LP PDL only vs con-ventional therapy. Superficial chemical peels in 6 patients (2 control and 4 ALA-LP PDL)	Face/ Cetaphil cleanser	1–6 (monthly)	19: 1 ALA + blue, 14 ALA + LP PDL, 4 control (2 LP PDL only and 2 conven-tional therapy)	LP PDL (595 nm, 7–7.5 J/cm^2, 6–10 ms, 10 mm spot size, blue light	ALA + LP PDL: 77% clearance rate per treatment vs LP PDL only:32% vs conventional therapy: 20%	13 months
Wiegell[156] (2006)	16.8% MAL, 3 hours under occlusion/ treatment × control group	Face/ Curettage	2 (2 weeks apart)	31 (19 treatment vs 12 control)	Noncoherent red (630 nm), 37 J/cm^2	MAL-PDT: 68% reduction of inflammatory lesions vs 0% in control	12 weeks
Wiegell[157] (2006)	Split-face 20% ALA vs 16.8% MAL, 3 hours under occlusion	Face/Not mentioned	1	15	Noncoherent red (630 nm), 37 J/cm^2, 34 mW/cm^2	59% reduction of inflammatory lesions for both MAL and ALA	12 weeks

Contd...

Contd...

Hörfelt[158] (2006)	16.8% MAL, 3 hours under occlusion/ Split-face treatment × control group	Face/ Nodular lesions were prepared using a cannula (1–2 mm)	2 (2 weeks apart)	30	Noncoherent red (630 nm), 37 J/cm^2	MAL-PDT-side: 54% clearance of inflammatory vs Control-side: 20%	10 weeks after last treatment
Gold[159] (2007)	20% ALA, 15–30 minutes	Face/ Cleanser	4 (2 weeks apart)	15	IPL (420–950 nm), 5–7 J/cm^2, 30–50 ms	54.5% reduction of inflammatory lesions	11 weeks
Akara-phanth[160] (2007)	10% ALA in acne spots, 1 hour/ Split-face blue light + ALA vs blue light alone	Face/Not mentioned	4 (1 week apart)	20	Blue LED (409–410 nm), 48 J/cm^2, 40 mW/cm^2	Blue + ALA: 71.1% reduction of inflammatory lesions vs Blue light alone: 56.7%; (no statistical difference)	16
Yeung[161] (2007)	16.8% MAL, 30 minutes/ Split-face MAL + IPL, IPL alone or control (ratio of 1:2:1); all patients used 0.1% adapalene during the study	Face/Soap followed by alcohol scrub	4 (3 weeks apart)	23 (11 with MAL-PDT)	IPL (530–750 nm), 7–9 J/cm^2	MAL-PDT: 65% reduction of inflammatory lesions vs IPL: 23% vs Control: 88% (no statistical difference)	3 months after last treatment
Hörfelt[166] (2007)	20% ALA, 3 hours/Split-area with different light doses	Face and back/Not mentioned	1	14 (9 Cheek, 5 Back)	Noncoherent red (600–730 nm), 50 mW/cm^2, 50 or 30 J/cm^2 (cheek); 50 or 70 J/cm^2 (back)	No difference in clinical results between the two doses for face and back, 8/9 patients with face acne had some improvement	10 (cheek) and 20 weeks (back)
Oh[162] (2009)	20% ALA/ Split-face 30 minutes or 3 hours incubation ALA-IPL vs IPL only	Face/Soap and 70% alcohol	3 (4 weeks apart)	20	IPL cutoff filter 590 nm, 12–15 J/cm^2	Clearance of 89.5% (3 hours), 83% (30 min) and 74% (IPL only). Long incubation group and IPL only group were statistically different	12 weeks after last treatment

Contd...

Contd...

Yin[163] (2010)	5%, 10%, 15% and 20% ALA, 1.5 hours occlusion/ Split-face ALA-PDT vs Placebo-Red light	Face/70% isopropyl alcohol	4 (10 days apart)	180	Red light (633 ± 3 nm), 126 J/cm^2	Statistically significantly more patient treated with 20% ALA achieved complete clearance, no statistical difference between 15 and 20% at 12 weeks or more	24 weeks

ALA: 5-aminolevulinic acid; IPL: Intense pulsed light; LED: Light emitting diodes; LP PDL: Long-pulsed pulsed-dye laser; PDT: Photodynamic therapy

Photodynamic Therapy with Blue Light

The blue light-PDT studies for acne treatment demonstrated a range of 25–75% decrease in inflammatory lesions[149,151,160] with the lower response (25% reduction) in patients treated with blue light alone (52P). A pilot study conducted by Taub[151] treated 18 patients with two to four treatments using short contact ALA 20% (15–30 minutes) followed by illumination with blue light or electro-optical synergy (ELOS) or both. Eleven of these patients had at least 50% improvement, and acne lesions have not recurred in 5 patients for at least 6 months of follow-up.

Goldman and Boyce[149] compared blue light with and without 20% ALA in 22 patients with mild to moderate acne. Patients were treated twice with short contact ALA-PDT/blue light (15 minutes incubation) at 2 week-interval, while patients in the blue light alone received two treatments at one-week interval. Reductions in papule count from baseline were 68% in patients treated with ALA-PDT/blue light vs 40% in the blue light alone group.

Photodynamic Therapy with Intense Pulsed Light

In 2004, Gold and colleagues[150] treated 15 patients with moderate to severe inflammatory acne with one hour of 20% ALA incubation followed by IPL (430–1,100 nm at 3–9 J/cm^2) for 4 treatments per week. The authors reported a 71.8% reduction in inflammatory lesions after 12 weeks. Subsequently, Gold and colleagues[159] evaluated 15 patients treated with 4 sessions of ALA-PDT, 2 weeks apart, using a pulsed light source (420–950 nm) and a short incubation of 15–30 minutes with 20% ALA. The total reductions of inflammatory and noninflammatory lesion counts were 54.5% and 37.5% respectively after 11 weeks.

Rojanamatin and Choawawanich[154] performed a split-face study in Thai patients, using intense pulsed light (550–700 nm) and 20% ALA. Fourteen patients received three sessions of IPL on one side and a combination of short contact (30 minutes incubation) ALA and IPL on the other side. There were very few adverse events and they observed a statistically significant improvement (87.7% vs 66.8%) in lesion counts 3 months after the last treatment for ALA-PDT and IPL only respectively.

Taub[165] compared the efficacies of intense pulsed light (680–850 nm), combination radiofrequency and intense pulsed light (580–980 nm) and blue light (417 nm) for activating ALA-induced PpIX for the treatment of acne vulgaris. All three groups used 30 minutes incubation with 20% ALA and received three treatments at 2 weeks intervals. They found IPL-PDT was superior to blue light, though the differences did not reach statistical significance. The author attributed these results to IPL's deeper penetration in the dermis compared to blue light.

Recently a randomized split-face treatment study[163] compared two different incubation times (30 minutes and 180 minutes) in 20 Korean patients with moderate to severe acne. Three sessions at 1 month intervals were performed. Twelve weeks after the third session, the reduction of inflammatory acne lesions was greater in the long incubation time group than the short incubation time group or the IPL-alone group, but this difference was statistically significant only between the long incubation group and the IPL-only group. The mean reduction of inflammatory acne lesions in the short incubation time was not statistically different from the IPL-alone group, suggesting that 30 minutes in not sufficient incubation time before PDT in acne patients. Finally, the prolonged incubation time did not result in more adverse effects than in the short incubation time group in this study.

Photodynamic Therapy with Pulsed-Dye Laser

Haedersdal and colleagues[166] compared MAL-PDL to PDL alone in 15 patients treated with 3 sessions at 2-week intervals. Twelve patients completed the study and were found to present significantly greater reduction in inflammatory lesions on the MAL-PDL side versus the PDL-alone side (80% vs 67% respectively) at 12 weeks after the final treatment. Alexiades-Armenakas[155] treated 14 patients with 20% ALA with 45 minutes incubation time followed by activation with PDL (595 nm, 7–7.5 J/cm^2, 10 ms, 10 mm spot size). Complete clearance was achieved in 100% (14/14 patients) with a mean of 2.9 treatments required to achieve complete clearance for a mean follow-up time of 6.4 months. Additionally, a decrease in erythema to acne scars was observed.

Photodynamic Therapy with Red Light Sources

Studies[145,152,156-158,162,164] investigating red light have demonstrated an overall range of 20–69% reduction of acne lesions. Hörfelt and colleagues[158] compared MAL-pretreated red light (3 hours occlusion, 635 nm, and 37 J/cm^2) therapy to red light treatment alone in 27 patients. After two treatment sessions, the authors found 54% and 20% reductions in inflammatory lesion on the red light plus MAL side and red light alone side respectively.

Wiegell and Wulf[157] conducted a randomized controlled investigator-blinded study with 15 patients to compare the efficacy and tolerability of ALA-PDT versus MAL-PDT. MAL and ALA were applied to each half of the face for 3 hours, followed by illumination with red light (635 nm, 34 mW/cm^2, 37 J/cm^2). Thirteen patients completed the study and presented at 12 weeks follow-up similar response rates for the two treatment regimens (59% reductions in inflammatory lesions). The two treatments were equally painful during illumination but ALA-PDT resulted in more prolonged and severe adverse effects after treatment.

A recent study conducted by Yin and colleagues[164] compared the efficacy and safety of different ALA concentrations in 180 Chinese patients. Patients received four sessions (10 days apart) using a variety of ALA concentrations (5%, 10%, 15% and 20%) with 1.5 hours occlusion on one side and placebo on the other side as control followed by irradiation with red light (633 ± 3 nm, 126 J/cm^2). The authors found a significant statistical difference among the four groups with different ALA concentration, with a clear positive correlation between global improvement scores and ALA concentration. However, there was no statistical difference in clinical outcomes between 15% and 20% ALA at 12 weeks of follow-up or more. Hyperpigmentation was positively correlated to the ALA concentration; therefore, the authors concluded 10% and 15% ALA for 1.5 hours, and red light source should provide ideal treatment for moderate to severe acne in patients with Fitzpatrick skin type III and IV.

Adverse Reactions and Summary of Findings for 5-Aminolevulinic Acid and Methyl Aminolevulinate-Photodynamic Therapy for Acne Vulgaris

Both ALA and MAL have shown effective with PDT for the treatment of acne. The most prevalent side effects reported in the studies were erythema, edema and pain at the time of the treatment. Other adverse reactions reported include: crusting,[149,160] photosensitivity following posttreatment sun exposure,[149,155] pustular eruptions,[156,166] and post-inflammatory hyperpigmentation.[153,161]

In conclusion, PDT has shown safety and efficacy in the treatment of inflammatory acne vulgaris with many effective light sources and photosensitizers. Unfortunately, PDT has been limited as the costs of the procedure must be borne by the patient. Clinicians should consider topical PDT in the treatment of acne particularly for those patients who are refractory to standard therapy, who have been on numerous medical therapies in the past and who are looking for clinical results to occur at a faster time interval. Further studies are warranted to establish consensus for optimal photosensitizer, ideal concentration, incubation time, activating light source and frequency of treatment.

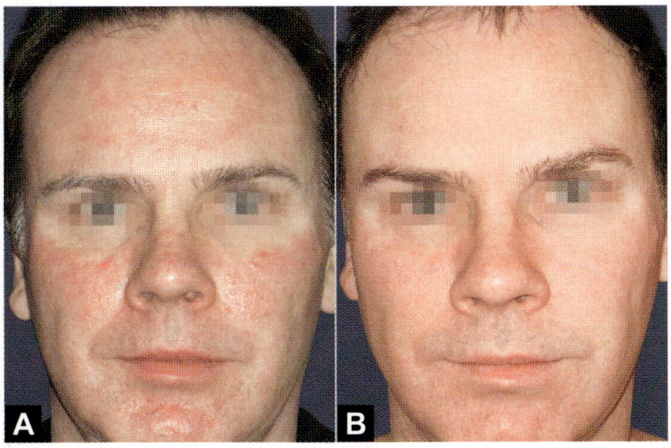

Figs 10.9A and B: Before and one month following multilaser aminolevulinic acid-photodynamic therapy in a middle-aged male with inflammatory acne vulgaris whom showed a significant improvement in inflammatory papules and pustules, facial erythema, fine lines, pore size and skin texture

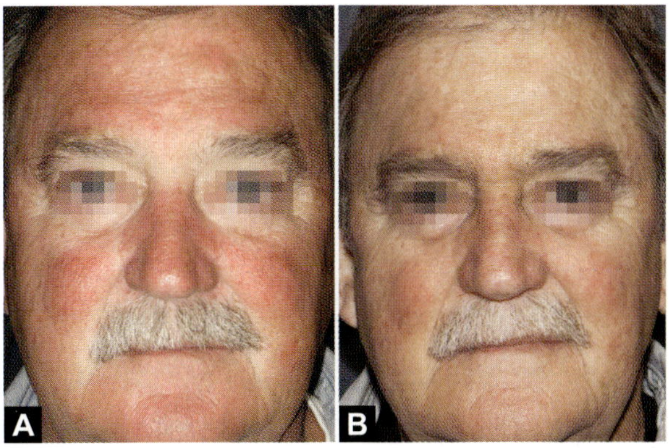

Figs 10.10A and B: Multiple aspects of acne rosacea are improved with aminolevulinic acid-photodynamic therapy. In this patient a combination of photodynamic therapy and intense pulsed light to treat facial erythema, telangiectasias and acneiform papules along with simultaneous illumination with red and blue lights for further reduction in acneiform lesions. Of note, the quality of the skin texture has improved with a reduction in the sebaceous quality of the skin

Aminolevulinic Acid-Photodynamic Therapy for Acne

The authors' treatment protocol using ALA-PDT for acne vulgaris involves the same steps described above for AKs except that they use longer incubation times (120–180 minutes). Of note, in teenagers the authors will often use 60 minutes incubation for their first treatment as the authors have anecdotally found they often have a decreased pain tolerance as compared to adults. Patients with a history of herpes simplex virus are prophylaxed with oral antivirals. One week prior to PDT patients are asked to discontinue the usage of topical retinoids, alpha hydroxy acids, beta hydroxy acids and benzoyl peroxides, and avoid chemical peels for one month prior. The authors recommend to hold PDT until the patient has been discontinued from oral retinoids for 12 months. Finally, after treatment a mineral based, noncomedogenic sunscreen is applied and patient is discharged home. Patients may resume topical acne medications once peeling is complete, approximately 5–7 days. The authors recommend a repeat treatment in 4 weeks. If there was little reaction following the initial PDT session, the incubation time should be increased. Figures 10.9 and 10.10 demonstrated clinical improvement in acne vulgaris following multilaser PDT. The authors also routinely utilize multilaser PDT in recalcitrant acne rosacea (see Fig. 10.6).

CLINICAL APPLICATIONS IN COSMETIC DERMATOLOGY

Photorejuvenation

Definition of Photoaging

Photoaging of the skin results from a combination of collective damage from ultraviolet exposure and the intrinsic aging process. The appearance can not only be concerning to the patient but also it can lead to precancerous conditions with the development of AKs.[65] Photodamaged skin is characterized by skin laxity, lines/wrinkles, hyperpigmentation, sallowness, erythema, tactile roughness, atrophy and telangiectasias.[34] Global photodamage scales have been developed for scoring the severity of skin involvement. Dover used a 5-point scale in evaluating several categories of photodamage including fine surface lines, mottled pigmentation, sallowness, tactile roughness, coarse wrinkling and global photodamage.[167] Working from this initial scale, others have added facial erythema, telangiectasias, sebaceous gland hyperplasia and facial AKs as separate categories in the evaluation of photodamage.[168,169]

Light Sources in Aminolevulinic Acid-Photodynamic Therapy Photorejuvenation

Many of the same lasers and light sources effective in ALA-PDT for the treatment of AKs have the added benefit of inducing photorejuvenative effects on the skin. Chromophores targeted during PDT treatment may include vessels, melanin and even collagen.[168] Blue light only allows for a photochemical effect in PDT with less tissue penetration than other light sources such as IPL and PDL. The latter sources penetrate deeply enough to target vessels, pigment and collagen.[88] The choice of which light source to use for ALA-PDT ultimately depends on such factors as the condition being treated, efficacy, cost of use and availability of equipment.

Treatment Results of Aminolevulinic Acid-Photodynamic Therapy and Methyl Aminolevulinate-Photodynamic Therapy in Photorejuvenation

Studies relating to the treatment of photodamage with ALA-PDT and MAL-PDT are organized in the section below according to the light source employed. A summary of these studies is provided in Table 10.6.

Table 10.6: Published clinical studies on aminolevulinic acid and methyl aminolevulinate-photodynamic therapy for photorejuvenation

Reference	*ALA Preparation*	*Location of Photodamage/Study Design*	*Incubation Period (Hours)*	*No. of Patients*	*Light Source (Emission λ, nm)*	*Response*	*Follow-up (Months)*
Ruiz-Rodriguez[65] (2002)	20% emulsion	Face and scalp, ≥1 AK and chronic photo-damage; 2 PDT sessions	4, occluded	17 (38 AKs)	IPL (590–1,200)	87% CR of AKs; excellent cosmesis	3
Goldman[53] (2003)	20% solution	Face, long-incubation PDT	15–20	32	Blue light (417)	94% CR of AKs; improved skin texture, pigmentation	3–6
Smith[66] (2003)	20% solution, 2 sessions	Face, scalp	1	35	Blue light (417) or PDL (595)	80% CR for AKs with blue light; 60% CR for PDL; both demonstrated improvement in global photodamage, tactile roughness, and hyper-pigmentation	1
Touma[9] (2004)	20% solution	Facial AK and mild-moderate photo-damage	1–3	17	Blue light (417)	Improvement in photo-damage markers, including skin quality, fine rhytides, and sallowness	1–5

Contd...

Contd...

Avram[170] (2004)	20% solution	Facial photo-damage (with AKs) treated with 1 ALA-IPL session	1	17	IPL	69% CR of AKs; improvement in telangiec-tasias, dys-pigmentation, skin texture	3
Alster[171] (2005)	20% solution	Split-face compari-son, IPL vs ALA-IPL	1–3	10	IPL (500–1,200)	ALA-IPL treated side showed greater improvement	6
Dover[167] (2005)	20% solution	Split-face compari-son, IPL vs ALA-IPL (5 treatment sessions)	0.5–1	20	IPL (515–1,200)	Greater improvement in ALA-IPL over IPL only for global photoaging, pigmentation, and fine lines only	1
Key[172] (2005)	20% solution	Face, subpurpuric doses of PDL	1	12	PDL (585)	Improvement in majority of photodamage parameters with ALA-PDL; no improvement with PDL alone	1
Lowe[173] (2005)	5–20% cream	Forearm, periorbital	0.5–2	6	Red light (633)	Mild improvement noted in photoaging	0.25
Marmur[174] (2005)	20% solution	Split-face compari-son, IPL vs ALA-IPL (1 treatment)	1	7	IPL	Microscopic changes demonstrated greater type I collagen on ALA-IPL side	N/A
Gold[169] (2006)	20% solution	Split-face com-parison, IPL vs ALA-IPL (3 treatment sessions)	0.5–1	16	IPL (550/570 cutoff filters—1,200)	ALA-IPL results superior to IPL alone	1–3
Serrano[175] (2009)	1–2% gel	Multiple application, low con-centration ALA-PDT to face, neck, hands (3 treatment sessions)	0.5–1	8/26 patients with photo-aging; 18/26 treated for acne, vitiligo	IPL (530–1,200) or yellow-red lamp (550–630)	90% of cases with hyper-pigmentation improvement; erythema (85%), skin texture (100%)	6

Contd...

Contd...

Park[176] (2010)	20% cream	Two ALA-PDT at one month interval, repeated (2 sessions) after one month if required.	4	14 with one-three AKs on the face and poto-damage	Red light (580–740 nm), dose of 100 J/cm^2, 100 mW/cm^2	82.6% CR of AKs one month after last treatment, microscopic analysis showed increased expression of type I and III procollagen, reduced elastotic material, decreased levels of MMP-1,-3 and -12	One month after last treatment
Clemen-toni[177] (2010)	20% solution	Face, pretreat-ment with a micro-needle roller followed by ALA-PDT	1	21	IPL (560 cutoff filter—1,200) and red LED light (630 nm)	Improvement in photo-damage markers, including fine lines, mottled pigmentation, sallowness, tactile rough-ness and telangiectasias	6
Xi et al.[178] (2011)	5–10% cream	Face, split-face compari-son, IPL vs ALA-IPL (3 treatment sessions) in Chinese patients	1	26	IPL (560 and 590 cutoff filter—1,200 nm)	Greater improvement in global score for photo-aging, fine lines and coarse wrink-les. PHI was higher on the ALA-IPL PDT side (22% vs 15% on the IPL-only side)	2
Reference	*MAL-PDT Study Design*	*Location of Photo-damage*	*Incubation Period (Hours)*	*No. of Patients*	*Light Source (Emission λ, nm)*	*Response*	*Follow-up (Months)*
Zane[168] (2007)	2 sessions, one month interval	Facial AK and severe photo-damage	3, occluded (2–3 tubes for each session)	20 (137 AKs)	Red LED (634 ± 3 nm, 37 J/cm^2)	88.3% CR of AKs, improvement of hyperpig-mented spots, sallowness, skin texture, and fine lines, erythema, telangiectasia, sebaceous gland hyper-trophy and deep wrinkles, showed no change	2 months after last treatment

Contd...

Contd...

Ruiz-Rodriguez[179] (2007)	2 sessions, 3 weeks apart	Perioral, pretreatment with fractional resurfacing (1,550 nm), one half followed by MAL-PDT	3, occluded	4	Red LED (634 ± 3 nm, 37 J/cm²)	Increased improvement in superficial wrinkles in 3 out of 4 patients on the combined treatment side	12 weeks after last treatment
Issa[180] (2010)	2 sessions, one month interval	Facial AK and photodamage (Glogau classification types II and III)	2, occluded (1/2 tube for each session)	14	Red LED (634 ± 3 nm, 37 J/cm²)	89.1% CR of AKs after 6 months; 10/14 patients: improvement of skin texture, wrinkles and firmness, and pigmentation; increase in collagen fibers density, and decrease in elastotic material assessed through morphometric exam 6 months after treatment	6

AKs: Actinic keratoses; ALA: 5-aminolevulinic acid; CR: Complete response; IPL: Intense pulsed light; LED: Light emitting diodes; PDL: Pulsed-dye laser; PDT: Photodynamic therapy

Photodynamic Therapy with Blue Light

Despite the shallow penetration of blue light, it still appears to improve the signs of photoaging following ALA-PDT. The first indication that blue light had photorejuvenative effects in PDT was with the phase II/III clinical trials for FDA approval of Levulan for nonhyperkeratotic AKs. In these studies, significant improvement in the signs of photoaging were noted after treatment.[48,68,181]

Goldman and Atkin[53] utilized a single session of ALA-PDT (1 hour occlusion) with a blue light source in 32 patients displayed a 72% improvement in skin texture and 59% improvement in skin pigmentation was found. Touma et al.[9] studied the effectiveness of ALA (short-contact, 1–3 hours) and blue light illumination in the treatment of AKs and diffuse photodamage. At 1 month and 5 months follow-up intervals, not only was there a significant reduction in AKs, but also there was marked improvement in photodamage parameters such as skin quality, fine wrinkling and sallowness were observed. Other markers of photodamage, such as pigmentary changes and coarse wrinkling, showed little to no improvement.

A final study by Smith and coworkers[66] as discussed in the AK section of this chapter, compared topical, low-concentration 5-FU to two forms of short-contact ALA-PDT—one arm with activation from a blue light source, the other with a PDL. While one patient in the 5-FU group discontinued due to a confluent erythematous reaction, all patients in the ALA-PDT group completed the study. In both ALA-PDT groups, patients experienced improvement in global photodamage, hyperpigmentation and tactile roughness. The ALA-PDL was more successful in treating pigmentation and blue light had lower response rates to global photoaging.

Photodynamic Therapy with Red Light

Many of the studies regarding red light PDT for the treatment of photoaging utilized MAL and have demonstrated excellent cosmetic results.[49,73] Zane and colleagues[168] evaluated MAL-PDT in 20 patients with two treatments (3 hour occlusion, red LED 37 J/cm^2) were performed at a one month interval. In addition to an 88.3% AK clearance rate, a global improvement was observed in mottled hyperpigmentation, fine lines and roughness of the skin. A clinical, histopathologic and morphometric study by Issa and colleagues[180] using MAL-PDT and red light (LED 635 nm, 37 J/cm^2) evaluated 14 patients treated with two sessions, 4 weeks apart. Clinical improvement in texture, firmness, wrinkle depth, skin coloration and AKs were observed, and histopathologic and morphometric studies were consistent, showing increased collagen fibers and decrease in the fragmented elastic fibers 6 months after treatment.

A histological and immunohistochemical analysis conducted by Park and colleagues[176] with ALA-PDT (twice at one month interval, using red light 580–740 nm, dose of 100 J/cm^2, 100 mW/cm^2) showed significant increase in type I and III procollagen expression. Elastotic material with fibrilin-1 and tropoelastin expression in the dermis decreased after treatment as well as the expression of matrix metalloproteinases-1, -3 and -12. Although the study was limited by the small sample size, those histological changes indicated restoration of photoaged skin with ALA-PDT.

Photodynamic Therapy with Intense Pulsed Light

Intense pulsed light treatments improve many of the signs of photoaging, including pigmentation in the form of solar lentigines, erythema and telangiectasias due to vascular ectasia/damage, as well as fine wrinkling.[36] Like the PDL, IPL treatments also promote neocollagenesis.[182] Although IPL alone has been proven effective in the treatment of photodamage, the addition of ALA to IPL treatment (ALA-IPL) appears to be more effective in treating photodamaged skin. Clinical examples of ALA-IPL treatment for photorejuvenation are illustrated in Figures 10.11 and 10.12.

In 2002, Ruiz-Rodriguez et al.[65] investigated the treatment of photodamage and AKs using two treatments of ALA-PDT with IPL as the light source for photorejuvenation. One month apart, treatments were well tolerated. At 3 months follow-up, 87% of AKs disappeared and marked cosmetic improvement was noted in wrinkling, coarse skin texture, pigmentary changes and telangiectasias. Avram and Goldman[170] evaluated the combined use of ALA-IPL for the treatment of photorejuvenation and AKs with one treatment session. Sixty-nine percent of the AKs responded to the use of ALA-IPL. Patients displayed a 69% AK clearance rate, a 55% improvement in telangiectasias, 48% improvement in pigment irregularities and 25% improvement in skin texture.

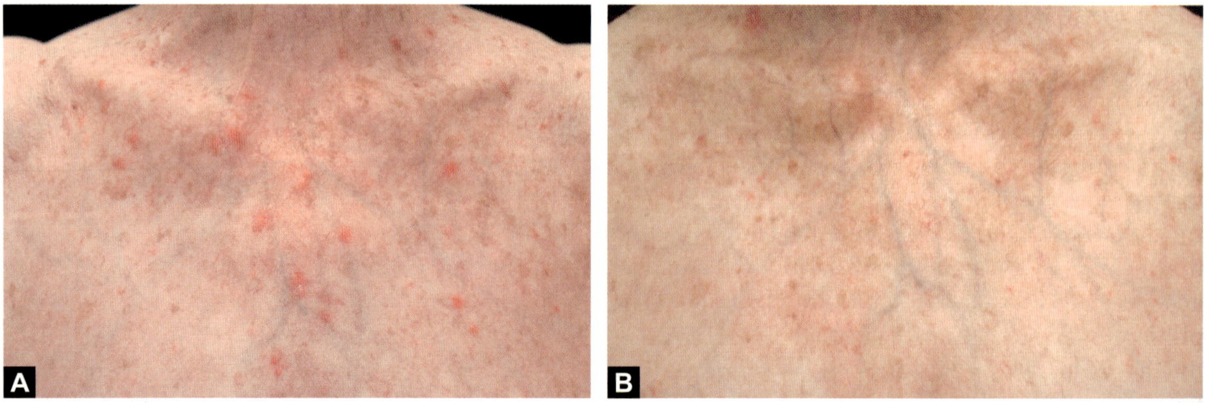

Figs 10.11A and B: (A) Multiple actinic keratoses (AKs) and extensive photodamage to a middle-aged female; (B) Following three treatments of multilaser aminolevulinic acid-photodynamic therapy utilizing pulsed-dye laser, intense pulsed light, and blue and red lights. Note the improvement in the presence of AKs, solar lentigines, sallowness and skin texture

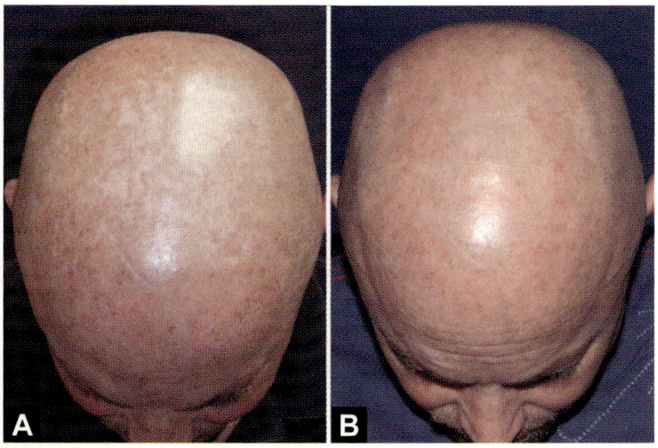

Figs 10.12A and B: Four treatments at yearly intervals of aminolevulinic acid-photodynamic therapy to the scalp. A combined reduction in photodamage and actinic keratoses is seen in the image at right taken four years following the last treatment

Alster and colleagues[171] also examined the use of IPL in ALA-PDT. Clinical improvement scores were noted to be higher on the side of the face treated with the combination of ALA-IPL. They concluded that the combination of topical 5 ALA + IPL is safe and more effective than IPL alone for the treatment of facial rejuvenation. A similar split-face study by Dover et al.[167] treated 20 subjects with 3 split-face treatments 3 weeks apart. They concluded, ALA-IPL resulted in greater improvement in global photoaging (80% vs 50%) and mottled pigmentation (95% vs 65%). Successful results were also noted for fine lines for the ALA-IPL side compared to the IPL side alone (55% vs 20%). Although tactile roughness and sallowness were noticeably better, pretreatment with ALA did not enhance the results of using IPL alone. Marmur et al.[174] demonstrated a greater increase in type I collagen was noted in the subjects receiving ALA-IPL as opposed to IPL alone.

Photodynamic Therapy with Pulsed-Dye Laser

Pulsed dye lasers have also been studied as a light source for photorejuvenation in ALA-PDT. PDL targets oxyhemoglobin as a chromophore according to the theory of selective photothermolysis. But thermal energy generated in the surrounding areas adjacent to targeted blood vessels may also result in photorejuvenative effects. Subpurpuric doses from the PDL alter dermal collagen and may improve skin texture.[36] Alexiades-Armenakas et al.[54] found ALA-PDT with the 595 nm PDL was successful in treating face and scalp AKs and photorejuvenation.

Key[172] treated 14 patients with long-incubation ALA (12 hours) followed by photoactivation using a PDL. Improvement was noted following ALA-PDL in terms of skin texture, tactile quality and brown spots, although the degree of vascularity and seborrheic keratoses were unaffected by treatment. The lack of improvement in blood vessel lesions in this study is curious given that PDL targets the vasculature.

Combination Therapy for Photorejuvenation

A combination of microneedling roller (108 m in width and 300 μm in depth) prior to ALA incubation (1 hour) to maximize epidermal penetration and irradiation of both red light (630 nm) and broadband pulsed light in a single treatment has been studied in 21 patients by Clementoni and colleagues.[177] At 6 months post treatment, 76.2% scored themselves an overall improvement greater than 75% and statistically significant improvement was observed in the global photoaging scores, fine lines, mottled pigmentation, sallowness, tactile roughness and telangiectasias at 3 months post treatment.

Enhanced efficacy of PDT after fractional resurfacing was observed by Ruiz-Rodriguez[179] in four patients treated in the perioral area. First the 1,550 nm fractional nonablative laser was applied periorally, immediately followed by MAL-PDT (3 hours occlusion, illumination with red LED 634 nm, 37 J/cm^2) on half of the perioral area. Two treatment sessions were administered, three weeks apart. Twelve weeks after the last treatment, a blinded investigator found increased improvement in superficial wrinkles in 3 out of 4 patients on the combined treatment side as compared to the 1,550 fractional laser alone. A recent study by Haedersdal and colleagues has demonstrated enhanced delivery of topical MAL deeply into in vivo porcine skin with ablative fractional CO_2 laser.[183]

Summary of Findings for ALA-PDT in Actinic Keratoses Treatment and Photorejuvenation

These results show the potential usefulness of a variety of lasers and light sources in the treatment of AKs and in the improvement of photodamage and photorejuvenation utilizing 5-ALA and MAL based PDT treatments. Current studies have been focused on novel photosensitizer drugs and reformulations of ALA, such as nanoemulsions or patch-based applicators, with 5-ALA patch PDT appearing to be superior to cryosurgery in the treatment of mild to moderate AK.[184] Beyond the treatment of AKs, ALA and MAL-PDT offer beneficial cosmetic outcomes in photorejuvenation.

Aminolevulinic Acid-Photodynamic Therapy for Photorejuvenation

For photorejuvenation, the authors use the identical protocol as they have previously described above for the treatment of AKs. Treatment is repeated in 4–8 weeks. If little reaction was noted following the initial PDT, the authors recommend to increase the incubation time, gently increase the fluence on IPL settings, or re-evaluate your skin preparation technique. Finally, the authors counsel their patients to expect 3–4 sessions of PDT when treating photorejuvenation, especially when sebaceous hyperplasia is present. These recommendations are consistent with the recommendations of the American Society of Photodynamic Therapy.[25]

PRACTICAL CONSIDERATIONS IN PHOTODYNAMIC THERAPY

Patient Selection for Aminolevulinic Acid-Photodynamic Therapy

Thoughtful selection of eligible patients for ALA-PDT benefits both physician and patient. Patients should be carefully screened at an initial clinical consultation for inclusion and exclusion criteria for PDT. Physicians should gauge, whether a patient has an accurate understanding and realistic expectations of the procedure. This will maximize patient results, reduce patient anxiety and ensure the PDT is conducted smoothly on the day of the procedure. A comprehensive consent that explains the risks, benefits and complications of therapy as well as treatment alternatives should be reviewed with patients carefully prior to treatment.

Exclusion Criteria

Patients should be screened for important exclusion criteria prior to undergoing PDT. A history of photosensitivity including porphyria, photodermatoses and photosensitizing medication use should preclude treatment.[53,61,168] Many studies have excluded patients from treatment if they have undergone treatment with systemic retinoids, chemotherapeutic agents or immunotherapy in the past 6 months.[48,61,173] Pregnant or nursing women and individuals with an active infection should not undergo treatment.[48,71] Jefferies et al. recommended patients refrain from topical retinoids, alpha hydroxy acids and chemical peels approximately 1 month prior to treatment.[61]

Safety, Adverse Effects and Complications of Photodynamic Therapy

Expected side effects following PDT are related to the phototoxic nature of treatment and are usually mild in nature. Pain and burning may be experienced during light irradiation. The precise mechanism of pain is not fully elucidated but likely involves nerve stimulation and/or tissue damage.[185] Shorter incubation times decrease the severity of side effects. Expected phototoxic side effects include erythema, edema, stinging/burning, pruritus and crusting. Pigmentary changes, whealing and vesiculation may also occur.[28,49,71] Erythema and mild crusting occur in most patients following treatment, usually resolving in 1–2 weeks (Figs 10.13A to H).[82] Hypopigmentation is rare, and hyperpigmentation, with an incidence as high as 27% following ALA-PDT,[71] is usually mild in nature. More pronounced reactions are correlated with disease burden. Typically, repeat treatments are less painful than previous ones.

In patients with extensive phototoxic reactions, especially in cases when patients are exposed to UV radiation in the 24–36 hours following treatment, topical therapy may be necessary to address erythema, edema and crusting. Topical steroid creams and ice packs may be used on the treated area until the symptoms subside. All patients should be screened for a history of cold sores and appropriate HSV prophylaxis begun prior to treatment in such cases.[5]

Pain management, especially with shorter incubation times (e.g. 1 hour), is usually a nonissue. Reassurance to the patient and "talk-esthesia" by a caring member of the clinical staff is usually more than adequate to comfort any patient anxiety and pain. However, the use of cooling fans, Avene Thermal Water Spray, forced air cooling systems, Xylocaine spray, and even oral non-narcotic pain medication have been used successfully to mitigate pain during ALA-PDT.[9,71,82]

A review study by Warren and colleagues[185] of 43 articles consisting of clinical PDT trials (2000–2008)

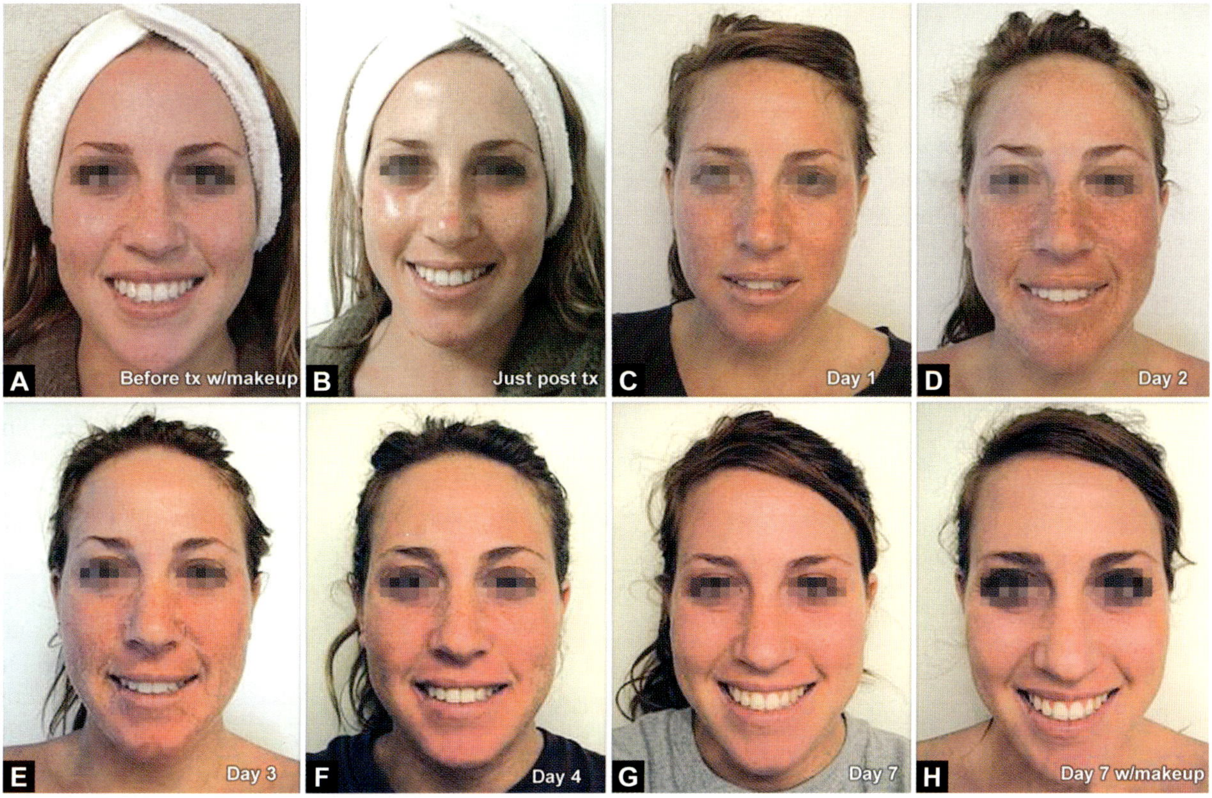

Figs 10.13A to H: Healing progression over 1 week in a young adult female with acne vulgaris following multilaser aminolevulinic acid-photodynamic therapy. Erythema and edema predominate in the first 2–3 days, followed by crusting and peeling which resolve in most instances within 1–2 weeks

that used ALA or MAL was performed to summarize the effectiveness of interventions to reduce ALA-PDT related pain and to explore contributing factors to pain induction. Their consensus opinion is that, in general, topical anesthetics do not work and cooling the skin with either ice water or with a high-airflow cooling device (such as Zimmer Medizin Systems, Irvine, CA) represents the best topical intervention to control the pain during PDT. They also found that pain intensity is associated with lesion size and location; certain diagnoses, particularly plaque-type psoriasis, appear to generate the highest PDT-related pain scores. Inconsistent results were encountered for the correlation of pain with light source, wavelength of light, fluence rate and total light dose.

Although the use of forced airflow cooling device (ACD) appears to be effective in reducing pain during PDT, a recent nonrandomized retrospective observational controlled study conducted by Tyrrell and colleagues[186] demonstrated that patients using ACD throughout treatment presented significantly less PpIX photobleaching than the control group. The one hundred lesions (in 100 patients) investigated in this study included: 39 AK, 29 sBCC and 32 SCCIS. After comparing the data from 50 patients who utilized the ACD throughout irradiation with the 50 patients not requiring any pain relief, the authors found 82% complete response in the non-ACD group versus only 68% complete response in the ACD group (including all three lesion types). As demonstrated by previous studies,[187,188] the level of PpIX photobleaching correlates to cell death, and therefore, tumor clearance rates and might be the reason that utilization of the ACD during light irradiation lowers the potential efficacy of the treatment. Furthermore, AK lesions using the ACD were more susceptible to reduced PpIX photobleaching when compared with PpIX accumulation indicating a potential reduction in treatment efficacy. It is proposed that the low temperature of air used may cause local vasoconstriction, reducing reactive oxygen species production and thus limiting clinical effectiveness.

Patients should be counseled to practice strict photoprotection for 24–36 hours following treatment.

Titanium dioxide and zinc oxide-containing sunblocks are preferred, in addition to protective clothing and sunglasses. Excessive UV radiation from sunlight, as well as intense spotlights, photocopy machines, photographic flashlights and medical examining lights/lamps should be avoided during the period of photosensitivity. Indoor light is usually not a concern, but patients should avoid bright sources of light, even while indoors.[28]

Not unexpectedly, if patients require a second treatment, the adverse effects as well as treatment pain are usually much less than those experienced with the initial treatment. The authors believe that the decrease is due to the resolution of most of the clinical and subclinical photodamage which occurs during the initial treatment.

CONCLUSION

Photodynamic therapy is a safe and effective treatment for nonhyperkeratotic lesions. Although FDA approved for use with a blue and red light source, other laser and light sources have demonstrated promise in the treatment of AKs during PDT. Shorter incubation times maintain AK clearance rates but decrease the occurrence of phototoxic adverse events. With careful patient selection, PDT allows selective field treatment of precancerous skin lesions with improvement in overall photodamage. Patient satisfaction is high and cosmetic results can be excellent. Strong evidence confirms the high efficacy of topical PDT in BD, sBCC, thin nBCC and acne following lesion preparation, as demonstrated by recent comparison studies.

REFERENCES

1. Kennedy JC, Pottier RH, Pross DC, et al. Photodynamic therapy with endogenous protoporphyrin IX: basic principles and present clinical experiences. J Photochem Photobiol B. 1990;6:143-8.
2. Peng Q, Warloe T, Berg K, et al. 5-Aminolevulinic acid-based photodynamic therapy. Clinical research and future challenges. Cancer. 1997;79:2282-308.
3. Soret JL. Recherches sur l'absorption des rayons ultra violets par diverses substances. Arch Sci Phys Nat. 1883;10:430-85.
4. Calzavara-Pinton PG, Venturini M, Sala R. Photodynamic therapy: Update 2006. Part 1: Photochemistry and photobiology. J Eur Acad Dermatol Venereol. 2007;21:293-302.
5. Nootheti PK, Goldman MP. Aminolevulinic acid-photodynamic therapy for photorejuvenation. Dermatol Clin. 2007;25:35-45.
6. Ericson MB, Sandberg C, Stenquist B, et al. Photodynamic therapy of actinic keratosis at varying fluence rates: Assessment of photobleaching, pain and primary clinical outcome. Br J Dermatol. 2004;151:1204-12.
7. Nakaseko H, Kobayashi M, Akita Y, et al. Histological changes and involvement of apoptosis after photodynamic therapy for actinic keratoses. Br J Dermatol. 2003;148:122-7.
8. Wolf P, Rieger E, Kerl H. Topical photodynamic therapy with endogenous porphyrins after application of 5-aminolevulinic acid. J Am Acad Dermatol. 1993;28:17-21.
9. Touma D, Yaar M, Whitehead S, et al. A trial of short incubation, broad-area photodynamic therapy for facial actinic keratoses and diffuse photodamage. Arch Dermatol. 2004;140:33-40.
10. Tsai T, Ji HT, Chiang PC, et al. ALA-PDT results in phenotypic changes and decreased cellular invasion in surviving cancer cells. Lasers Surg Med. 2009;41:305-15.
11. Gad F, Viau G, Boushira M, et al. Photodynamic therapy with 5-aminolevulinic acid induces apoptosis and caspase activation in malignant T cells. J Cutan Med Surg. 2001;5:8-13.
12. Kuzelova K, Grebenova D, Pluskalova M, et al. Early apoptotic features of K562 cell death induced by 5-aminolaevulinic acid-based photodynamic therapy. J Photochem Photobiol B. 2004;73:67-78.
13. Noodt BB, Berg K, Stokke T, et al. Apoptosis and necrosis induced with light and 5-aminolaevulinic acid derived protoporphyrin IX. Br J Cancer. 1996;74:22-9.
14. Webber J, Luo Y, Crilly R, et al. An apoptotic response to photodynamic therapy with endogenous protoporphyrin in vivo. J Photochem Photobiol B. 1996; 35:209-11.
15. Dougherty TJ, Gomer CJ, Henderson BW, et al. Photodynamic therapy. J Natl Cancer Inst. 1998; 90:889-905.
16. Henderson BW, Dougherty TJ. How does photodynamic therapy work? Photochem Photobiol. 1992; 55:145-57.
17. Wieman TJ, Fingar VH. Photodynamic therapy. Surg Clin North Am. 1992;72:609-22.
18. Klausner JM, Paterson IS, Kobzik L, et al. Oxygen free radicals mediate ischemia-induced lung injury. Surgery. 1989;105:192-9.
19. Doukas J, Hechtman HB, Shepro D. Vasoactive amines and eicosanoids interactively regulate both polymorphonuclear leukocyte diapedesis and albumin permeability in vitro. Microvasc Res. 1989; 37:125-37.
20. Krosl G, Korbelik M, Dougherty GJ. Induction of immune cell infiltration into murine SCCVII tumor by photofrin-based photodynamic therapy. Br J Cancer. 1995;71:549-55.

21. Gollnick SO, Liu X, Owczarczak B, et al. Altered expression of interleukin 6 and interleukin 10 as a result of photodynamic therapy in vivo. Cancer Res. 1997;57:3904-9.
22. Korbelik M. Induction of tumor immunity by photodynamic therapy. J Clin Laser Med Surg. 1996; 14:329-34.
23. Canti G, Lattuada D, Nicolin A, et al. Antitumor immunity induced by photodynamic therapy with aluminium phthalocyanine and laser light. Anticancer Drugs. 1994;5:443-7.
24. MacCormack MA. Photodynamic therapy in dermatology: An update on applications and outcomes. Semin Cutan Med Surg. 2008;27:52-62.
25. Nestor MS, Gold MH, Kauvar ANB, et al. The use of photodynamic therapy in dermatology: Results of a consensus conference. J Drugs Dermatol. 2006; 5:140-54.
26. Product information (package insert): Levulan (R) Kerastick (TM) (aminolevulinic acid HCl) for topical solution, 20%. DUSA Pharmaceuticals, Inc., Wilmington, MA, USA; 2009.
27. Fotinos N, Campo MA, Popowycz F, et al. 5-aminolevulinic acid derivatives in photomedicine: Characteristics, application and perspectives. Photochem Photobiol. 2006;82:994-1015.
28. Kalka K, Merk H, Mukhtar H. Photodynamic therapy in dermatology. J Am Acad Dermatol. 2000;42: 389-413.
29. Gaullier JM, Berg K, Peng Q, et al. Use of 5-aminolevulinic acid esters to improve photodynamic therapy on cells in culture. Cancer Res. 1997;57:1481-6.
30. Borelli C, Herzinger T, Merk K, et al. Effect of subcutaneous infiltration anesthesia on pain in photodynamic therapy: a controlled open pilot trial. Dermatol Surg. 2007;33:314-8.
31. Kasche A, Luderschmidt S, Ring J, et al. Photodynamic therapy induces less pain in patients treated with methyl aminolevulinate compared to aminolevulinic acid. J Drugs Dermatol. 2006;5:353-6.
32. Goldberg DJ. Photodynamic therapy in skin rejuvenation. Clin Dermatol. 2008;26:608-13.
33. Nakano A, Tamada Y, Watanabe D, et al. A pilot study to assess the efficacy of photodynamic therapy for Japanese patients with actinic keratosis in relation to lesion size and histological severity. Photodermatol Photoimmunol Photomed. 2009;25:37-40.
34. Zakhary K, Ellis DAF. Applications of aminolevulinic acid-based photodynamic therapy in cosmetic facial plastic practices. Facial Plast Surg. 2005;21:110-16.
35. Clark C, Bryden A, Dawe R, et al. Topical 5-aminolevulinic acid photodynamic therapy for cutaneous lesions: outcome and comparison of light sources. Photodermatol Photoimmunol Photomed. 2003; 19:134-41.
36. DeHoratius DM, Dover JS. Nonablative tissue remodeling and photorejuvenation. Clin Dermatol. 2007;25:474-9.
37. Markham T, Collins P. Topical 5-aminolaevulinic acid photodynamic therapy for extensive scalp actinic keratoses. Brit J Dermatol. 2001;145:502-4.
38. Kalisiak MS, Rao J. Photodynamic therapy for actinic keratoses. Dermatol Clin. 2007;25:15-23.
39. Marks R. Epidemiology of nonmelanoma skin cancer and solar keratoses in Australia: A tale of self-immolation in Elysian fields. Australas J Dermatol. 1997;38:S26-9.
40. Diepgen TL, Mahler V. The epidemiology of skin cancer. Br J Dermatol. 2002;146:1-6.
41. Osborne JE. Skin cancer screening and surveillance. Br J Dermatol. 2002;146:745-54.
42. Marks R, Rennie G, Selwood TS. Malignant transformation of solar keratoses to squamous cell carcinoma. Lancet. 1988;1:795-7.
43. Glogau RG. The risk of progression to invasive disease. J Am Acad Dermatol. 2000;42(1 Pt 2):23-4.
44. Lehmann P. Methyl aminolaevulinate-photodynamic therapy: A review of clinical trials in the treatment of actinic keratoses and nonmelanoma skin cancer. Brit J Dermatol. 2007;156:793-801.
45. Berking C, Herzinger T, Flaig MJ, et al. The efficacy of photodynamic therapy in actinic cheilitis of the lower lip: A prospective study of 15 patients. Dermatol Surg. 2007;33:825-30.
46. Ortonne JP. From actinic keratoses to squamous cell carcinoma. Br J Dermatol. 2002;146:S20-S23.
47. Hurwitz RM, Monger LE. Solar keratosis: an evolving squamous cell carcinoma. Benign or malignant? Dermatol Surg. 1995;21:184.
48. Jeffes EW, McCullough JL, Weinstein GD, et al. Photodynamic therapy of actinic keratoses with topical aminolevulinic acid hydrochloride and fluorescent blue light. J Am Acad Dermatol. 2001;45: 96-104.
49. Szeimies RM, Karrer S, Radakovic-Fijan S, et al. Photodynamic therapy using topical methyl 5-aminolevulinate compared with cryotherapy for actinic keratosis: A prospective, randomized study. J Am Acad Dermatol. 2002;47:258-62.
50. Gold MH. Pharmacoeconomic analysis of the treatment of multiple actinic keratoses. J Drugs Dermatol. 2008;7:23-5.
51. Kurwa HA, Yong-Gee SA, Seed PT, et al. A randomized paired comparison of photodynamic therapy and topical 5-fluorouracil in the treatment of actinic keratoses. J Am Acad Dermatol. 1999;41:414-8.
52. Tierney EP, Eide MJ, Jacobsen, et al. Photodynamic therapy for actinic keratoses: Survey of patient perceptions of treatment satisfaction and outcomes. J Cosm Laser Ther. 2008;10:81-6.
53. Goldman MP, Atkin DH. ALA/PDT in the treatment of actinic keratosis: spot versus confluent therapy. J Cosmetic Laser Ther. 2003;5:107-10.
54. Alexiades-Amenakas MR, Geronemus RG. Laser-mediated photodynamic therapy of actinic keratoses. Arch Dermatol. 2003;139;1313-20.

55. Dijkstra AT, Majoie IML, van Dongen JWF, et al. Photodynamic therapy with violet light and topical δ-aminolaevulinic acid in the treatment of actinic keratosis, Bowen's disease and basal cell carcinoma. J Eur Acad Dermatol Venereol. 2001;15:550-4.
56. Morton CA, Whitehurst C, Moseley H, et al. Development of an alternative light source to lasers for photodynamic therapy: Clinical evaluation in the treatment of pre-malignant non-melanoma skin cancer. Lasers Med Sci. 1995;10:165-71.
57. Fijan S, Honigsmann H, Ortel B. Photodynamic therapy of epithelial skin tumors with delta-aminolaevulinic acid and desferrioxamine. Br J Dermatol. 1995;133;282-8.
58. Szeimies RM, Karrer S, Sauerwald A, et al. Photodynamic therapy with topical application of 5-aminolevulinic acid in the treatment of actinic keratoses: An initial clinical study. Dermatol. 1996; 192:246-51.
59. Fink-Puches R, Hofer A, Smolle J, et al. Primary clinical response and long-term follow-up of solar keratoses treated with topically applied 5-aminolevulinic acid and irradiation by different wave bands of light. J Photochem Photobiol. 1997;41:145-51.
60. Fritsch C, Stege H, Saalmann G, et al. Green light is effective and less painful than red light in photodynamic therapy of facial solar keratoses. Photodermatol Photoimmunol Photomed. 1997;13:181-5.
61. Jeffes WJ, McCullagh JL, Weinstein GD, et al. Photodynamic therapy of actinic keratosis with topical 5-aminolaevulinic acid. Arch Dermatol. 1997;133:727-32.
62. Karrer S, Bäumler W, Abels C, et al. Long-pulse dye laser for photodynamic therapy: Investigations in vitro and in vivo. Lasers Surg Med. 1999;25:51-9.
63. Itoh Y, Nineomiya Y, Henta T, et al. Topical delta-aminolevulinic acid-based photodynamic therapy for Japanese actinic keratoses. J Dermatol. 2000; 27:513-8.
64. Varma S, Wilson H, Kurwa HA, Gambles B, et al. Bowen's disease, solar keratoses and superficial basal cell carcinomas treated by photodynamic therapy using a large-field incoherent light source. Br J Dermatol. 2001;144:567-74.
65. Ruiz-Rodriguez R, Sanz-Sánchez T, Córdoba S. Photodynamic photorejuvenation. Dermatol Surg. 2002;28:742-4.
66. Smith S, Piacquadio D, Morhenn V, et al. Short incubation PDT versus 5-FU in treating actinic keratoses. J Drugs Dermatol. 2003;2:629-35.
67. Dragieva G, Hafner J, Dummer R, et al. Topical photodynamic therapy in the treatment of actinic keratoses and Bowen's disease in transplant recipients. Transplantation, 2004;17:115-21.
68. Piacquadio DJ, Chen DM, Farber HF, et al. Photodynamic therapy with aminolevulinic acid topical solution and visible blue light in the treatment of multiple actinic keratoses of the face and scalp: Investigator-blinded, phase 3, multicenter trials. Arch Dermatol. 2004;140:41-6.
69. Gilbert D. Treatment of actinic keratoses with sequential combination of 5-fluorouracil and photodynamic therapy. J Drugs Dermatol. 2005;4:161-3.
70. Kim HS, Yoo JY, Cho KH, et al. Topical photodynamic therapy using intense pulsed light for treatment of actinic keratosis: Clinical and histopathologic evaluation. Dermatol Surg. 2005;31:33-7.
71. Tschen EH, Wong DS, Pariser DM, et al. Photodynamic therapy using aminolaevulinic acid for patients with nonhyperkeratotic actinic keratoses of the face and scalp: Phase IV mulicentre clinical trial with 12-month follow up. Brit J Dermatol. 2006; 155:1262-9.
72. Freeman M, Vinciullo C, Francis D, et al. A comparison of photodynamic therapy using topical methyl aminolevulinate (Metvix) with single cycle cryotherapy in patients with actinic keratosis: a prospective, randomized study. J Dermatolog Treat. 2003;14:99-106.
73. Pariser DM, Lowe NJ, Stewart DM, et al. Photodynamic therapy with topical methyl aminolevulinate for actinic keratosis: results of a prospective randomized multicenter trial. J Am Acad Dermatol. 2003;48:227-32.
74. Dragieva G, Prinz BM, Hafner J, et al. A randomized controlled clinical trial of topical photodynamic therapy with methyl aminolaevulinate in the treatment of actinic keratosis in transplant patients. Br J Dermatol. 2004;151:196-200.
75. Tarstedt M, Rosdahl I, Berne B, et al. A randomized multicenter study to compare two treatment regimens of topical methyl aminolevulinate (Metvix)-PDT in actinic keratosis of the face and scalp. Acta Derm Venereol. 2005;85:424-8.
76. Morton CA, Campbell S, Gupta G, et al. Intraindividual, right-left comparison of topical methyl aminolaevulinate-photodynamic therapy and cryotherapy in subjects with actinic keratoses: a multicentre, randomized controlled study. Br J Dermatol. 2006;155:1029-36.
77. Perrett CM, McGregor JM, Warwick J, et al. Treatment of posttransplant premalignant skin disease: a randomized intrapatient comparative study of 5-fluorouracil cream and topical photodynamic therapy. Br J Dermatol. 2007;156(2):320-8.
78. Kaufmann R, Spelman L, Weightman W, et al. Multicentre intraindividual randomized trial of topical methyl aminolaevulinate photodynamic therapy vs cryotherapy for multiple actinic keratoses on the extremities. Br J Dermatol. 2008;158:994-9.
79. Palm MD, Goldman MP. Safety and efficacy comparison of blue versus red light sources for photodynamic therapy using methyl aminolevulinate in photodamaged skin. J Drugs Dermatol. 2011;10: 53-60.

80. Ross EV, Anderson RR. Laser-tissue interactions. In: Goldman MP (Ed.). Cutaneous and Cosmetic Laser Surgery. Philadelphia: Elsevier; 2006. p. 1-26.
81. Ormrod D, Jarvis B. Topical aminolevulinic acid HCl photodynamic therapy. Am J Clin Dermatol. 2000;2:133-9.
82. Moseley H, Ibbotson S, Woods J, et al. Clinical and research applications of photodynamic therapy in dermatology: Experience of the Scottish PDT centre. Lasers Surg Med. 2006;38:403-16.
83. Vatve M, Ortonne JP, Birch-Machin MA, et al. Management of field change in actinic keratosis. Br J Dermatol. 2007;157 (Suppl 2):21-4.
84. Szeimies RM, Matheson RT, Davis SA, et al. Topical Methyl aminolevulinate photodynamic therapy using red light-emitting diode light for multiple actinic keratoses: a randomized study. Dermatol Surg. 2009;35:586-92.
85. Serra-Guillen C, Nagore E, Hueso L, et al. A randomized comparative study of tolerance and satisfaction in the treatment of actinic keratosis of the face and scalp between 5% imiquimod cream and photodynamic therapy with methylaminolaevulinate. Br J Dermatol. 2011;164:429-33.
86. Martin G. Prospective, case-based assessment of sequential therapy with topical fluorouracil cream 0.5% and ALA-PDT for the treatment of actinic keratosis. J Drugs Dermatol. 2011;10(4):372-8.
87. Shaffelburg M. Treatment of actinic keratoses with sequential use of photodynamic therapy and imiquimod 5% cream. J Drugs Dermatol. 2009; 8:35-9.
88. Uebelhoer NS, Dover J. Photodynamic therapy for cosmetic applications. Dermatol Ther. 2005;18: 242-52.
89. Lee WR, Tsai RY, Fang CL, et al. Microdermabrasion as a novel tool to enhance drug delivery via the skin: an animal study. Dermatol Surg. 2006;32:1013-22.
90. Katz BE, Truong S, Maiwald DC, et al. Efficacy of microdermabrasion preceding ALA application in reducing the incubation time of ALA in laser PDT. J Drugs Dermatol. 2007;6:140-2.
91. Albert MR, Weinstock MA. Keratinocyte carcinoma. CA Cancer J Clin. 2003;53:292-302.
92. Szeimies RM, Morton CA, Sidoroff A, et al. Photodynamic therapy for nonmelanoma skin cancer. Acta Derm Venereol (Stockh). 2005;85:483-90.
93. Morton CA, Brown SB, Collins S, et al. Guidelines for topical photodynamic therapy: report of a workshop of the British Photodermatology Group. Br J Dermatol. 2002;146:552-67.
94. Morton CA, Whitehurst C, Moseley H, et al. Comparison of photodynamic therapy with cryotherapy in the treatment of Bowen's disease. Br J Dermatol. 1996;135:766-71.
95. Salim A, Leman JA, McColl JH, et al. Randomized comparison of photodynamic therapy with topical 5-fluorouracil in Bowen's disease. Br J Dermatol. 2003;148:539-43.
96. Morton CA, Whitehurst C, Moore JV, et al. Comparison of red and green light in the treatment of Bowen's disease by photodynamic therapy. Br J Dermatol. 2000;143:767-72.
97. Leman JA, Mackie RM, Morton CA. Recurrence rates following aminolaevulinic acid photodynamic therapy for intraepidermal squamous cell carcinoma compare favourably with outcome following conventional modalities. Br J Dermatol. 2002;147(Suppl 62):35.
98. Morton CA, Whitehurst C, McColl JH, et al. Photodynamic therapy for large or multiple patches of Bowen disease and basal cell carcinoma. Arch Dermatol. 2001;137(3):319-24.
99. Morton C, Horn M, Leman J, et al. Comparison of topical methyl aminolevulinate photodynamic therapy with cryotherapy or fluoracil for treatment of squamous cell carcinoma in situ. Arch Dermatol. 2006;142:729-35.
100. Morton CA, Horn M, Leman J, et al. A randomized, placebo-controlled, European study comparing MAL-PDT with cryotherapy and 5-fluorouracil in subjects with Bowen's disease. J Eur Acad Dermatol Venereol. 2004;18(Suppl 2):415.
101. Thestrup-Pedersen K, Ravnborg L, Reymann F. Morbus Bowen. A description of the disease in 617 patients. Acta Derm Venereol. 1988;68:236-9.
102. Morton CA, McKenna KE, Rhodes LE, et al. Guidelines for topical photodynamic therapy: update. Br J Dermatol. 2008;159(6):1245-66.
103. Braathen LR, Szeimies RM, Basset-Seguin N, et al. Guidelines on the use of photodynamic therapy for nonmelanoma skin cancer: an international consensus. International Society for Photodynamic Therapy in Dermatology, 2005. J Am Acad Dermatol. 2007;56(1):125-43.
104. McCormack CJ, Kelly JW, Dorevitch AP. Differences in age and body site distribution of the histological subtypes of basal cell carcinoma. A possible indicator of differing causes. Arch Dermatol. 1997;133:593-6.
105. Calzavara-Pinton PG. Repetitive photodynamic therapy with topical delta-aminolaevulinic acid as an appropriate approach to the routine treatment of superficial non-melanoma skin tumours. J Photochem Photobiol B. 1995;29:53-7.
106. Wennberg AM, Lindholm LE, Alpsten M, et al. Treatment of superficial basal cell carcinomas using topically applied delta-aminolaevulinic acid and a filtered xenon lamp. Arch Dermatol Res. 1996;288(10):561-4.
107. Fink-Puches R, Soyer HP, Hofer A, et al. Long-term follow-up and histological changes of superficial nonmelanoma skin cancers treated with topical delta-aminolevulinic acid photodynamic therapy. Arch Dermatol. 1998;134:821-6.

108. Haller JC, Cairnduff F, Slack G, et al. Routine double treatments of superficial basal cell carcinomas using aminolaevulinic acid-based photodynamic therapy. Br J Dermatol. 2000;143:1270-5.
109. Soler AM, Angell-Petersen E, Warloe T, et al. Photodynamic therapy of superficial basal cell carcinoma with 5-aminolevulinic acid with dimethylsulfoxide and ethylediaminetetraacetic acid: a comparison of two light sources. J Photochen Photobiol. 2000;71:724-9.
110. Wang I, Bendsoe N, Klinteberg CA, et al. Photodynamic therapy vs cryosurgery of basal cell carcinomas: results of a phase III clinical trial. Br J Dermatol. 2001;144(4):832-40.
111. Soler AM, Warloe T, Berner A, et al. A follow-up study of recurrence and cosmesis in completely responding superficial and nodular basal cell carcinomas treated with methyl 5-aminolaevulinate-based photodynamic therapy alone and with prior curettage. Br J Dermatol. 2001;145:467-71.
112. Horn M, Wolf P, Wulf HC, et al. Topical methyl aminolevulinate photodynamic therapy in patients with basal cell carcinoma prone to complications and poor cosmetic outcome with conventional therapy. Br J Dermatol. 2003;149:1242-9.
113. Vinciullo C, Elliott T, Francis D, et al. Photodynamic therapy with topical methyl aminolaevulinate for 'difficult-to-treat' basal cell carcinoma. Br J Dermatol. 2005;152:765-72.
114. Surrenti T, De Angelis L, Di Cesare A, et al. Efficacy of photodynamic therapy with methylaminolevulinate in the treatment of superficial and nodular basal cell carcinoma: an open-label trial. Eur J Dermatol. 2007;17:412-5.
115. Basset-Seguin N, Ibbotson SH, Emtestam L, et al. Topical methyl aminolaevulinate photodynamic therapy versus cryotherapy for superficial basal cell carcinoma: a 5 year randomized trial. Eur J Dermatol. 2008;18:547-53.
116. Szeimies RM, Ibbotson S, Murrell DF, et al. A clinical study comparing methyl aminolevulinate photodynamic therapy and surgery in small superficial basal cell carcinoma (8-20 mm), with a 12-month follow-up. J Eur Acad Dermatol Venereol. 2008;22:1302-11.
117. Fantini F, Greco A, Del Giovane C, et al. Photodynamic therapy for basal cell carcinoma: clinical and pathological determinants of response. J Eur Acad Dermatol Venereol. 2011;25(8):896-901.
118. Vinciullo C, Elliott T, Gebauer K, et al. MAL-PDT in patients with basal cell carcinoma: results of an Australian multicenter study. Poster presented to the International Skin Cancer Conference 2004, Zurich, Switzerland, July 22-24, 2004.
119. Thissen MR, Neumann MH, Schouten LJ. A systematic review of treatment modalities for primary basal cell carcinomas. Arch Dermatol. 1999;135:1177-83.
120. Rowe DE, Carroll RJ, Day CI Jr. Long term recurrence rates in previously untreated (primary basal cell carcinoma): implications for subject follow-up. J Dermatol Surg Oncol. 1989;15:315-28.
121. Tierney E, Barker A, Ahdout J, et al. Photodynamic therapy for the treatment of cutaneous neoplasia, inflammatory disorders and photoaging. Dermatol Surg. 2009;35:725-46.
122. Blume JE, Oseroff AR. Aminolevulinic acid photodynamic therapy for skin cancers. Dermatol Clin. 2007;25:5-14.
123. Thissen MR, Schroeter CA, Neumann HA. Photodynamic therapy with delta-aminolaevulinic acid for nodular basal cell carcinoma using a prior debulking technique. Br J Dermatol. 2000;142:338-9.
124. Kuijpers DI, Thissen MR, Thissen CA, et al. Similar effectiveness of methyl aminolevulinate and 5-aminolevulinate in topical photodynamic therapy for nodular basal cell carcinoma. J Drugs Dermatol. 2006;5:642-5.
125. Tope WD, Menter A, El-Azhary RA, et al. Comparison of topical methyl aminolevulinate photodynamic therapy versus placebo photodynamic therapy in nodular BCC. J Eur Acad Dermatol Venereol. 2004;18(Suppl 2):413-4.
126. Foley P, Freeman M, Siller G, et al. MAL-PDT or placebo cream in nodular basal cell carcinoma: results of an Australian double-blind randomized multicenter study. Poster presented at the International Skin Cancer Conference 2004, Zurich, July 22-24, 2004.
127. Rhodes LE, de Rie M, Enstrom Y, et al. Photodynamic therapy using topical methyl aminolevulinate vs surgery for nodular basal cell carcinoma: results of a multicenter randomized prospective trial. Arch Dermatol. 2004;140:17-23.
128. Rhodes LE, de Rie M, Leifsdottir R, et al. Five-year follow-up of a randomized, prospective trial of topical methyl aminolevulinate photodynamic therapy vs surgery for nodular basal cell carcinoma. Arch Dermatol. 2007;143:1131-6.
129. Szeimies RF. Methyl aminolevulinate-photodynamic therapy for basal cell carcinoma. Dermatol Clin. 2007;25:89-94.
130. Christensen E, Skogvoll E, Viset T, et al. Photodynamic therapy with 5-aminolaevulinic acid, dimethylsulfoxide and curettage in basal cell carcinoma: a 6-year clinical and histological follow-up. J Eur Acad Dermatol Venereol. 2009:23:58-66.
131. Foley P, Freeman M, Menter A, et al. Photodynamic therapy with methyl aminolevulinate for primary nodular basal cell carcinoma: results for two randomized studies. Int J Dermatol. 2009;48:1236-45.
132. Tierney E, Petersen J, Hanke CW. Photodynamic diagnosis of tumor margins using methyl aminolevulinate before Mohs micrographic surgery. J Am Acad Dermatol. 2011;64(5):911-8.

133. Lee CY, Kim KH, Kim YH. The efficacy of photodynamic diagnosis in defining the lateral border between a tumor and a tumor-free area during mohs micrographic surgery. Dermatol Surg. 2010;36: 1704-10.
134. Oseroff A. PDT as a cytotoxic agent and biological response modifier: Implications for cancer prevention and treatment in immunosuppressed and immunocompetent patients. J Invest Dermatol. 2006;126:542-4.
135. de Graaf YGL, Kennedy C, Wolterbeek R, et al. Photodynamic therapy does not prevent cutaneous squamous-cell carcinoma in organ-transplant recipients: Results of a randomized-controlled trial. J Invest Dermatol. 2006;126:569-74.
136. Harper JC. An update on the pathogenesis and management of acne vulgaris. J Am Acad Dermatol. 2004;51(1 Suppl):s36-8.
137. Herane MI, Ando I. Acne in infancy and acne genetics. Dermatology. 2003;206:24-8..
138. Strauss JS, Leyden JJ, Lucky AW, et al. A randomized trial of the efficacy of a new micronized formulation versus a standard formulation of isotretinoin in patients with severe recalcitrant nodular acne. J Am Acad Dermatol. 2001;45:187-95.
139. Layton AM, Knaggs H, Taylor J, et al. Isotretinoin for acne vulgaris—10 years later: a safe and successful treatment. Br J Dermatol. 1993;129:292-6.
140. Quereux G, Volteau C, N'Guyen JM, et al. Prospective study of risk factors of relapse after treatment of acne with oral isotretinoin. Dermatology. 2006;212:168-76.
141. Zouboulis CC. The truth behind this undeniable efficacy— recurrence rates and relapse risk factors of acne treatment with oral isotretinoin. Dermatology. 2006;212:99-100.
142. Zane LT, Leyden WA, Marqueling AL, et al. A population-based analysis of laboratory abnormalities during isotretinoin therapy for acne vulgaris. Arch Dermatol. 2006;142(8):1016-22.
143. DiGiovanna JJ, Langman CB, Tschen EH, et al. Effect of a single course of isotretinoin therapy on bone mineral density in adolescent patients with severe, recalcitrant, nodular acne. J Am Acad Dermatol. 2004;51:709-17.
144. Wysowski DK, Pitts M, Beitz J. An analysis of reports of depression and suicide in patients treated with isotretinoin. J Am Acad Dermatol. 2001;45:515-9.
145. Hongcharu W, Taylor CR, Chang Y, et al. Topical ALA-photodynamic therapy for the treatment of acne vulgaris. J Invest Dermatol. 2000;115:183-92.
146. Pollock B, Turner D, Stringer MR, et al. Topical aminolaevulinic acid-photodynamic therapy for the treatment of acne vulgaris: a study of clinical efficacy and mechanism of action. Br J Dermatol. 2004;151:616-22.
147. Ashkenazi H, Malik Z, Harth Y, et al. Eradication of Propionibacterium acnes by its endogenic porphyrins after illumination with high intensity blue light. FEMS Immunol Med Microbiol. 2003;35:17-24.
148. Itoh Y, Ninomiya Y, Tajima S, et al. Photodynamic therapy of acne vulgaris with topical delta-aminolaevulinic acid and incoherent light in Japanese patients. Br J Dermatol. 2001;144:575-9.
149. Goldman MP, Boyce SM. A single-center study of aminolevulinic acid and 417 nm photodynamic therapy in the treatment of moderate to severe acne vulgaris. J Drugs Dermatol. 2003;2:393-4.
150. Gold MH, Bradshaw VL, Boring M, et al. The use of a novel intense pulsed light and heat source and ALA-PDT in the treatment of moderate to severe inflammatory acne vulgaris. J Drugs Dermatol. 2004;3:S15-6.
151. Taub AF. Photodynamic therapy for the treatment of acne: a pilot study. J Drugs Dermatol. 2004;3:S10-14.
152. Hong SB, Lee MH. Topical aminolevulinic acid–photodynamic therapy for the treatment of acne vulgaris. Photodermatol Photoimmunol Photomed. 2005;21:322-5.
153. Santos MAV, Belo VG, Santos G. Effectiveness of photodynamic therapy with topical 5-aminolevulinic acid and intense pulsed light versus intense pulsed light alone in the treatment of acne vulgaris: comparative study. Dermatol Surg. 2005; 31:910-15.
154. Rojanamatin J, Choawawanich P. Treatment of inflammatory facial acne vulgaris with intense pulsed light and short contact of topical 5-aminolevulinic acid: a pilot study. Dermatol Surg. 2006;32:991-7.
155. Alexiades-Armenakas M. Long-pulsed dye laser-mediated photodynamic therapy combined with topical therapy for mild to severe comedonal, inflammatory, or cystic acne. J Drugs Dermatol. 2006;5:45-56.
156. Wiegell SR, Wulf HC. Photodynamic therapy of acne vulgaris using methyl aminolaevulinate: a blinded, randomized, controlled trial. Br J Dermatol. 2006; 154:969-76.
157. Wiegell SR, Wulf HC. Photodynamic therapy using 5-aminolevulinic acid versus methyl aminolevulinate. J Am Acad Dermatol. 2006;54:647-51.
158. Hörfelt C, Funk J, Frohm-Nilsson M et al. Topical methyl aminolaevulinate photodynamic therapy for treatment of facial acne vulgaris: results of a randomized, controlled study. Br J Dermatol. 2006;155:608-13.
159. Gold MH, Biron JA, Boring M, et al. Treatment of moderate to severe inflammatory acne vulgaris:

photodynamic therapy with 5-aminolevulinic acid and a novel advanced fluorescence technology pulsed light source. J Drugs Dermatol. 2007;6: 319-22.

160. Akaraphanth R, Kanjanawanitchkul W, Gritiya-rangsan P. Efficacy of ALA–PDT vs blue light in the treatment of acne. Photodermatol Photoimmunol Photomed. 2007;23:186-90.
161. Yeung CK, Shek SY, Bjerring P, et al. A comparative study of intense pulsed light alone and its combination with photodynamic therapy for the treatment of facial acne in Asian skin. Lasers Surg Med. 2007;39:1-6.
162. Oh SH, Ryu DJ, Han EC, et al. A comparative study of topical 5-aminolevulinic acid incubation times in photodynamic therapy with intense pulsed light for the treatment of inflammatory acne. Dermatol Surg. 2009;35:1918-26.
163. Yin R, Hao F, Deng J, et al. Investigation of optimal aminolaevulinic acid concentration applied in topical aminolaevulinic acid-photodynamic therapy for treatment of moderate to severe acne: a pilot study in Chinese subjects. Br J Dermatol. 2010; 163:1064-71.
164. Taub AF. A comparison of intense pulsed light, combination radiofrequency and intense pulsed light, and blue light in photodynamic therapy for acne vulgaris. J Drugs Dermatol. 2007;6:1010-6.
165. Haedersdal M, Togsverd-Bo K, Wiegell SR, et al. Long-pulsed dye laser versus long-pulsed dye laser-assisted photodynamic therapy for acne vulgaris: a randomized controlled trial. J Am Acad Dermatol. 2008;58:387-94.
166. Hörfelt C, Stenquist B, Larkö O, et al. Photodynamic therapy for acne vulgaris: a pilot study of the dose-response and mechanism of action. Acta Derm Venereol. 2007;87:325-9.
167. Dover JS, Bhatia AC, Stewart B, et al. Topical 5-aminolevulinic acid combined with intense pulsed light in the treatment of photoaging. Arch Dermatol. 2005;141:1247-52.
168. Zane C, Capezzera R, Sala R, et al. Clinical and echographic analysis of photodynamic therapy using methylaminolevulinate as sensitizer in the treatment of photodamaged facial skin. Lasers Surg Med. 2007;39:203-209.
169. Gold MH, Bradshaw VL, Boring MM, et al. Split-face comparison of photodynamic therapy with 5-aminolevulinic acid and intense pulsed light versus intense pulsed light alone for photodamage. Dermatol Surg. 2006;32:795-803.
170. Avram DK, Goldman MP. Effectiveness and safety of ALA-IPL in treating actinic keratoses and photodamage. J Drugs Dermatol. 2004;3:S36-39.
171. Alster TS, Tanzi EL, Welch EC. Photorejuvenation of facial skin with topical 20% 5-aminolevulinic acid and intense pulsed light treatment: A split-face comparison study. J Drugs Dermatol. 2005;4:35-8.
172. Key DJ. Aminolevulinic acid-pulsed dye laser photodynamic therapy for the treatment of photoaging. Cosmet Dermatol. 2005;18:31-6.
173. Lowe NJ, Lowe P. Pilot study to determine the efficacy of ALA-PDT photorejuvenation for the treatment of facial ageing. J Cosmetic Laser Ther. 2005;7:159-62.
174. Marmur ES, Phelps R, Goldberg DJ. Ultrastructural changes seen after ALA-IPL photorejuvenation: a pilot study. J Cosmet Laser Ther. 2005;7:21-4.
175. Serrano G, Lorente M, Reyes M, et al. Photodynamic therapy with low-strength ALA, repeated applications and short contact periods (40–60 minutes) in acne, photoaging, and vitiligo. J Drugs Dermatol. 2009;8:562-8.
176. Park MY, Sohn S, Lee E, et al. Photorejuvenation induced by 5-aminolevulinic acid photodynamic therapy in patients with actinic keratosis: a histologic analysis. J Am Acad Dermatol. 2010;62(1): 85-95.
177. Clementoni MT, B-Roscher M, Munavalli GS. Photodynamic photorejuvenation of the face with a combination of microneedling, red light, and broadband pulsed light. Lasers Surg Med. 2010;42:150-9.
178. Xi Z, Shuxian Y, Zhong L, et al. Topical 5-aminolevulinic acid with intense pulsed light versus intense pulsed light for photodamage in chinese patients. Dermatol Surg. 2011;37:31-40.
179. Ruiz-Rodriguez R, López L, Candelas D, et al. Enhanced efficacy of photodynamic therapy after fractional resurfacing: fractional photodynamic rejuvenation. J Drugs Dermatol. 2007;6(8):818-20.
180. Issa MCL, Pineiro-Maceira J, Vieira MTC, et al. Photorejuvenation with topical methyl aminolevulinate and red light: a randomized, prospective, clinical, histopathologic, and morphometric study. Dermatol Surg. 2010;36:39-48.
181. Jeffes EW. Levulan: the first approved topical photosensitizer for the treatment of actinic keratosis. J Dermatol Treat. 2002;13:S19-S23.
182. Goldberg DJ. New collagen formation after dermal remodeling with intense pulsed light sources. J Cutan Laser Ther. 2000;2:59-61.
183. Haedersdal M, Sakamoto FH, Farinelli WA, et al. Fractional CO(2) laser-assisted drug delivery. Lasers Surg Med. 2010;42:113-22.

184. Szeimies RM, Stockfleth E, Popp G, et al. Long-term follow-up of photodynamic therapy with self-adhesive 5-aminolaevulinic acid patch: 12 months data. Br J Dermatol. 2010;162:410-4.
185. Warren CB, Karai LJ, Vidimos A, et al. Pain associated with aminolevulinic acid-photodynamic therapy of skin disease. J Am Acad Dermatol. 2009;61(6):1033-43.
186. Tyrrell J, Campbell SM, Curnow A. The effect of air cooling pain relief on protoporphyrin IX photobleaching and clinical efficacy during dermatological photodynamic therapy. J Photochem Photobiol B. 2011;103(1):1-7.
187. Tyrrell J, Campbell SM, Curnow A. The relationship between protoporphyrin IX photobleaching during real-time dermatological methyl-aminoluvinate photodynamic therapy (MAL-PDT) and subsequent clinical outcome. Lasers Surg Med. 2010;42:613-19.
188. Ascencio M, Collinet P, Farine MO, et al. Protoporphyrin IX fluorescence photobleaching is a useful tool to predict the response of rat ovarian cancer following hexaminolevulinate photodynamic therapy. Lasers Surg Med 2008;40:332-41.

CHAPTER

11

Intense Pulsed Light

Arisa E Ortiz, E Victor Ross

INTRODUCTION

Intense pulsed light (IPL) devices use flashlamps, computer-controlled power supplies, and band-pass filters to produce pulsed polychromatic high-intensity broadband light. The emission spectrum of IPL sources ranges in the visible to near-infrared (IR) range (400–1,200 nm), while pulse durations and intervals vary widely amongst different devices. The basic principle of IPL devices is similar to laser devices, which are based on the theory of selective photothermolysis.[1] While lasers are monochromatic, the main chromophores in the skin (hemoglobin, melanin and water) have broad absorption peaks and do not require monochromaticity for selective heating. In many dermatologic applications that require millisecond (ms) or longer pulse deliveries to large skin areas, IPLs are sufficient or even preferable to laser devices for many dermatologic applications.[2]

In contrast to IPL devices, lasers use a xenon flashlamp as an energy source to excite a laser medium. Intense pulsed light units use a flashlamp directly much like a slide projector that emits white light, which is then converted to a narrower range of colors by an external filter.[3] Flashlamps are high-intensity xenon gas-discharge lamps that produce bright light when an electrical current passes through the gas. These lamps convert electrical energy that is stored in capacitor banks into optical energy in a pulsed mode. Newer IPL systems use partial discharge technology, which ensures a more even energy flow.[4] The lamp is cooled by circulating water around a quartz envelope. The quartz envelope filters out harmful far-ultraviolet (UV) output. The lamp output is focused toward the distal end of the handpiece and is usually coupled into the skin surface via a sapphire or quartz block. Some IPL units use multiple flashlamps to eliminate "hotspots" in the beam.[3] This also prolongs lamp life. Cooling of the skin surface may be achieved by cryogen spray, forced refrigerated air or contact cooling on the distal end of the handpiece depending on the particular IPL device.

A major advantage of IPL devices is their therapeutic versatility given their ability to combine various wavelengths, fluences, pulse durations and pulse intervals in order to treat a wide spectrum of skin conditions. By varying filtration, lamp types or current density, an IPL can be configured for different emission spectra.[3] The ability to deliver multiple wavelengths simultaneously allows for the target of multiple chromophores, such as hemoglobin, melanin and water, using the same light exposure. In general, an IPL unit is more cost efficient than purchasing multiple lasers, or combination laser units that offer the same therapeutic range. The possible wavelength ranges of IPLs are, however, limited. For example, there are no commercially available systems that are comparable to carbon dioxide (CO_2) or erbium-doped yttrium aluminum garnet (YAG) devices for ablative resurfacing.

The complexity of selecting appropriate parameters (i.e. cutoff filters and wavelength) for these devices makes them more operator dependent. However, newer modifications have reduced adverse events, making them less operator dependent and more user friendly. The advantage that IPL offers in therapeutic versatility also contributes to its reduced selectivity. The side effect profile may be increased due to greater risk of nonspecific thermal damage with the use of multiple wavelengths. For example, unwanted hair reduction may be observed in male patients being treated for skin rejuvenation for several months. In the hands of a skilled user, IPL devices have a good safety profile and are intrinsically more eye-safe than lasers due to the beam divergence. However, the potential eye damage from the lamp filament cannot be dismissed. Several reports of eye damage have been reported after IPL treatment (discussed below), particularly when treatment occurred within or just outside the orbit.[5] Therefore, appropriate eye protection is always recommended.

Although IPLs typically have a slow repetition rate (0.3–2 Hz), they have large spot sizes, which allows for greater skin coverage per pulse and rapid treatment.[6] In general, for most devices, as the fluence increases, more time is required for lamp recovery and recharging and the pulse repetition decreases accordingly. Larger handpieces tend to be more bulky, making maneuverability over irregular skin surfaces more difficult. This is especially true for discrete lesion treatment. There is not always an option to adjust the spot size, because IPLs cannot be focused to achieve higher intensities. It is physically impossible for the light intensity at the skin surface to exceed that delivered by the source lamp.[3]

Treatment settings between various manufacturers or even successive device models are generally not interchangeable due to variances in fluences. For example, changes in lamp pumping affect the pulse profile, and spectral emission creating a domino effect, with simple changes of fluence impacting other treatment parameters. Various devices emit different wavelength ranges and spectral shapes allowing for different depth of light penetration and absorption by human skin with the same macropulse duration, nominal filtration and fluence. Different companies use various techniques for measuring fluences, such as "effective fluence". Thus, the fluence that is given on the instrument panel might not be equivalent to the energy density at the tip.

The reason for this variability is partially due to the fact that IPL devices, unlike lasers, are largely unregulated. Lasers are governed by strict standards that manufacturers must adhere to. In contrast, IPL devices are only required to comply with technical performance data and operating tolerances under electrical safety standards. Without a standard on key performance characteristics, there is no guidance in place for manufacturers to determine optimal performance characteristics. A comparison of key IPL parameters in 18 different IPL devices found variance between what the device displayed on the screen monitor as the maximum fluence and the actual measured fluence.[7] This discrepancy could be a result of a difference in the method used by the manufacturer to determine fluence. However, there was also a poor correlation found between the measured pulse duration and the system-displayed values.[7] Discrepancies between measured parameters and manufacturer claims underscore the importance of a national standard and the need for legislation to produce standard measurement procedures. As it stands, the lack of a standard amongst IPL devices makes it difficult to compare fluences between devices or even between different models of the same device. Therefore, the authors stress that the parameters suggested in this chapter are suggestions for use with only certain devices and are not meant to provide guidance for all IPL devices.

Unlike lasers, IPLs are also more variable from pulse to pulse, or even during a pulse due to the instantaneous "pumping" voltage of the capacitors. During the course of a pulse, the beginning and end portions are less energetic, while the middle of the pulse is more energetic, termed "spectral jitter". Newer devices use sophisticated computer control systems to minimize this phenomenon.

Another drawback of IPLs is that the handpiece must be in direct contact with the skin for effective treatment because of rapid beam divergence. Therefore, the immediate tissue response is difficult to observe. Direct contact of the IPL device over firmer surfaces (i.e. dorsum of the nose) can also result in vessel compression leading to ineffective treatment of telangiectasia. One exception to this is the Solis IPL (Iridex, San Jose, CA) (no longer manufactured, but available on the aftermarket). In this design, the lamp is approximately 1 cm above the skin surface, and cryogen spray cooling (CSC) is delivered through multiple ports along the perimeter of the plastic enclosure. Light scatter is mitigated by reflectors positioned throughout the interior of the handpiece housing.[3]

VARIOUS DEVICE MODELS AND DEVICE MODIFICATIONS

As IPL sources gain popularity, devices are becoming more sophisticated with newer modifications to improve upon previous shortcomings.

The Omnilight (American Medical Bio Care Inc, Newport, CA) uses fluorescent polymers to convert shorter wavelengths into more advantageous visible light. The benefit of using fluorescent dyes is the ability to reduce the lamp voltage, which increases the lifespan of the lamp while maintaining a high output of desirable spectra. Unusable light is either converted through fluorescence or directed back toward the lamp. The remainder of the energy is absorbed by a polymer wafer, which results in heating and degradation of the wafer (~100 pulses prior to wafer degradation).

Prior to integrated cooling, a thick layer of cooling gel between the quartz crystal and the skin was required for surface cooling. This led to variability of skin tissue effects from pulse to pulse due to the rapid beam divergence of IPLs even a few millimeters between the handpiece and skin surface. A slight variation of pressure exerted by the operator would lead to variations in fluence (i.e. firmer pressure leads to a higher fluence and more robust tissue effects). The addition of integrated cooling allows for more reproducible dosimetry. Newer generation IPLs contain sapphire rather than quartz for epidermal cooling. While sapphire is more expensive, it has a much higher thermal conductivity and thermal diffusivity than quartz. With improved epidermal protection, devices that use sapphire have the potential to use higher light doses such as in hair removal and vessel ablation.

ProWave and LimeLight (Cutera, Burlingame, CA) create different emission spectra by varying current density and filtering. This device promotes the treatment of darker skin with the use of a lower sapphire tip temperature and longer pulse duration. These changes are made electronically, avoiding the need to exchange handpieces and/or filter assembly.

AcuTip (Cutera, Burlingame, CA) has a smaller 6 mm spot size that allows for treatment of discrete brown and red dyschromic lesions. This "small" spot size is achieved by using a long cylindrical sapphire waveguide and high performance reflectors. Another IPL device has the option of a 4 mm adaptor tip (Fig. 11.1) for their MaxG™ handpiece (Palomar Medical Technologies, Inc, Burlington, MA). The BBL™ (Sciton, Inc, Palo Alto, CA) also has adapter tip in three different sizes for harder to reach areas. If smaller spot sizes are not available, a white plastic "mask" with small holes (Palomar Medical Technologies, Inc, Burlington, MA, and Alma Lasers, Buffalo Grove, IL) can be added to other adapters to achieve a smaller area of irradiation. A problem that arises with using a "mask" is that cooling is compromised because it prevents direct contact of the cooling mechanism with the skin.

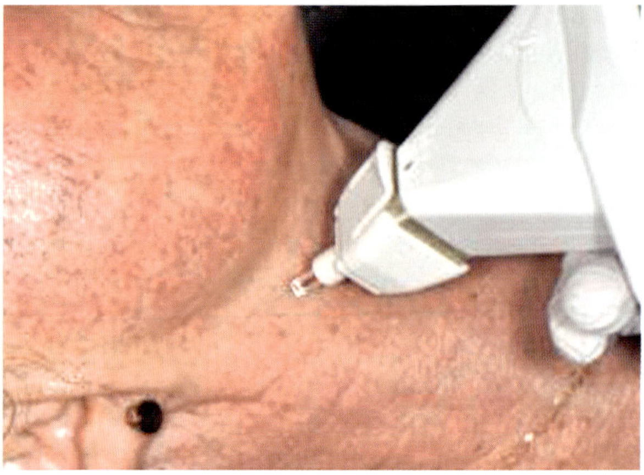

Fig. 11.1: Four millimeter adapter piece
Courtesy: E Victor Ross, Director, Laser and Cosmetic Dermatology Center, Scripps Clinic, Carmel Valley, CA

Regardless of their limitations, IPL sources are widely used for their versatility and their overall safety when used appropriately by experienced users. By selecting the appropriate combination of wavelengths, pulse durations, pulse intervals and fluences, IPL devices can treat a wide range of skin conditions. In this chapter, we shall discuss the current literature on IPL for the treatment of these various skin disorders.

PIGMENTED LESIONS

Intense pulsed light is an effective therapy for the treatment of melanocytic hyperpigmentation. The localization of the pigment determines the appropriate therapeutic wavelength. Wavelengths between 630 nm and 1100 nm will preferentially absorb melanin over hemoglobin, while achieving deep dermal penetration. Lower cutoff filters can be used for the treatment of superficial pigmentation and higher cutoff filters can be used for lesions deeper in the dermis.

When treating solar lentigines, it is important to distinguish them from melanocytic nevi, pigmented actinic keratoses and malignant melanoma. Once the diagnosis has been established, treatment with IPL may ensue. The mechanism of action of IPL for the treatment of solar lentigines was evaluated with reflectance-mode confocal microscopy and optical coherence tomography.[8] Melanosomes in the epidermal basal layer were observed to rapidly migrate to the skin surface after therapy. The melanosomes are then eliminated as the microcrusts are removed from the skin surface. However, melanocytes were left intact and resumed high activity after treatment. Therefore, additional therapy with hydroquinone or quality-switched (QS) laser irradiation may be necessary to suppress residual active melanocytes.

It is important to emphasize that while IPL devices have been reported to be effective in the treatment of pigmented lesions, IPLs are best considered for so called higher contrast lesions (where the pigment difference between the background skin and lesion is large). Intense pulsed light devices have pulse durations in the millisecond range, which make them less effective for low-contrast pigmented lesions, than QS laser devices, which operate in the nanosecond range. However, the longer pulse duration also allows for gentle heating (yet less localized) that decreases the risk of postinflammatory hyperpigmentation (PIH).

Treatment of nevomelanocytic lesions is controversial and should not be treated with light-based devices unless their benign nature is certain. Recurrence is also very common. The treatment of nevomelanocytic nevi is controversial because residual melanocytes may be left untreated, particularly in the deeper, nonpigmented portion of the lesion.[9] IPL devices and lasers may also cause superficial scarring, which could potentially mask an underlying malignant process. The effects of laser and light irradiation on the cellular biologic response of nevomelanocytes and their potential for malignant transformation, which is an inherent risk even without treatment, remains unclear. However, there have been reports of melanoma diagnosed after treatment of pigmented lesions with ablative lasers and pigment-targeting lasers.[10-12] The authors stress the importance of clinical examination and skin biopsies when indicated prior to light-based treatment of pigmented lesions. The treatment of dysplastic nevi should be avoided and is better removed by standard excision.

Intense pulsed light is also used in the treatment of melasma. However, the authors caution the use of IPL in the treatment of melasma because of the potential to worsen the condition and the likelihood that it will recur. One study reported a 51–100% improvement of melasma with four treatments at three-week intervals using an IPL device (Lumenis One; Lumenis, Inc., Santa Clara, CA) in Chinese patients. The settings used were a fluence of 13–17 J/cm^2, 560–590 nm filters or 590 nm, 615 nm and 640 nm filters, a triple pulse with a 3–4 ms pulse duration, and a 25–40 ms pulse delay. Epidermal melasma responded better to treatment compared to melasma that also involved the dermis.[13] Another study evaluating the safety and efficacy of an IPL device (Deka M.E.L.A. s.r.l., Calenzano-Florence, Italy) in the treatment of melasma reported "excellent" results in 47% of patients.[14] Three to five treatments were administered every 40–45 days using a wavelength of 550 nm, a pulse duration of 5–10 ms, a 10–20 ms pulse delay and a fluence of 6–14 J/cm^2 depending on the localization of the melasma (i.e. dermal vs epidermal) and the Fitzpatrick phototype.

While IPL is a reasonable treatment option for melasma with very little side effects, improvement is modest and recurrence is common. As first line therapy, we recommend strict sun protection and bleaching agents.

In our experience, the following IPL settings in Table 11.1 are a possible approach to pigmented lesions.

VASCULAR LESIONS

Many vascular lesions have been successfully treated with IPLs. As with laser treatment, the mechanism of action of IPLs is based on their selective absorption by hemoglobin. Intense pulsed light targets oxyhemoglobin at 542 nm, 577 nm and 940 nm. When thermal energy raises the blood temperature high enough, coagulation within the blood vessels leads to destruction and replacement by fibrous granulation tissue. The appropriate endpoint of vascular lesions is the immediate dark blue to gray color change of the vessel or disappearance. The former represents coagulation of the vessel and the latter represents vessel stenosis with immediate contraction and disappearance clinically, which confirms that the appropriate photophysical parameters are being used.

Table 11.1: Suggested parameters for pigment reduction*

	Skin Type	*Fluence (J/cm²)*		*Pulse Width (ms)*	*Filter (nm)*	*Cooling (°C)*
BBL™ (Sciton, Inc, Palo Alto, CA)	I–II	12		10	515	25
	III–IV	9		20	515	10–25
	V	7		30	515	10–25
	VI	N/A		N/A	N/A	N/A
StarLux® (Palomar Medical Technologies, Inc, Burlington, MA)	I–II	Face	34–50	10–20	MaxG™ Handpiece	
		Chest	32–38	30		
	III	Face	32–44	30		
		Chest	28–36	30		
	IV	Face	28–36	30		
		Chest	26–32	30		
	I–II	Face, arm, body	25–27	15	MaxY™ Handpiece	
		Chest, neck, legs, hands	23–27	15		
	III	Face, arm, body	17–27	20		
		Chest, neck, legs, hands	21–27	15		
	IV	Face, arm, body	24–36	40		
		Chest, neck, legs, hands	15–27	20		

*In combination devices, only intense pulsed light settings are addressed

Pulsed-dye lasers (PDL) have been considered the gold standard in the treatment of port-wine stains (PWS). However, complete clearance of the PWS is infrequently achieved.[15] Complete clearance of PWS is only achieved in approximately 20% of cases due to PWS blood vessel reformation.[16] Thus, PWS require multiple treatment sessions to achieve maximal lightening. Pulsed-dye laser sources are inadequate to treat nodular components in PWS because most of the energy is deposited in superficial vessels, decreasing the light available to target deeper vessels due to a shadowing effect.[17] Port-wine stains lesions are especially difficult to treat in adults and darker skin types. Thus, new devices or treatment strategies are sought-after that will improve the treatment of PWS.

Intense pulsed light theoretically has an advantage over laser treatment since IPL produces variable pulse durations along with multiple split light pulses causing additional heating to treat vessels of different diameters. Variable wavelengths emitted by IPL potentially targets the full range of the hemoglobin absorption peaks (540–940 nm) for destruction of both superficial and deep components of the PWS.[18] IPL has been shown to be effective in PWS resistant to PDL. PWS resistant to PDL were treated with an IPL (Ellipse Flex system with a MKII vascular applicator; Danish Dermatologic Development A/S, Hørsholm, Denmark).[19] All patients received four IPL treatments at 2-month intervals with pulse durations ranging from 8 ms to 30 ms, wavelength of 555–950 nm (median wavelength of 705 nm), 10 mm × 48 mm spot size and fluences ranging 13–22 J/cm². About 46.7% of patients had more than 50% reduction of their lesions. However, 53.3% of patients did not respond to IPL. This was attributed to PWS in the V_2 distribution of the face, which is more unresponsive to IPL.

A split-face comparison of IPL with dye lasers for the treatment of previously untreated PWS found that IPL (Ellipse Flex PPT; Danish Dermatologic

Development A/S, Hørsholm, Denmark) did significantly better than treatment with the short-pulsed dye laser.[20] However, IPL and long-pulsed dye laser treatment did not differ significantly. The IPL settings used were a wavelength range of 555–950 nm, pulse duration of 8–14 ms, 10 mm × 48 mm spot size and a fluence of 11–16.7 J/cm². There was a higher risk of epidermal damage with the IPL compared to the PDL equipped with a dynamic cooling device (DCD). A comparison of PDL, IPL, neodymium (Nd):YAG, alexandrite, and potassium titanyl phosphate (KTP) laser with previously PDL-treated capillary malformations, found the alexandrite laser to be the most effective.[21] However, treatment with the alexandrite laser resulted in hyperpigmentation and scarring likely due to its deeper penetration and lower specificity for oxyhemoglobin. IPL (Lumina; Lynton Lasers, Cheshire, England) had additional fading of previously PDL-resistant lesions using a 550–1,100 nm filter, fluence of 28–34 J/cm², and a 10 mm × 10 mm spot size set to deliver two pulses with a 10 ms delay.[21] On the other hand, in another side-to-side comparison study of PDL and IPL for the treatment of PWS, PDL achieved better clearance than IPL.[22]

Intense pulsed light works reasonably well for PWS. However, PDL remains our first choice for most newborn PWS, particularly in type III–V skin where DCD confers a high level of epidermal protection. PDL is also preferred when purpuric settings are necessary. The role of purpura in PWS treatment remains controversial. In a recent study performed by one of the authors (E Victor Ross), purpuric settings with IPL (3 ms) resulted in slightly greater clearing than nonpurpuric settings after an equal number of sessions; however, the risk of PIH was greater (Figs 11.2A to D). Therefore, for very light PWS, purpuric settings are best (0.45 ms vs 1.5 ms). In these cases, PDL is preferred because IPL cannot achieve very short (0.45 ms) pulse durations.

Intense pulsed light can also be used in the treatment of rosacea. In one study, IPL was found to be effective in treating erythematotelangiectatic rosacea. After four treatments with an IPL device (Quantum SR; Lumenis, London, UK) at 3-week intervals, patients had significant reduction in erythema (46%) and telangiectasia (55%), which was maintained through 6-month follow-up visits.[23] IPL settings used were an 8 mm × 34 mm spot size, wavelength range of 515–1,200 nm with a 560 nm cutoff filter, a fluence of 24–32 J/cm², and a double pulse of 2.4 ms and 4 ms, 5 ms or 6 ms depending on the skin type, with a 15 ms delay.[23]

Another study showed positive and lasting results of an IPL device in the treatment of erythema and the vascular lesions associated with rosacea. Patients achieved a 77.8% mean clearance of vascular facial telangiectases after an average of four treatments using an IPL system (PhotoDerm VL; ESC Medical Systems Ltd, Yokneam, Israel) with an 8 mm × 35 mm spot size, a wavelength range of 515–1,200 nm (most commonly 550 nm), a pulse duration ranging 4.3–6.5 ms (mean 4.8 ms), and a fluence varying from 25 J/cm² to 35 J/cm² (mean 30.4 J/cm²).[24] These results were maintained for an average of 51.6 months. The best clearance was found on the forehead, with the most treatments required on the nose.[24]

The authors have had good results treating vascular lesions with IPL (Figs 11.3A and B). When compared to PDL, IPL therapy is comparable for reduction of erythema and telangiectasia.[25] In fact, the different filter settings available in IPL systems potentially allow for the treatment of a broader range of vessel size and depth, and the opportunity to treat various targets with a single device. A "duel" among IPL, a 532 nm laser and a 595 nm laser found comparable results in reduction of ectasias in addition to hyperpigmented macules in one pass.[6] An advantage of the IPL was a larger spot size that allowed for more efficient treatment time. Treatments with IPL were relatively painless compared to laser treatment, which usually require some form of anesthesia.

Also, there is a new appreciation for modulation of lamp pumping to optimize outcomes for vascular disorders. For example, by elongating the pulse duration (around 100 ms or a train of two–three pulses over a similar or longer time period), a typical spectrum red shifts so that deeper larger vessels are preferentially heated. In this way a larger venous lake or larger 1 mm nasal vessel tends to close more completely than if a shorter pulse were delivered (Figs 11.4A and B).[26]

Intense pulsed light is not preferred over PDL in the treatment of erythema in dark skin patients (Fitzpatrick skin type IV and higher) because the cooling is not adequate for epidermal protection compared to the DCD available with PDL. In all patients, IPL devices must be used by highly trained

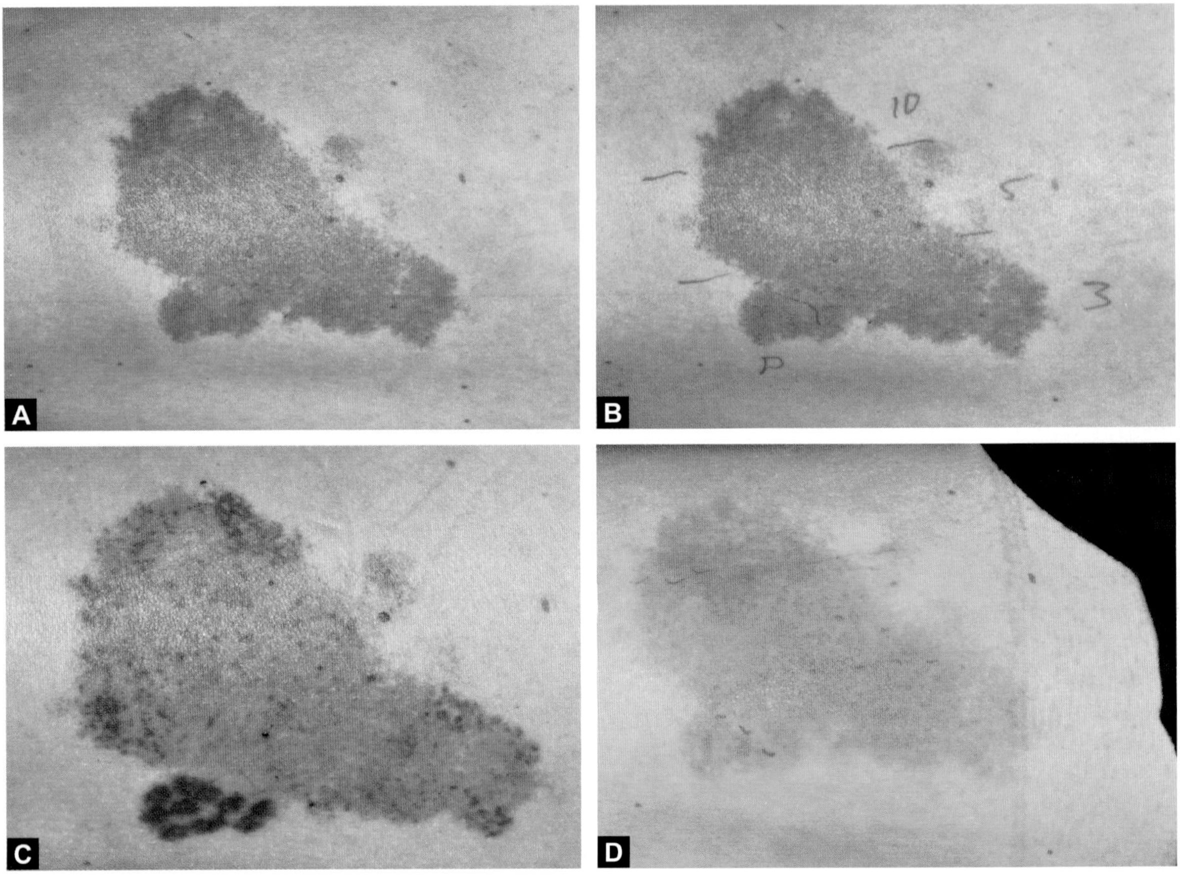

Figs 11.2A to D: (A) Port-wine stains (PWS) prior to treatment; (B) PWS prior to treatment with variable pulse durations (top, 10 ms; middle, 5 ms; bottom, 3 ms). The P in corner of the diagram refers to a PDL test site (8J/cm^2, 3 ms, 7 mm spot, + cryogen spray); (C) Immediately after treatment. Purpura achieved with 3 ms pulse duration (bottom); (D) Three months after fourth treatment. PWS after treatment with intense pulsed light. Notice greater improvement with purpuric settings (bottom, 3 ms)
Courtesy: E Victor Ross, Director, Laser and Cosmetic Dermatology Center, Scripps Clinic, Carmel Valley, CA

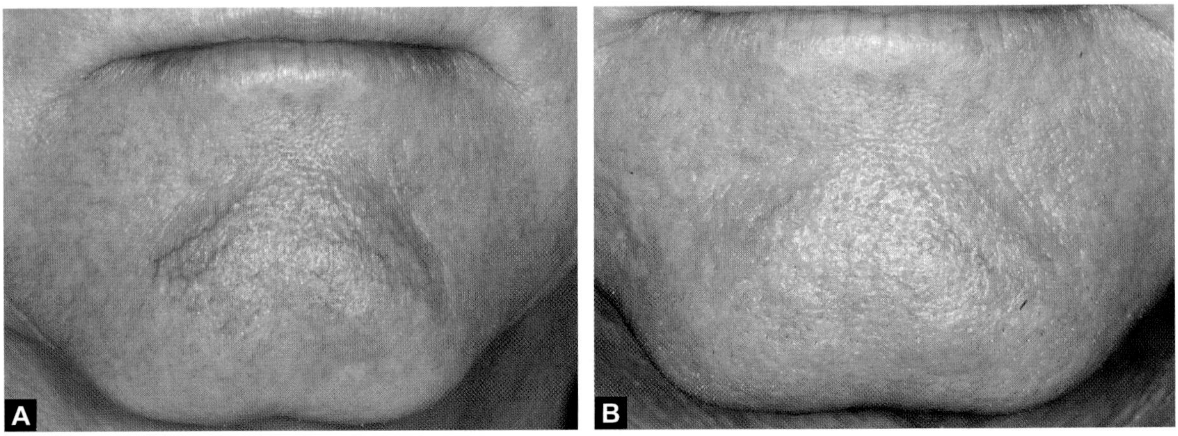

Figs 11.3A and B: (A) Telangiectasia on the chin before treatment; (B) Telangiectasia on the chin after one treatment (MaxG™ handpiece, 32 J/cm^2, 10 ms).
Courtesy: E Victor Ross, Director, Laser and Cosmetic Dermatology Center, Scripps Clinic, Carmel Valley, CA

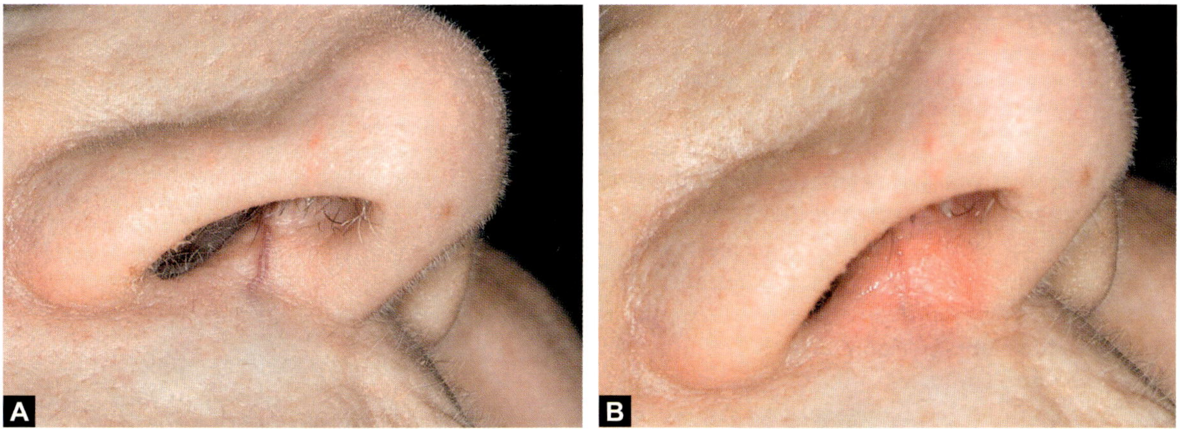

Figs 11.4A and B: (A) Large nasal vessel before treatment; (B) Resolution of nasal vessel after treatment (MaxG™ handpiece, 34 J/cm^2, 10 ms)
Courtesy: E Victor Ross, Director, Laser and Cosmetic Dermatology Center, Scripps Clinic, Carmel Valley, CA

individuals that select appropriate parameters (i.e. pulse duration, pulse delay) required for vessel occlusion without causing bulla or scar formation.

In the authors' experience, the following IPL settings in Table 11.2 are a possible approach to vascular lesions.

PHOTOREJUVENATION

Photoaged skin is characterized by rhytides, pigmentary changes, telangiectases and skin thinning. Wrinkles develop after long-term exposure to UV radiation from the sun, which leads to collagen

<table>
<tr><th colspan="7">Table 11.2: Suggested parameters for treating vascular lesions*</th></tr>
<tr><td rowspan="5">BBL™ (Sciton, Inc, Palo Alto, CA)</td><td>Skin Type</td><td colspan="2">Fluence (J/cm²)</td><td>Pulse Width (ms)</td><td>Filter (nm)</td><td>Cooling (°C)</td></tr>
<tr><td>I–II</td><td colspan="2">12</td><td>10</td><td>560</td><td>25</td></tr>
<tr><td>III–IV</td><td colspan="2">10</td><td>20</td><td>560</td><td>20</td></tr>
<tr><td>V</td><td colspan="2">10</td><td>30</td><td>590</td><td>15</td></tr>
<tr><td>VI</td><td colspan="2">N/A</td><td>N/A</td><td>N/A</td><td>N/A</td></tr>
<tr><td rowspan="11">StarLux® (Palomar Medical Technologies, Inc, Burlington, MA)</td><td rowspan="4">I–II</td><td>Vessels >0.3 mm</td><td>30–50</td><td>10–20</td><td rowspan="11">MaxG™ Handpiece</td><td rowspan="11"></td></tr>
<tr><td>Vessels <0.3 mm</td><td>30–46</td><td>10</td></tr>
<tr><td>Chest and neck vessels</td><td>30–46</td><td>30</td></tr>
<tr><td>Rosacea</td><td>30–42</td><td>10</td></tr>
<tr><td rowspan="4">III</td><td>Vessels >0.3 mm</td><td>26–42</td><td>10–20</td></tr>
<tr><td>Vessels <0.3 mm</td><td>34–46</td><td>10</td></tr>
<tr><td>Chest and neck vessels</td><td>28–34</td><td>30</td></tr>
<tr><td>Rosacea</td><td>30–42</td><td>10</td></tr>
<tr><td rowspan="3">IV</td><td>Vessels >0.3 mm</td><td>32–38</td><td>20</td></tr>
<tr><td>Vessels <0.3 mm</td><td>32–42</td><td>15</td></tr>
<tr><td>Chest and neck vessels</td><td>26–32</td><td>30</td></tr>
<tr><td colspan="7">*In combination devices, only intense pulsed light settings are addressed</td></tr>
</table>

and elastic fiber breakdown by oxygen radicals. The decrease in volume and dermal structural support causes redundant epidermis to wrinkle. IPL has shown to improve photodamaged skin. Finer, more superficial wrinkles tend to respond better than deeper furrows. However, these results are inconsistent and more impressive data exists for the use of IPL in the treatment of vascular lesions and pigmentation associated with photodamage. The mechanism of rhytide and skin texture improvement with IPL treatment is possibly due to the increase of both type one and three collagens after therapy, replacing volume and structural support.[27] Increased fibroblast activity and uniform arrangement of collagen fibers has also been documented with transmission electron microscopy.[27] Heating of collagen fibers leads to their contracture and may account for tightening of the skin and improvement in texture secondarily observed in many studies.[28] The improvement of wrinkles is likely better treated with laser modalities, although, IPL offers a reasonable alternative with a low side-effect profile.

In a randomized, split-face study comparing an IPL device (Ellipse Flex; Danish Dermatologic Development A/S, Hørsholm, Denmark) with a long-pulsed dye laser (LPDL) (V-beam Perfecta, 595 nm, Candela Laser Corporation, Wayland, MA) for facial rejuvenation, LPDL was the preferred treatment due to superior vessel clearance and less pain.[29] Three treatments were administered at 3-week intervals with LPDL and IPL (530–750 nm PR applicator or 555–950 nm VL applicator, spot size 10 mm × 48 mm, pulse duration 2 × 2.5 ms, delay 10 ms or 8–20 ms, fluence 6–20 J/cm^2). Irregular pigmentation and skin texture had comparable improvement between the two devices without much improvement in rhytides. The 555–950 nm VL applicator has shown better improvement of irregular pigmentation, while the 530–750 nm PR applicator is better for treatment of telangiectasia and diffuse erythema.[30]

Another split-face comparison evaluated the PDL (Perfecta; Candela, Wayland, MA) with a compression handpiece versus an IPL device (StarLux; Palomar Medical Technologies, Burlington, MA) for photorejuvenation favored PDL for vascular lesions.[31] However, both treatments were highly effective for the treatment of dyschromia secondary to photorejuvenation. Three treatments at 3–4-week intervals with IPL were administered with fluences ranging between 32 J/cm^2 and 40 J/cm^2, pulse durations of 10–20 ms at 0.5 Hz with no overlap. Final treatments were at 36 J/cm^2 with a pulse width of 10 ms.

Poikiloderma of Civatte is a type of photoaging on the neck, lower anterior neck, and the "V" area of the chest associated with erythema, reticulate pigmentation and telangiectasia. With increasing procedures done for facial rejuvenation, it is important to also consider treatment of the chest in order to avoid a sharp line of demarcation between a newly rejuvenated neckline with an untreated neck and chest. The chest is an area of special concern when treating photodamaged skin due to the thinness of the epidermis and dermis, and the decreased number of pilosebaceous units compared to the face. Therefore, minimally invasive treatments may be preferred to avoid adverse events. IPL may be a modality of choice for this indication due to its potential to simultaneously treat telangiectasia, erythema, pigmented lesions and skin texture using its ability to transmit a broad spectrum of wavelengths.[32] A large published series showed 80% clearance of poikiloderma of Civatte with three treatment sessions at 3-week intervals using an IPL device (Vasculight Plus; ESC/Sharplan, Yokneam, Israel).[33] A 515 nm cutoff was used for more superficial lesions and a 590 nm filter was used for larger telagiectasias and dermal pigment. A single, double or triple pulse was delivered at pulse durations from 2.5 ms to 3.5 ms with a 10 ms pulse delay for small, superficial structures and 3.5–4.5 ms pulse duration with a 30 ms delay for targeting larger diameter vessels. Fluence depended on the skin type, with lower fluences used in darker skin types to prevent epidermal damage. However, the authors prefer using the PDL for treatment of poikiloderma in darker skin patients.

In general, three to five sessions are necessary to optimize results. To avoid pinstriping when using an IPL device with a rectangular tip handpiece, the direction of the handpiece should be alternated between a horizontal manner and a vertical manner between treatment sessions.

HAIR REMOVAL

There are many published reports documenting effective treatment of hair removal with IPLs.[34]

However, there are few randomized controlled trials to prove their efficacy. A benefit to using IPL over laser hair removal is a large spot size available with IPL units. The larger spot size makes treating larger surfaces, such as the back, more efficient. The mechanism of IPLs for hair reduction is similar to laser hair reduction. Light delivered with each pulse (ms) is absorbed by melanin within melanosomes located in the hair matrix and within keratinocytes located in the hair shaft.[35,36] The heat absorbed by melanin then diffuses from the follicular matrix to the surrounding nonpigmented follicular epithelium and perifollicular dermis creating sufficient thermal injury to the follicle.[37] This results in miniaturization of the follicle, making them clinically unapparent for a variable duration of time. Similar to laser hair removal, darker, coarser hair responds better than lighter, finer hair due to better energy absorption of the former[38] (Figs 11.5A and B).

Since melanin is also found in the epidermis, it is important to selectively target the melanin in the follicular epithelium. This can be challenging since melanin's peak absorption is best at lower wavelengths, while reaching the hair follicle requires deeper penetration. Thus, cooling mechanisms, such as cryogen spray or contact cooling, are employed to protect the epidermal melanin from thermal injury.

A split-face comparison study of facial hair removal in women with polycystic ovarian syndrome with an alexandrite laser (GentleLase; Candela, Wayland, MA) using 10–30 J/cm^2, with a 15 mm spot and 3 ms pulse duration compared to an IPL device (Lumina; Lynton Lasers, Cheshire, UK) using wavelengths ranging from 650 nm to 1,100 nm, fluences from 16 J/cm^2 to 42 J/cm^2 and three pulses at 55 ms with a 20 ms delay, showed that laser hair removal is more efficacious and preferred by patients.[39] In contrast, a split-face study comparing the effectiveness of an IPL device (Ellipse Relax Light 1000; Danish Dermatologic Development A/S, Hørsholm, Denmark) to a ruby laser (Epitouch; ESC Sharplan, Tel Aviv, Israel) for hair reduction determined that the IPL was 3.94 times more effective for hair removal.[40] After three treatments, patients achieved an average hair count reduction of 49.3% with the IPL (600–950 nm, 10 mm × 48 mm spot size, 18.5 J/cm^2) versus 21.3% with the ruby laser (694 nm, 5 mm spot, 0.9 ms pulse duration).

Another study comparing the efficacy of IPL technology with either a red filter (StarLux Rx; Palomar Medical Technologies, Inc, Burlington, MA), or yellow filter (StarLux Y; Palomar Medical Technologies, Inc., Burlington, MA) versus an 810 nm diode laser (LightSheer; Lumenis, Inc, Santa Clara, CA) and a 755 nm alexandrite laser (GentleLase; Candela, Wayland, MA) for hair removal on the back or thigh found no statistical difference in efficacy among the four devices.[41] Treatment with the IPL with a red filter was administered with a wavelength of 650–1,200 nm, 12 mm × 28 mm spot size, contact cooling, fluence of 65 J/cm^2 and a pulse width of 100 ms. Treatment with the IPL with a yellow filter was administered at 525–1,200 nm, 16 mm × 46 mm spot size, contact cooling, a fluence of 35 J/cm^2 and a pulse width of 100 ms. No difference was found

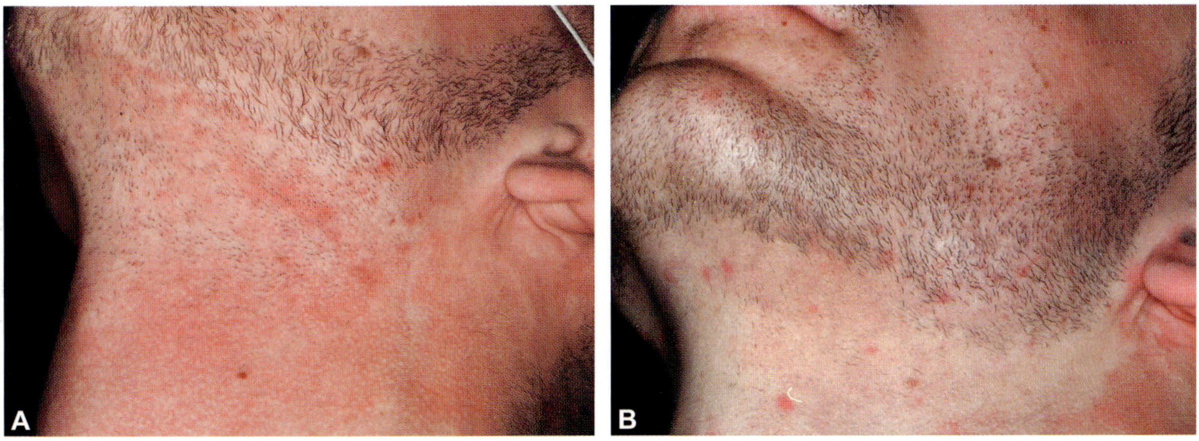

Figs 11.5A and B: (A) Hair on male neck prior to treatment; (B) Good hair reduction after intense pulsed light treatment (Omnilight, 10 J/cm^2, American Medical Bio Care, Inc, Newport Beach, CA)
Courtesy: E Victor Ross, Director, Laser and Cosmetic Dermatology Center, Scripps Clinic, Carmel Valley, CA

in the treatment efficacy among the four devices. However, the IPL devices were associated with less pain compared to the alexandrite laser.

While some studies have shown safe and effective treatment of hair removal even in Fitzpatrick skin types III–V with no significant complications,[42] other studies have reported side effects with IPL hair removal. Although less likely in the hands of a well-trained user, the most frequent side effects reported are burning, PIH or postinflammatory hypopigmentation, bulla, erosion, leukotrichia, folliculitis and rarely scar formation.[43] Darker skin types are at greater risk of dyschromic side effects and this should be accounted for when selecting the appropriate fluence and pulse duration for these patients. Some manufacturers have created special handpieces for darker skin (MaxR™; Palomar Medical Technologies, Inc, Burlington, MA) or have electronically modulated the spectrum and pulse duration to spare the epidermis (ProWave Mode C; Cutera, Burlingame, CA).

As with laser hair removal, paradoxical hypertrichosis can also occur with IPL photoepilation and may even be more common.[44,45] The pathogenesis of this phenomenon is not well understood. It is postulated that subtherapeutic thermal energies delivered to follicles at the periphery of the treatment area may induce terminal anagen hair growth. Therefore, cooling of nontreatment areas may prevent paradoxical hair stimulation. The most important risk factor for paradoxical hypertrichosis with IPL treatment seems to be the presence of fine hair prior to treatment.[45] Caution is advised when treating hirsute females with IPL photoepilation. These patients should be warned of the possibility of multiple sessions required for effective treatment. In general, hirsute patients should be treated more frequently and at higher energies for optimal treatment.

In our experience, the following IPL settings in Table 11.3 are a possible approach in achieving hair reduction.

PHOTODYNAMIC THERAPY

Photodynamic therapy (PDT) is commonly used for the treatment of actinic keratosis (AK) and nonmelanoma skin cancers, such as basal cell carcinomas.[46,47] PDT works by applying a sensitizer, such as 5-aminolevulinic acid (ALA) or its methyl ester form, which induces the endogenous porphyrin and protoporphyrin IX (PpIX). PpIX acts as a photosensitizer that is activated by polychromic light. PpIX absorbs light energy that leads to the generation of toxic oxygen species in the form of free radicals and cytotoxic singlet oxygen.[48] This process irreversibly damages the cells in the target tissue. IPL is particularly useful for photodynamic therapy (PDT) because it targets the major absorption bands for PpIX including 410 nm, 504 nm, 538 nm, 576 nm and 630 nm.

The first report of PDT with IPL for the treatment of AKs and photorejuvenation resulted in complete clearing of 89% of AK lesions.[49] Several subsequent studies investigating ALA-PDT with IPL have shown improvement of mottled hyperpigmentation and global photoaging with more modest improvement in fine lines.[50,51]

An IPL device (Energist Ultra VPL; Energist Ltd, Swansea, UK) was compared to LED in the treatment of AKs and was found to be an efficient alternative with complete remission and significantly less pain.[52] IPL treatments were delivered at 610–950 nm, two pulse trains, each 15 pulses of 5 ms, delay of 20 ms and a fluence of 40 J/cm^2 per pulse train.

Conflicting evidence was found in another study that compared the clinical and histopathological

Table 11.3: Suggested parameters for hair reduction*

	Skin Type	*Fluence (J/cm^2)*			*Pulse Width (ms)*	*Filter (nm)*
		Dark Hair	*Medium Hair*	*Light Hair*		
BBL™ (Sciton, Inc, Palo Alto, CA)	I–II	5–10	7–15	10–20	15–20	590
	III–IV	5–10	7–15	10–20	20–30	640
	V	5–12	7–18	30–50	30–50	695
	VI	N/A	N/A	N/A	N/A	N/A

* In combination devices, only intense pulsed light settings are addressed

evidence of ALA-PDT with an IPL device (Ellipse Flex; Danish Dermatologic Development A/S, Hørsholm, Denmark) for the treatment of AKs.[53] Treatments were administered at 555–950 nm, spot size of 10 mm × 48 mm, a pulse duration of 20–30 ms, and a fluence of 12–16 J/cm² for two passes. While clinical clearance after a single treatment was 50%, histologic clearance was only 42%. Therefore, clinical appearance of resolution is not always consistent with histologic resolution, and long-term monitoring of these lesions is important. However, ALA-PDT with IPL has been shown to improve the clearance of AKs compared with IPL alone.[54]

ACNE

Targeting acne with light-based devices can be achieved either via destruction of blood vessels that supply sebaceous glands to decrease the sebum secretion rate, destruction of *Propionibacterium acnes* through absorption of porphyrins (PpIX, Coproporphyrin III) produced by *P. acnes* (absorption peaks: 400 nm, 510 nm, 542 nm, 578 nm, 630 nm and 665 nm) leading to generation of reactive oxygen species with ensuing bactericidal effects or through the use of a topically applied photosensitizer, which accumulates in the sebaceous glands and leads to their destruction.[55] IPL has the advantage of targeting absorption peaks of both porphyrin and hemoglobin making it a suitable treatment for acne.

A study comparing an IPL device (Danish Dermatologic Development A/S, Hørsholm, Denmark) alone with IPL combined with PDT [methyl aminolevulinate cream (MAL)], compared to just adapalene 0.1% gel alone for the treatment of moderate acne in skin type IV or V showed a 38% significant reduction of noninflammatory lesions in the MAL-PDT group compared to 43% in the IPL only group at 12 weeks.[56] IPL treatments were administered with a 10 mm × 48 mm spot size, wavelength range of 530–750 nm, pulse duration of 2 × 2.5 ms, 10 ms delay and a fluence of 7–9 J/cm². The adapalene control group had an increase of 15% of noninflammatory lesions. However, 25% of patients in the PDT group withdrew from the study due to procedure-associated discomfort.

Different light sources were compared for effectiveness of ALA-PDT in treating moderate to severe acne. ALA-PDT with IPL resulted in more long-lasting improvement compared to bipolar radiofrequency combined with IPL or blue light activation.[57]

Other studies have shown no significant improvement of IPL over benzoyl peroxide gel alone.[58] Like treatment with antibiotics, prolonged treatments with light are required to reduce *P. acnes* levels and maintain improvement of acne. IPL is a good alternative for treatment of acne if patients cannot tolerate oral antibiotics or other conventional therapies.

OTHER

Intense pulsed light has a broad therapeutic range and has very few side effects, making it a good treatment option for many skin conditions. As physicians become more comfortable with their use, IPL is being tested in a variety of new indications, such as scars. IPL has been shown to be effective on surgically induced scar.[59] The mechanism of action in scar improvement was suggested to be due to a reduction of vascular proliferation, which is essential to collagen overgrowth. A study evaluating the efficacy of IPL in improving keloids and hypertrophic scar from burns, trauma, surgery and acne found overall clinical improvement in 92.5% of patients with 31.2% of them having excellent improvement.[60] Intense pulsed light has also been successfully tried in the treatment of angiokeratomas in Fabry disease.[61] After 10 sessions, the lesions almost completely cleared without any scars or significant complaints, without recurrence at a 12-month follow-up.

COMPLICATIONS

Although IPL is generally perceived to be a safe and easy-to-use therapy, it is not without risk. The complexity of IPL procedures is largely underestimated. In fact, IPL technology requires a great deal of experience given the wide range of possible parameter combinations of wavelength, pulse duration, pulse frequency and fluence. The increase in popularity of IPL devices is attributed to its broad clinical applications and aggressive advertising. As IPL sources become increasingly popular, a greater number of treatments are being performed by inexperienced nonmedical professionals and even untrained physicians. The result of the nonphysician practice of these procedures is an increase in complications being reported nationally.[62] The rise in serious complications caused by nonphysician practice underscores the importance of improving the Food and Drug Administration (FDA) regulation on who is able to use these devices.

Preventable errors should be distinguished from adverse effects or complications. Commonly reported side effects that are within reason include transient erythema, lasting up to 2 days, and edema. When not used within appropriate parameters, more severe complications are seen. Potential side effects include blistering, bruising, crusting, erythema, dyspigmentation, scar or infection. Scarring is almost always a result of treatment with excessive fluence.[63] Preventable errors stem from a lack of training, insufficient documentation, inaccurate patient information, misdiagnosis, lack of a test treatment or incorrect operation of light sources.[64]

Complications may be avoided by appropriate selection of parameters based on skin type, along with pretreatment test doses in inconspicuous sites. Test doses are important to evaluate for appropriate clinical endpoints. In Figure 11.6, the right circle received a fluence of 24 J/cm^2, 15 ms pulse duration and 5°C cooling (LuxYs™ handpiece; Palomar Medical Technologies, Inc, Burlington, MA) using a mask, which resulted in a diffusely pink circle representing an overly brisk response. While, the left box received a fluence of 22 J/cm^2 with the same pulse duration and cooling, resulting in appropriate erythema of only the pigmented lesions. Patients should return 4–6 weeks after the test dose to evaluate for any

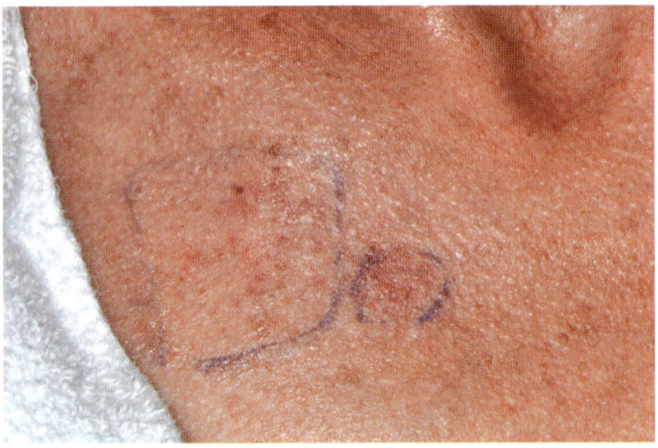

Fig. 11.6: Test areas 1 hour after treatment
Courtesy: E Victor Ross, Director, Laser and Cosmetic Dermatology Center, Scripps Clinic, Carmel Valley, CA

unwanted effects prior to treatment of entire areas to determine appropriate settings.

One common mistake we see is the use of overly aggressive settings, which can result in a striped appearance, referred to as "striping" (Fig. 11.7A). This can generally be improved with further treatment (Fig. 11.7B). Another common mistake we have seen is the use of IPL or laser devices with millisecond pulse durations to remove tattoos, which may result in scarring (Fig. 11.8). With the growing number of tattoo removal procedures being executed every year, more side effects are being seen. Tattoo removal requires very short (nanosecond) pulse durations given that the chromophore (tattoo pigment) is small. When inexperienced practitioners use IPL devices which have millisecond pulse durations, this results in excessive nonspecific heating, blistering and scarring of the tissues.[65] Even when treating conditions, when a millisecond pulse duration would be appropriate, one should avoid tattoos in the treatment area to avoid these risks.

A complication reported after inappropriate IPL use was a severe blistering eruption.[66] This patient was a 21-year-old female looking for treatment of a 10-year history of redness on her medial and lateral cheeks. She presented to a "skin care center" where she was diagnosed with rosacea by a nonphysician. She was treated with an IPL device without a test-spot treatment. The parameters used for this treatment are unknown and likely represent excessively high fluence tissue injury given the immediate vesiculation and bullae formation after treatment. She also developed significant edema with visual field obstruction.

While IPLs are more intrinsically eye-safe than lasers, eye injuries have been reported from IPL treatment.[5,67] After treatment of pigmented lesions of the upper eyelids without eye protection at a beauty salon, the patient developed bilateral irreversible anterior uveitis and ocular iritis.[68] Another case of iris photoablation from treatment of the upper eyelid without ocular protection resulted in pupil asymmetry.[69] It is also important to keep in mind the eye-safety of the operator. Lightspeed goggles (Glendale Inc., Smithfield, RI) are protective and darken only upon light exposure decreasing obscured vision of the operator.

It is important for practitioners to have a high level of training and experience with these devices in

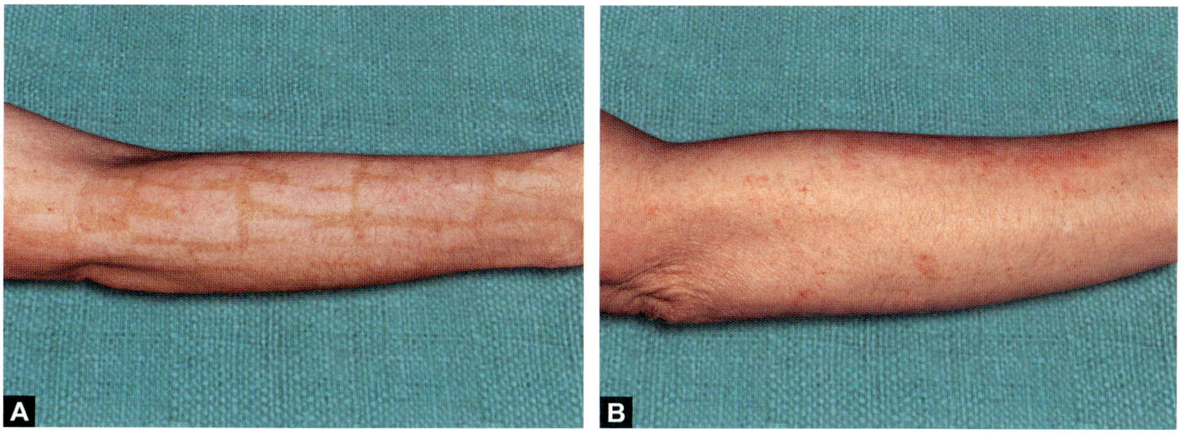

Figs 11.7A and B: (A) "Striping" due to aggressive intense pulsed light settings; (B) Great improvement of "striping" after treatment with a long-pulsed alexandrite laser
Courtesy: E Victor Ross, Director, Laser and Cosmetic Dermatology Center, Scripps Clinic, Carmel Valley, CA

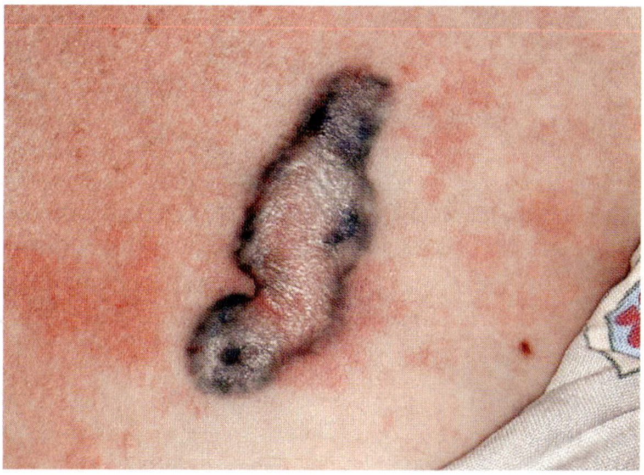

Fig. 11.8: Scarring secondary to attempted tattoo removal with intense pulsed light
Courtesy: E Victor Ross, Director, Laser and Cosmetic Dermatology Center, Scripps Clinic, Carmel Valley, CA

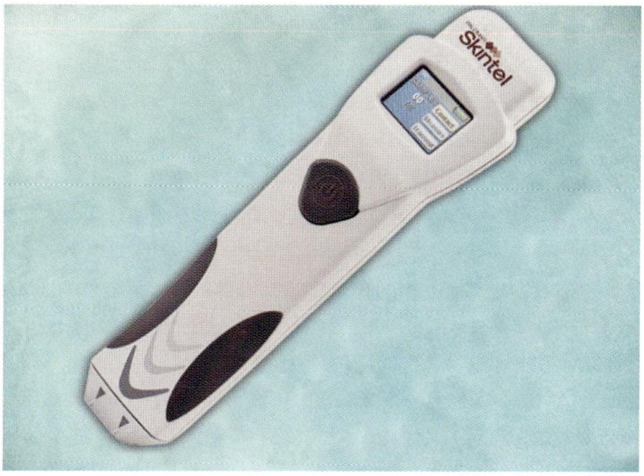

Fig. 11.9: The Skintel™ Reader
Courtesy: Palomar Medical Technologies, Inc, Burlington, MA

order to reduce the risk of complications. However, it may be impossible to completely eliminate side effects all together. Perhaps an oral or written board exam should be required prior to operating IPL and other light-based devices.

WHAT'S NEW?

As IPL devices continue to gain popularity, newer technologies are designed to make these devices more user friendly. Skintel™ Reader (Palomar Medical Technologies, Inc, Burlington, MA) (Fig. 11.9) is an accessory to an IPL device designed to objectively measure the melanin content in the skin. The melanin reader guides selection of appropriate treatment settings to improve safety by minimizing operator error and optimizing treatment settings. It also provides guidance in tracking changes in an individual's sun exposure. Rather than subjective "eyeball" assessment of background epidermal melanin content, the operator takes three sample readings with the Skintel™ Reader on clear skin, which is then averaged into a Melanin Index Value. This value is communicated wirelessly to the IPL system. The operator then chooses a suitable pulsewidth using the Skintel™ Test Spot Tables and proceeds to enter a test spot fluence based on assessment of the client's skin and the Skintel™ Value. This technology adds an element of treatment confidence and allows the user to be less dependent on the more subjective Fitzpatrick Skin Type. More importantly, guidance in setting selection has the potential to reduce the risk of complications, particularly in less experienced users.

In the horizon, new devices are for home use. Devices appropriate for home-use need to be cost-effective for mass production, easy to use without any training, eye-safe, while still achieving effective results. There is a growing market for at home hair removal devices, and numerous IPL devices are now available. Several studies show significant hair reduction with home-use IPL devices.[70-72] However, these devices require extended treatment times and increased frequency of use compared to in-office devices.

There is a trend toward cheaper, more convenient treatments through home-use devices. A newer portable IPL device (Silk'n, Home Skinovations Ltd, Kfar Saba, Israel) is safe for home-use without a cooling mechanism or eye protection. This device was shown to be effective in 37.8–53.6% hair reduction 6 months after three treatments with erythema as the only side effect.[70]

A concern with home-use devices is that additional safety measures with skin-sensor technologies are required to prevent use on darker skin types. Accurate complication rates may not be reflected in previous studies, because they are carefully monitored rather than regular consumer use outside of a clinical trial. Comparing three leading IPL hair removal devices: iPulse Personal (CyDen Ltd, Swansea, UK) Silk'n SensEpil (Home Skinovations Ltd, Yokneam, Israel), and SatinLux/Lumea (Philips, Eindhoven, Netherlands), ocular safety may be compromised if their primary safety mechanisms fail or if users intentionally defeat safeguards.[73] The results of home devices are impressive, but still inferior to office-base devices. Therefore, it is unlikely that home devices will replace in-office procedures.

CONCLUSION

Intense pulsed light has been shown to be effective in a variety of skin conditions. Most studies comparing laser to IPL show similar effectiveness with less risk of complications. In some cases, IPL may even be more effective than lasers especially when there is more than one target that needs to be treated. There is no question that the range of settings inherent to these devices makes them more versatile than laser devices. This is advantageous to the skilled dermatologist, but can lead to grave error in the hands of the unqualified user. Due to their economical pricing and lack of governmental regulation, IPL systems are commonly purchased for use in beauty salons and "medispas", which unfortunately, puts these devices in possession of untrained users. If used in the appropriate manner, these devices are really the "jack of all trades". However, long-term, large controlled and blinded comparative trials are lacking.

REFERENCES

1. Anderson RR, Parrish JA. Selective photothermolysis: precise microsurgery by selective absorption of pulsed radiation. Science. 1983;220(4596):524-7.
2. Anderson RR. Dermatologic history of the ruby laser: the long story of short pulses. Arch Dermatol. 2003;139(1):70-4.
3. Ross EV. Laser versus intense pulsed light: Competing technologies in dermatology. Lasers Surg Med. 2006;38(4):261-72.
4. Cartier H. Use of intense pulsed light in the treatment of scars. J Cosmet Dermatol. 2005;4(1):34-40.
5. Sutter FK, Landau K. Ocular complication of PhotoDerm VL therapy for facial port-wine stain. Dermatol Surg. 2003;29(1):111-2.
6. Ross EV, Smirnov M, Pankratov M, et al. Intense pulsed light and laser treatment of facial telangiectasias and dyspigmentation: some theoretical and practical comparisons. Dermatol Surg. 2005;31(9 Pt 2):1188-98.
7. Town G, Ash C, Eadie E, et al. Measuring key parameters of intense pulsed light (IPL) devices. J Cosmet Laser Ther. 2007;9(3):148-60.
8. Yamashita T, Negishi K, Hariya T, et al. Intense pulsed light therapy for superficial pigmented lesions evaluated by reflectance-mode confocal microscopy and optical coherence tomography. J Invest Dermatol. 2006;126(10):2281-6.
9. Grevelink JM, van Leeuwen RL, Anderson RR, et al. Clinical and histological responses of congenital melanocytic nevi after single treatment with Q-switched lasers. Arch Dermatol. 1997;133(3): 349-53.
10. Dummer R. About moles, melanomas, and lasers: the dermatologist's schizophrenic attitude toward pigmented lesions. Arch Dermatol. 2003; 139(11):1405-6.
11. Gottschaller C, Hohenleutner U, Landthaler M. Metastasis of a malignant melanoma 2 years after carbon dioxide laser treatment of a pigmented lesion: case report and review of the literature. Acta Derm Venereol. 2006;86(1):44-7.
12. Lee EH, Busam KJ. Desmoplastic melanoma presenting after laser treatment: a case report and tale of caution. Dermatol Surg. 2011;37(11):1689-92.
13. Li YH, Chen JZ, Wei HC, et al. Efficacy and safety of intense pulsed light in treatment of melasma in Chinese patients. Dermatol Surg. 2008;34(5): 693-700.

14. Zoccali G, Piccolo D, Allegra P, et al. Melasma treated with intense pulsed light. Aesthetic Plast Surg. 2010;34(4):486-93.
15. Landthaler M, Hohenleutner U. Laser therapy of vascular lesions. Photodermatol Photoimmunol Photomed. 2006;22(6):324-32.
16. Katugampola GA, Lanigan SW. Five years' experience of treating port wine stains with the flash-lamp-pumped pulsed dye laser. Br J Dermatol. 1997;137(5):750-4.
17. Lucassen GW, Verkruysse W, Keijzer M, et al. Light distributions in a port wine stain model containing multiple cylindrical and curved blood vessels. Lasers Surg Med. 1996;18(4):345-57.
18. Raulin C, Schroeter CA, Weiss RA, et al. Treatment of port-wine stains with a noncoherent pulsed light source: a retrospective study. Arch Dermatol. 1999;135(6):679-83.
19. Bjerring P, Christiansen K, Troilius A. Intense pulsed light source for the treatment of dye laser resistant port-wine stains. J Cosmet Laser Ther. 2003;5(1): 7-13.
20. Babilas P, Schreml S, Eames T, et al. Split-face comparison of intense pulsed light with short- and long-pulsed dye lasers for the treatment of port-wine stains. Lasers Surg Med. 2010;42(8):720-7.
21. McGill DJ, MacLaren W, Mackay IR. A direct comparison of pulsed dye, alexandrite, KTP and Nd:YAG lasers and IPL in patients with previously treated capillary malformations. Lasers Surg Med. 2008;40(6):390-8.
22. Faurschou A, Togsverd-Bo K, Zachariae C, et al. Pulsed dye laser vs. intense pulsed light for port-wine stains: a randomized side-by-side trial with blinded response evaluation. Br J Dermatol. 2009;160(2):359-64.
23. Papageorgiou P, Clayton W, Norwood S, et al. Treatment of rosacea with intense pulsed light: significant improvement and long-lasting results. Br J Dermatol. 2008;159(3):628-32.
24. Schroeter CA, Haaf-von Below S, Neumann HA. Effective treatment of rosacea using intense pulsed light systems. Dermatol Surg. 2005;31(10):1285-9.
25. Neuhaus IM, Zane LT, Tope WD. Comparative efficacy of nonpurpuragenic pulsed dye laser and intense pulsed light for erythematotelangiectatic rosacea. Dermatol Surg. 2009;35(6):920-8.
26. Weiss RA, Ross EV, Tanghetti EA, et al. Characterization of an optimized light source and comparison to pulsed dye laser for superficial and deep vessel clearance. Lasers Surg Med. 2011;43(2):92-8.
27. Feng Y, Zhao J, Gold MH. Skin rejuvenation in Asian skin: the analysis of clinical effects and basic mechanisms of intense pulsed light. J Drugs Dermatol. 2008;7(3):273-9.
28. Weiss RA, Weiss MA, Beasley KL. Rejuvenation of photoaged skin: 5 years results with intense pulsed light of the face, neck, and chest. Dermatol Surg. 2002;28(12):1115-9.
29. Jorgensen GF, Hedelund L, Haedersdal M. Long-pulsed dye laser versus intense pulsed light for photodamaged skin: a randomized split-face trial with blinded response evaluation. Lasers Surg Med. 2008;40(5):293-9.
30. Bjerring P, Christiansen K, Troilius A, et al. Facial photo rejuvenation using two different intense pulsed light (IPL) wavelength bands. Lasers Surg Med. 2004;34(2):120-6.
31. Galeckas KJ, Collins M, Ross EV, et al. Split-face treatment of facial dyschromia: pulsed dye laser with a compression handpiece versus intense pulsed light. Dermatol Surg. 2008;34(5):672-80.
32. Peterson JD, Goldman MP. Rejuvenation of the aging chest: a review and our experience. Dermatol Surg. 2011;37(5):555-71.
33. Rusciani A, Motta A, Fino P, et al. Treatment of poikiloderma of Civatte using intense pulsed light source: 7 years of experience. Dermatol Surg. 2008; 34(3):314-9.
34. Cameron H, Ibbotson SH, Dawe RS, et al. Within-patient right-left blinded comparison of diode (810 nm) laser therapy and intense pulsed light therapy for hair removal. Lasers in medical science. 2008;23(4):393-7.
35. Dierickx CC, Grossman MC, Farinelli WA, et al. Permanent hair removal by normal-mode ruby laser. Arch Dermatol. 1998;134(7):837-42.
36. Grossman MC, Dierickx C, Farinelli W, et al. Damage to hair follicles by normal-mode ruby laser pulses. J Am Acad Dermatol. 1996;35(6):889-94.
37. Altshuler GB, Anderson RR, Manstein D, et al. Extended theory of selective photothermolysis. Lasers Surg Med. 2001;29(5):416-32.
38. Gold MH, Bell MW, Foster TD, et al. Long-term epilation using the EpiLight broad band, intense pulsed light hair removal system. Dermatol Surg. 1997;23(10):909-13.
39. McGill DJ, Hutchison C, McKenzie E, et al. A randomised, split-face comparison of facial hair removal with the alexandrite laser and intense pulsed light system. Lasers Surg Med. 2007;39(10):767-72.
40. Bjerring P. Clinical comparison of hair reduction using the newest generation IPL and a first generation ruby laser. J Cutan Laser Ther. 2000;2(4):211.
41. Amin SP, Goldberg DJ. Clinical comparison of four hair removal lasers and light sources. J Cosmet Laser Ther. 2006;8(2):65-8.
42. Feng YM, Zhou ZC, Gold MH. Hair removal using a new intense pulsed light source in Chinese patients. J Cosmet Laser Ther. 2009;11(2):94-7.
43. Radmanesh M, Azar-Beig M, Abtahian A, et al. Burning, paradoxical hypertrichosis, leukotrichia and folliculitis are four major complications of

intense pulsed light hair removal therapy. J Dermatolog Treat. 2008;19(6):360-3.
44. Radmanesh M. Paradoxical hypertrichosis and terminal hair change after intense pulsed light hair removal therapy. J Dermatolog Treat. 2009; 20(1):52-4.
45. Willey A, Torrontegui J, Azpiazu J, et al. Hair stimulation following laser and intense pulsed light photo-epilation: review of 543 cases and ways to manage it. Lasers Surg Med. 2007;39(4):297-301.
46. Jeffes EW, McCullough JL, Weinstein GD, et al. Photodynamic therapy of actinic keratoses with topical aminolevulinic acid hydrochloride and fluorescent blue light. J Am Acad Dermatol. 2001;45(1):96-104.
47. Lehmann P. Methyl aminolaevulinate-photodynamic therapy: a review of clinical trials in the treatment of actinic keratoses and nonmelanoma skin cancer. Br J Dermatol. 2007;156(5):793-801.
48. Peng Q, Berg K, Moan J, et al. 5-Aminolevulinic acid-based photodynamic therapy: principles and experimental research. Photochem Photobiol. 1997; 65(2):235-51.
49. Ruiz-Rodriguez R, Sanz-Sanchez T, Cordoba S. Photodynamic photorejuvenation. Dermatol Surg. 2002;28(8):742-4.
50. Avram DK, Goldman MP. Effectiveness and safety of ALA-IPL in treating actinic keratoses and photodamage. J Drugs Dermatol. 2004;3(1 Suppl):S36-9.
51. Dover JS, Bhatia AC, Stewart B, et al. Topical 5-aminolevulinic acid combined with intense pulsed light in the treatment of photoaging. Arch Dermatol. 2005;141(10):1247-52.
52. Babilas P, Schreml S, Szeimies RM, et al. Intense pulsed light (IPL): a review. Lasers Surg Med. 2010; 42(2):93-104.
53. Kim HS, Yoo JY, Cho KH, et al. Topical photodynamic therapy using intense pulsed light for treatment of actinic keratosis: clinical and histopathologic evaluation. Dermatol Surg. 2005;31(1):33-6.
54. Gold MH, Bradshaw VL, Boring MM, et al. Split-face comparison of photodynamic therapy with 5-aminolevulinic acid and intense pulsed light versus intense pulsed light alone for photodamage. Dermatol Surg. 2006;32(6):795-801.
55. Gold MH. Acne and PDT: new techniques with lasers and light sources. Lasers in medical science. 2007;22(2):67-72.
56. Yeung CK, Shek SY, Bjerring P, et al. A comparative study of intense pulsed light alone and its combination with photodynamic therapy for the treatment of facial acne in Asian skin. Lasers Surg Med. 2007;39(1):1-6.
57. Taub AF. A comparison of intense pulsed light, combination radiofrequency and intense pulsed light, and blue light in photodynamic therapy for acne vulgaris. J Drugs Dermatol. 2007;6(10):1010-6.
58. Chang SE, Ahn SJ, Rhee DY, et al. Treatment of facial acne papules and pustules in Korean patients using an intense pulsed light device equipped with a 530- to 750-nm filter. Dermatol Surg. 2007;33(6):676-9.
59. Bellew SG, Weiss MA, Weiss RA. Comparison of intense pulsed light to 595-nm long-pulsed pulsed dye laser for treatment of hypertrophic surgical scars: a pilot study. J Drugs Dermatol. 2005;4(4): 448-52.
60. Erol OO, Gurlek A, Agaoglu G, et al. Treatment of hypertrophic scars and keloids using intense pulsed light (IPL). Aesthetic plastic surgery. 2008; 32(6):902-9.
61. Morais P, Santos AL, Baudrier T, et al. Angiokeratomas of Fabry successfully treated with intense pulsed light. J Cosmet Laser Ther. 2008;10(4):218-22.
62. Friedman PM, Jih MH, Burns AJ, et al. Nonphysician practice of dermatologic surgery: the Texas perspective. Dermatol Surg. 2004;30(6):857-63.
63. Adamic M, Troilius A, Adatto M, et al. Vascular lasers and IPLS: guidelines for care from the European Society for Laser Dermatology (ESLD). J Cosmet Laser Ther. 2007;9(2):113-24.
64. Greve B, Raulin C. Professional errors caused by lasers and intense pulsed light technology in dermatology and aesthetic medicine: preventive strategies and case studies. Dermatol Surg. 2002;28(2):156-61.
65. Wenzel S, Landthaler M, Baumler W. Recurring mistakes in tattoo removal. A case series. Dermatology. 2009;218(2):164-7.
66. Sperber BR, Walling HW, Arpey CJ, et al. Vesiculobullous eruption from intense pulsed light treatment. Dermatol Surg. 2005;31(3):345-8.
67. Moreno-Arias GA, Castelo-Branco C, Ferrando J. Side-effects after IPL photodepilation. Dermatol Surg. 2002;28(12):1131-4.
68. Pang AL, Wells K. Bilateral anterior uveitis after intense pulsed light therapy for pigmented eyelid lesions. Dermatol Surg. 2008;34(9):1276-9.
69. Javey G, Schwartz SG, Albini TA. Ocular complication of intense pulsed light therapy: iris photoablation. Dermatol Surg. 2010;36(9):1466-8.
70. Alster TS, Tanzi EL. Effect of a novel low-energy pulsed-light device for home-use hair removal. Dermatol Surg. 2009;35(3):483-9.
71. Mulholland RS. Silk'n--a novel device using Home Pulsed Light for hair removal at home. J Cosmet Laser Ther. 2009;11(2):106-9.
72. Emerson R, Town G. Hair removal with a novel, low fluence, home-use intense pulsed light device. J Cosmet Laser Ther. 2009;11(2):98-105.
73. Town G, Ash C. Are home-use intense pulsed light (IPL) devices safe? Lasers in medical science. 2010;25(6):773-80.

CHAPTER

12

Noninvasive Skin Tightening and Body Contouring

Andrew A Nelson, Mathew M Avram

INTRODUCTION

Mankind has long been obsessed with achieving the so-called "perfect body"; in differing times and different circumstances, the ideal body has evolved. Currently, in our image-obsessed culture, many people possess a strong desire to lose weight to achieve their perfect body. Unfortunately, obesity is an epidemic in our culture and weight loss is a challenging goal for many. While traditional dieting and exercise remain the best way to lose weight and maintain the weight loss, this may not work for all patients. Even patients who have achieved weight loss may continue to have small "problem areas". As a result, patients are increasingly turning to their physicians desiring new technologies to help achieve body contouring and the ideal body.

Historically, liposuction was the only means to achieve body contouring. And while liposuction remains the gold standard, it is an invasive procedure with associated pain, bruising, and downtime. Modern medicine has witnessed a dramatic movement towards minimal or no downtime procedures, as patients have become increasingly unwilling to tolerate prolonged healing or recovery times. The field of body contouring has rapidly evolved in the last several years with the introduction of numerous new technologies including lasers, radiofrequency devices, ultrasound devices and cryolipolysis. These noninvasive devices have been reported to have multiple beneficial effects including: improving the appearance of excess adipose tissue, reducing the overall volume of fat, reducing waist and thigh circumference, improving the appearance of cellulite and skin tightening. While these technologies are relatively new, and their potential utility must ultimately be determined by well done randomized scientific studies, the initial results and possibilities are incredibly exciting.

DETERMINING YOUR PATIENT'S CURRENT STATUS AND TREATMENT GOALS

The first step in determining which treatment option is best for your patient is to first assess your patient and discuss their therapeutic goal. Depending on your patient's status, as well as their "problem areas" and goals, certain devices may be a better option.

The classic definition for obesity is based on a patient's body mass index (BMI) (It is calculated as a person's weight in kilograms divided by the square of his/her height in meters). This is a quick and easy calculation for patients and physicians. Obese patients are defined as those patients having a BMI greater than 30. Typically, obese patients (BMI > 30) are not good candidates for noninvasive body contouring and likely would benefit more from bariatric or other surgical interventions to help achieve meaningful weight loss. Thus, the simple BMI calculation may help to determine those patients who are not ideal candidates for noninvasive body contouring. Unfortunately, the BMI is also an oversimplification, as it does not necessarily take into account the patient's mixture of muscle and adipose tissue, or their overall body type. Many patients who present for noninvasive body sculpting may be in very good shape overall with a normal BMI, but feel plagued by only a few small problem areas, such as the thighs or flanks. Therefore for these patients, the authors utilize measurements such as thigh circumference, waist circumference, skin fold thickness, visual assessment, and photographic comparisons pre- and post procedure in our practice; these assessments more typically reflect the patient's ultimate clinical presentation and outcome.

It is also important to differentiate between fat and cellulite when assessing your patient. Excess fat and obesity are due to an overabundance of structurally normal adipocytes. In contrast, cellulite is best considered as a structural abnormality of adipocytes. How then does normal fat become cellulite? This remains an area of ongoing research, but it is thought that cellulite may result from hormonal changes. Cellulite is rare in prepubertal females and males of any age, but is so common in postpubertal females that some researchers classify cellulite as a female secondary sexual characteristic. Estrogens are thought to stimulate lipogenesis while inhibiting lipolysis, thereby contributing to cellulite formation. Furthermore, it is believed that certain body areas have less effective lymphatic and vascular circulation, thereby contributing to the development of cellulite in these "high-risk areas". Ultrasound and magnetic resonance imaging (MRI) studies have documented the significant structural alterations between normal adipose tissue and abnormal cellulite structure. In normal adipose tissue, the fibrous septae between the lobules of adipose tissue are arranged in an overlapping criss-cross pattern, creating greater strength of the tissue. Cellulite, on the other hand, has fibrous septae that are arranged parallel to each other, and perpendicular to the skin surface. This weaker structure allows for the focal herniation of adipose tissue, which ultimately contributes to the classic undulating, lumpy, "cottage cheese" appearance of cellulite. It remains unclear whether the presence of excess adipose tissue increases the risk of the development of cellulite. As a result of the differences between excess normal adipose tissue and structurally abnormal cellulite, the authors believe that excess fat and cellulite should be considered distinct entities and treated as such. Certain devices that may be effective for treating cellulite may not treat excess adipose tissue, and vice versa.

Once the patient has been evaluated and their treatment goals discussed, the patient and the treating physician can begin to effectively discuss the noninvasive body contouring options. Determining the best treatment option for your patient is dependent on clinical presentation, treatment goals, and most importantly—the patient's preferences.

PHYSICAL TREATMENT OF FAT AND CELLULITE

Noninvasive Devices

Endermologie (LPG Systems, Valence, France) is an FDA (United States Food and Drug Administration) cleared device, which improves the appearance of cellulite through massage and kneading of the affected skin. The device combines positive and negative pressure created between two rollers to physically manipulate the patient's skin. The technique is thought to stimulate blood and lymphatic flow, thereby altering the architecture of the fat and improving the appearance of cellulite. It is less clear if Endermologie has any effect on reducing unwanted excess adipose tissue. Modest clinical improvements in cellulite have been documented in clinical studies. A study by Güleç of 33 women who were treated with Endermologie for 15 sessions, demonstrated a statistically significant improvement in the appearance of cellulite as assessed by a visual scale; however, few of the patients (5 of the 33 patients) actually demonstrated clinical improvement.[1] A recent study by Collis et al. compared twice weekly treatment with Endermologie to a combination treatment of aminophylline cream and Endermologie; the authors concluded that Endermologie is not an effective treatment of cellulite, although 10 out of 35 patients with Endermologie-treated legs reported that their cellulite appearance clinically improved.[2] In summary, Endermologie may result in modest improvements in the clinical appearance of fat and cellulite; however, it is likely that ongoing treatments would be necessary to maintain the improvement.

Radiofrequency Devices

Radiofrequency (RF) devices pass sinusoidal, alternating current (AC) through tissue thereby causing ionic flow and ultimately heat from molecular friction. In essence, the tissue itself is the source of the heat, instead of the actual device. Radiofrequency is therefore thought to create localized heat in the targeted tissue mass, while limiting the collateral spread of energy, neuromuscular reactions, or electrolysis. Adipocytes have high tissue resistance and relatively low heat transfer coefficients; as a result, adipose tissue can be readily heated by RF technologies and the heat will be relatively localized to the adipocytes. Recently, many RF devices have been advertised to improve the appearance of fat and cellulite.

The VelaSmooth and VelaShape (Syneron Medical Ltd, Irvine, CA) devices combine physical manipulation similar to Endermologie (massage and suction), with bipolar RF energy and broadband infrared light (700–2000 nm) to treat excess fat and cellulite. It has been proposed that these devices heat subcutaneous tissue and fat, resulting in increased blood flow and lipolysis in the treatment areas, thereby improving the appearance of fat and cellulite. In a randomized clinical study by Nootheti et al., patients were treated twice weekly for 6 weeks with either the VelaSmooth device or another laser device for cellulite (TriActive, Cynosure Inc, Westford, MA).[3] Seventy-five percent of patients were observed to have an improvement, when comparing pre- and post-treatment photographs, but the results were modest. Patients were also observed to have a decrease in the upper and lower thigh circumference, as well as an improvement in the appearance of cellulite (Figs 12.1 and 12.2). However, no statistically significant differences in the efficacies of the two devices were observed and no placebo group was included in the study. Bruising is a common side-effect following treatment with the VelaSmooth device, likely related to the vacuum pressure and physical manipulation of the tissue rather than the RF technology itself.

Unipolar, volumetric RF devices with more diffuse, deep heating are also being studied for the treatment of fat and cellulite. Thirty patients were treated by Goldberg et al. with a unipolar RF device (Accent, Alma Lasers US, Buffalo Grove, IL) every other week for a total of 6 treatment sessions; a decrease in mean leg circumference of 2.45 cm was observed, although the study was limited due to a lack of placebo or untreated controls.[4]

Recently, a novel RF device combining controlled radiofrequency heating and high voltage ultrashort electrical pulses has been developed to treat adipose tissue (BodyFX, InMode Inc, Richmond Hill, Canada). The BodyFX system utilizes a vacuum system and traditional RF heating to warm the tissue and adipocytes to the range of 43–45°C. This heats the triglyceride droplet within the adipocyte and begins thermal adipocyte apoptosis. The BodyFX device then delivers high voltage RF pulsing, which electroporates the cell membrane, basically poking a hole in the adipocyte membrane, leading to apoptosis of the adipocyte. These two mechanisms act synergistically to achieve greater levels of adipocyte apoptosis and greater clinical improvement. In initial studies, BodyFX has been shown to reduce circumferential measurements of treated areas, as well as improve

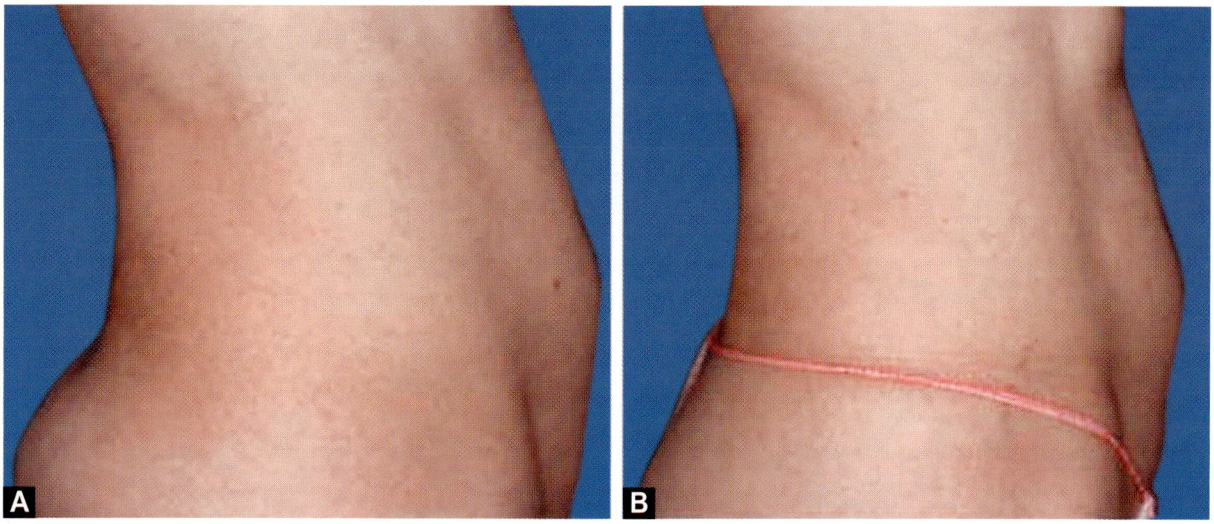

Figs 12.1A and B: Clinical improvement in the appearance of the abdomen of a 60-year-old woman before (A) and 3 months after (B) treatment with VelaShape. Baseline circumference: 87 cm; 3 month follow-up circumference: 84 cm
Source: Photos courtesy of Dr Lori Brightman. Reprinted with permission from: Kim J, Lask G, Nelson A (Eds). Comprehensive Aesthetic Rejuvenation: A Regional Approach. New York: Informa Healthcare; 2012

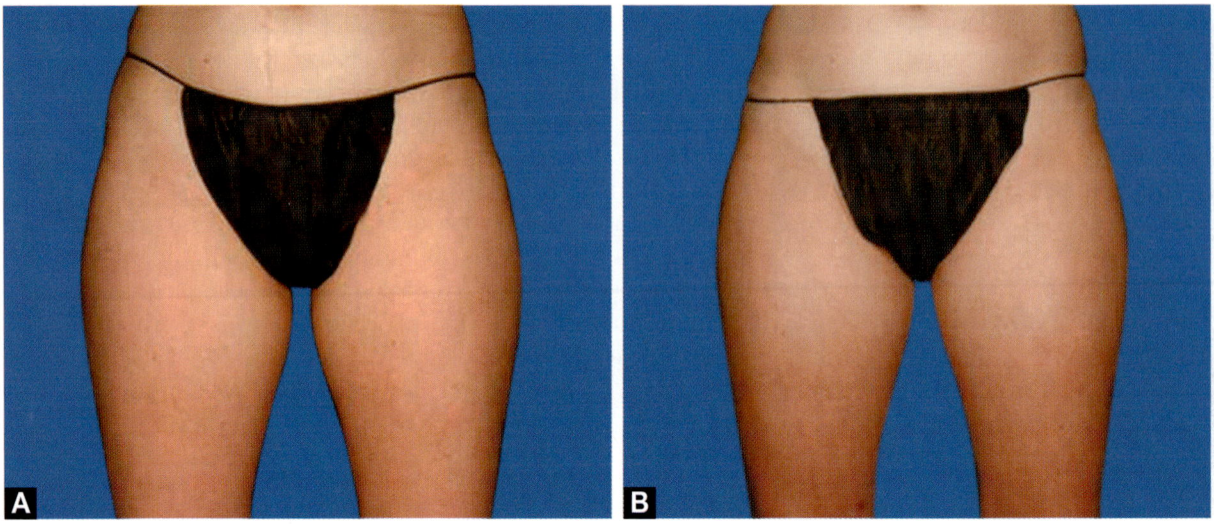

Figs 12.2A and B: Clinical improvement in the appearance of the thighs of a 41-year-old woman before (A) and 6 months after (B) treatments with VelaShape. Five treatments, radiofrequency level: 3, infrared level: 2. Vacuum level: 1, treatment duration: 3 minutes 53 seconds and 10 minutes 10 seconds. Mean baseline measurement: 58.5; mean 6-month follow-up measurement: 56.8 cm
Source: Photos courtesy of Dr Lori Brightman. Reprinted with permission from: Kim J, Lask G, and Nelson A (Eds). Comprehensive Aesthetic Rejuvenation: A Regional Approach. New York: Informa Healthcare; 2012

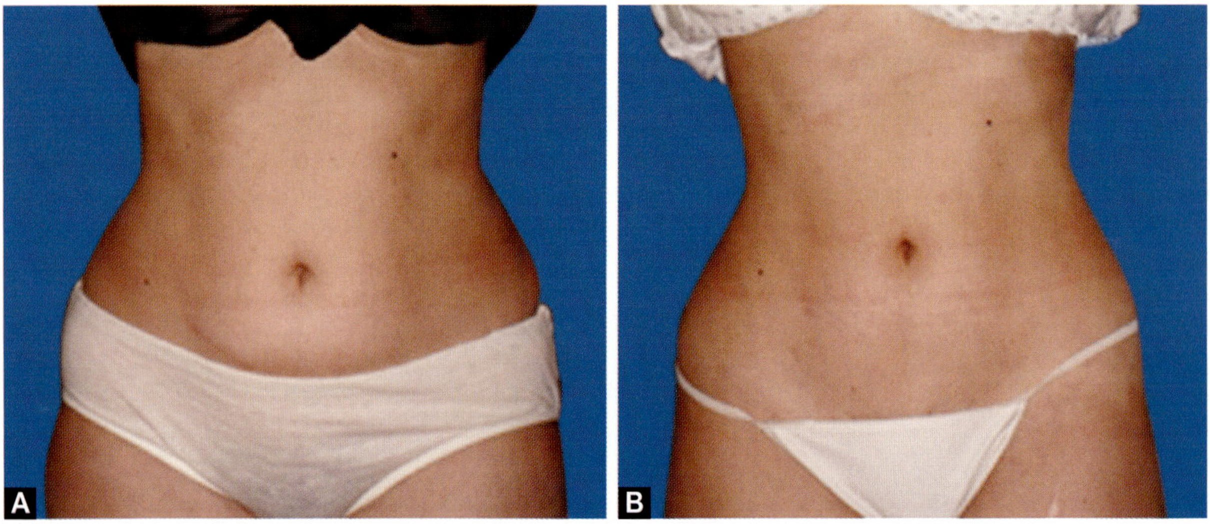

Figs 12.3A and B: Clinical improvement in abdominal circumference "muffin top" before (A) and 1 month after (B) 8 weekly treatments with the BodyFX device. Note that there is not only the reduction in subcutaneous adipose tissue, but there is tightening of the overlying skin as well
Source: Photos courtesy of Dr Stephen Mulholland

the appearance of cellulite (Figs 12.3 and 12.4). At this time, the BodyFX device has not been cleared by the United States Food and Drug Administration, although it is approved in Canada, Europe, Australia, and parts of Asia. The BodyFX device represents a very exciting option for the treatment of excess fat, as it combines the added benefit of tightening the treatment area through traditional RF.

These RF technologies represent safe and efficacious therapeutic options for patients, although further clinical studies are necessary to establish their exact roles.

Ultrasound Devices

The diagnostic utility of ultrasound devices has long been established; more recently, high intensity

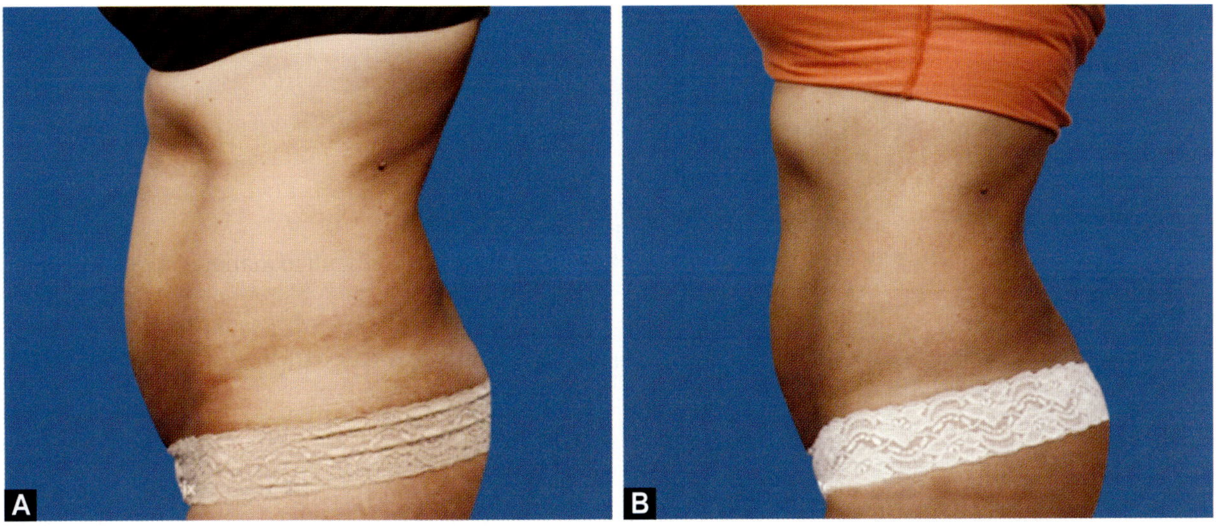

Figs 12.4A and B: Clinical improvement in abdominal circumference "muffin top", shown in profile view, before (A) and 1 month after (B) 8 weekly treatments with the BodyFX device. Note that there is not only the reduction in subcutaneous adipose tissue, but there is tightening of the overlying skin as well
Source: Photos courtesy of Dr Stephen Mulholland

focused ultrasound (HIFU) devices have been developed to treat adipocytes and the subcutis. The LipoSonix device (Medicis Technologies Corp, Scottsdale, AZ) was recently FDA cleared for noninvasive waist circumference reduction. Other ultrasound devices are not yet FDA cleared or commercially available in the United States for the treatment of fat and cellulite.

A recent study by Jewell et al. of the LipoSonix high intensity focused ultrasound (HIFU) device documented significant improvement following a single treatment session.[5] One hundred and eighty patients were randomized to one of two different doses of HIFU or to a sham treatment. Twelve weeks following the single treatment, the patients treated with the higher HIFU dose had achieved a statistically significant improvement in waist circumference compared to the sham group (–2.44 cm versus –1.43 cm). Patients were observed to have "improved" or "much improved" outcomes as assessed by physicians, and patients were satisfied with their treatments. Common adverse events following the treatment included pain, bruising and edema. However, no significant laboratory abnormalities were observed following treatment, including: lipid profiles, markers of inflammation, coagulation, liver or renal function, hematologic assessments, or blood chemistry.

Another novel ultrasound technology, the Ultrashape Contour I (Ultrashape Ltd, Tel Aviv, Israel) is being used in Europe and the United Kingdom for the treatment of excess adipose tissue. A recent prospective, nonrandomized, controlled trial of 164 patients was conducted by Teitelbaum et al., to determine the efficacy of the device.[6] A total of 137 patients underwent one Ultrashape treatment to the abdomen, thighs, or flanks. Twelve weeks after the treatment, circumference reductions of the abdomen (mean reduction: 2.3 cm), thighs (mean reduction: 1.8 cm), and flanks (mean reduction: 1.6 cm) were observed. The majority of the improvement in measured circumference was noted to occur within the first two weeks following treatment.

Ultrasound technologies represent a new and evolving area within the field of noninvasive fat treatment. Ultrasound technologies can also be incorporated into invasive liposuction procedures, known as ultrasound-assisted liposuction (UAL). While this is an effective treatment method, it requires an invasive liposuction procedure. More recently, novel noninvasive high intensity focused ultrasound technologies have been developed for improving the appearance of fat and cellulite. While these devices require further clinical study to determine their long-term efficacy and safety profile, they represent an exciting and promising opportunity within this field.

Lasers and Light Sources

Multiple novel light sources and laser technologies have been developed as therapeutic options for fat and cellulite. Historically, these laser devices were utilized as an adjunct with liposuction, known as laser-assisted liposuction (LAL). More recently, new noninvasive laser and light source devices have been marketed for the treatment of fat and cellulite. It is important to note that several devices which are advertised to improve fat and cellulite actually do not affect the adipocytes themselves, but rather, target the dermis in an attempt to stimulate collagen formation/remodeling. Devices with wavelengths in the near-infrared region, as well as intense pulsed light (IPL) sources, fall into this category. At the time of this writing, few laser devices are FDA cleared for the direct treatment of fat and cellulite.

The TriActive device (Cynosure Inc, Bedford, MA) combines deep tissue massage and suction (similar to Endermologie), with contact cooling and a low-intensity diode laser (808 nm). The TriActive device is thought to improve the appearance of cellulite by increasing lymphatic drainage, improving blood flow and tightening the skin in treated areas. Patients typically are treated with the device twice weekly, with progressive improvement following each treatment. In clinical studies, patients were noted to achieve objective reductions in hip and thigh circumference as well as subjective improvements in the appearance of cellulite, including a reduction in the appearance of skin dimpling, improvement in the overall contour of the limb, and improvement in overall skin texture (Figs 12.5A to D). TriActive treatments were generally well tolerated, although approximately 20% of patients developed mild bruising.

The SmoothShapes device (Eleme Medical, Merrimack, NH), combines two different wavelengths of laser with a physical massage system similar to Endermologie. The 915-nm diode wavelength liquefies fat, while the 650-nm wavelength improves fat membrane permeability, thereby allowing the adipocytes to be mobilized to the interstitium. A treatment session consists of multiple passes with the SmoothShapes device, and two to three treatment sessions are performed each week for best results. In clinical studies by Lach and Kulick, the SmoothShapes device results in reduction of the thickness of the subcutaneous fat pad, as assessed by MRI.[7,8] The device was well tolerated with no significant associated adverse events.

The VelaSmooth and VelaShape (Syneron Medical Ltd, Irvine, CA) devices, as discussed previously, combine physical manipulation, bipolar RF energy, and broadband infrared light (700–2000 nm) to facilitate a multimodality approach to fat and cellulite treatment. The efficacy of these devices was previously discussed in the section regarding radiofrequency. In the future, more devices may approach fat and cellulite treatment through this multimodality approach in an effort to achieve greater efficacy.

Recently, a low-level laser device (Zerona, Erchonia Inc, McKinney, TX) was FDA cleared for the noninvasive reduction of circumference of hips, waist and thighs. Zerona is a low-level diode laser (615 nm), which produces five independent beams. The center beam is fixed, while the four remaining beams can be individually adjusted allowing multiple body areas (abdomen, flank, thighs) to be treated simultaneously. The exact mechanism of action has not been fully elucidated, though it has been proposed that low-level laser therapy stimulates the

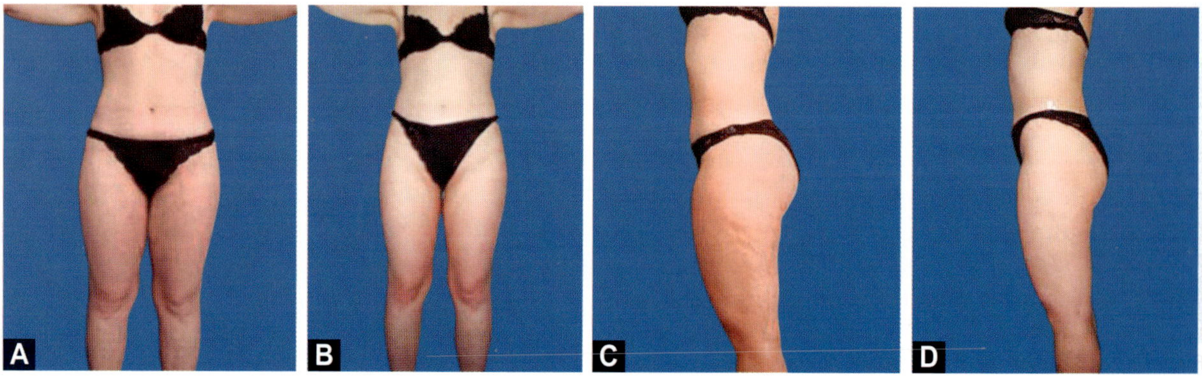

Figs 12.5A to D: Marked clinical improvement in appearance in thighs before (A and C) and after (B and D) 19 treatments with TriActive

Source: Photos courtesy of Andrea Pelosi, Milan. Reprinted with permission from: Kim J, Lask G, Nelson A (Eds). Comprehensive Aesthetic Rejuvenation: A Regional Approach. New York: Informa Healthcare; 2012

fat cell to emulsify; the liquefied fat is then mobilized via a temporary pore in the cell membrane from inside the cell to the interstitium, where the fat is ultimately absorbed into the lymphatic system. Typically, Zerona treatments are performed every other day for a total of six treatments, with each treatment lasting approximately 40 minutes. In a recent clinical trial, a total of 67 patients were randomized to either six treatments with the Zerona device or six "sham" treatments. At the completion of the study at 2 weeks, the "active" treatment group averaged a cumulative reduction of 3.54 inches compared to the "sham" group which averaged a cumulative reduction of just 0.68 inches. No significant adverse effects were observed in the study. Low-level laser therapies represent another potentially promising treatment option for excess adipose tissue.

Cryolipolysis

CoolSculpting (Zeltiq Aesthetics, Pleasanton, CA) is a relatively novel FDA cleared device for noninvasive fat reduction. CoolSculpting utilizes cryolipolysis technology (controlled cold exposure) to selectively cool fat, thereby causing adipocyte apoptosis. The treatment cycle lasts approximately 60 minutes, at the conclusion of which, the skin appears cool, firm and erythematous. Following the treatment, the physician massages the area gently to break up any crystallized adipocytes. Over the next several weeks to months, the adipocytes undergo apoptosis, are mobilized and ultimately eliminated by the body. Typical treatment areas include the flank "love handle", the back "back fat pads" or the abdomen "muffin top" (Figs 12.6A and B). In a recent clinical study, a significant reduction in the thickness of the fat in the treatment area was observed following a single CoolSculpting treatment (mean fat pad thickness reduction of 22.4%, as measured on ultrasound). Of the 32 patients in the study, all had achieved a significant visible contour improvement following a single treatment. The best results were in patients with localized, discrete fat bulges. Treatments are typically well tolerated, although patients may develop bruising as well as transient altered sensation, numbness or even pain in the treatment area. CoolSculpting represents a safe, novel and efficacious, noninvasive treatment option for fat.

CONCLUSIONS

The last few years have witnessed profound changes in the field of body contouring with the development of safe, effective and noninvasive technologies. These noninvasive devices have been reported to have multiple beneficial effects including: improving the appearance of excess adipose tissue, reducing the overall volume of fat, reducing waist and thigh circumference, improving the appearance of cellulite, and skin tightening. While liposuction and surgical procedures remain the gold standard for patients seeking large volume fat removal, many patients prefer these novel noninvasive therapies as simple, no downtime procedures to improve the appearance of limited fat and cellulite.

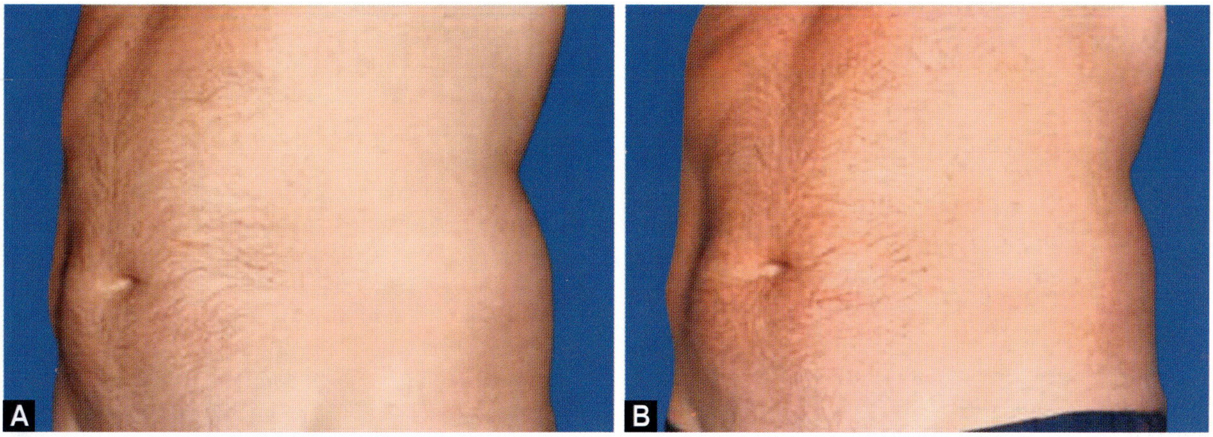

Figs 12.6A and B: Clinical improvement in the appearance of the abdomen of a 56-year-old man at baseline (A) and 2 months after (B) a single treatment with the CoolSculpting Breeze device vacuum, massage 60 minutes each. Baseline: 88 cm; FU 2-month circumference: 86 cm

Source: Photos courtesy of Dr Lori Brightman. Reprinted with permission from: Kim J, Lask G, Nelson A (Eds). Comprehensive Aesthetic Rejuvenation: A Regional Approach. New York: Informa Healthcare; 2012

Physical manipulation devices, radiofrequency devices, ultrasound devices, lasers and cryolipolysis have all been developed for the noninvasive treatment of fat and cellulite. Each technology has its own risks and benefits. Ultimately, rather than there being one single best technology for all patients, it is likely that different technologies will have specific patient types and situations in which they are best suited. As a result, it is important for physicians to assess each patient individually, discuss their current state and ultimate treatment goals, and choose a device accordingly. Ultimately, determining the best treatment option for your patient is dependent on clinical presentation, treatment goals, and most importantly, their patient's preferences. Following these principles, it is possible for patients to undergo safe, effective, noninvasive treatments to improve unwanted fat and cellulite.

SUMMARY

- Obesity is an epidemic; traditional exercise and dieting may not be effective for everyone. Many patients now turn to noninvasive technologies to achieve their ideal body.
- Noninvasive therapies represent safe, effective methods to treat limited areas of unwanted fat and cellulite. These technologies include: physical massage of the areas, radiofrequency, ultrasound, laser and cryolipolysis technologies.
- Physical massage of tissue is thought to improve the appearance of fat and cellulite by altering blood and lymphatic flow. Ongoing therapy may be necessary to maintain the improvement.
- Radiofrequency (RF) devices utilize alternating current to generate ionic flow and localized heat in adipocytes. Newer RF technologies also create holes in the adipocyte membrane (electroporation). These changes cause apoptosis of adipocytes, improving the appearance of fat and cellulite.
- High intensity focused ultrasound can also specifically target adipocytes, causing apoptosis, and thereby improving the appearance and thickness of the subcutaneous fat layer.
- Multiple laser devices, typically utilizing near-infrared wavelengths (in combination with physical manipulation), have been developed to improve the appearance of fat and cellulite by stimulating dermal collagen formation.
- Cryolipolysis is a technology which is thought to cause adipocyte apoptosis through controlled cold exposure (heat extraction), gradually improving the appearance and thickness of the fat layer over several months following the treatment.
- There are few head-to-head studies comparing these technologies, so it is not possible to determine an "ideal" device for all patients. It is likely that each technology may have a specific patient type or treatment area for which it is best suited.
- The best treatment option for your patient is best determined by discussing the options with the patient, their ultimate treatment goals and reaching an informed decision together.

REFERENCES

1. Güleç AT. Treatment of cellulite with LPG Endermologie. Int J Dermatol. 2009;48:265-70.
2. Collis N, Elliot LA, Sharpe C, et al. Cellulite treatment: a myth or reality: a prospective randomized, controlled trial of two therapies, Endermologie and aminophylline cream. Plast Reconstr Surg. 1999;104(4):1110-4.
3. Nootheti PK, Magpantay A, Yosowitz G, et al. A single center, randomized, comparative, prospective clinical study to determine the efficacy of the Velasmooth system versus the Triactive system for the treatment of cellulite. Lasers in Surgery and Medicine. 2006;38(10):908-12.
4. Goldberg DJ, Fazeli A, Berlin AL. Clinical, laboratory and MRI analysis of cellulite treatment with a unipolar radiofrequency device. Dermatol Surg. 2008;34(2):204-9.
5. Jewell ML, Baxter RA, Cox SE, et al. Randomized sham-controlled trial to evaluate the safety and effectiveness of a high-intensity focused ultrasound device for noninvasive body sculpting. Plast Reconstr Surg. 2011;128(1):253-62.
6. Teitelbaum SA, Burns JL, Kubota J, et al. Noninvasive body contouring by focused ultrasound: safety and efficacy of the Contour I device in a multicenter, controlled, clinical study. Plast Reconstr Surg. 2007; 120(3):779-89.
7. Lach R. Reduction of subcutaneous fat and improvement in cellulite appearance by dual-wavelength, low-level laser energy combined with vacuum and massage. J Cosmet Laser Ther. 2008;10(4):202-9.
8. Kulick MI. Evaluation of a noninvasive, dual-wavelength laser-suction and massage device for the regional treatment of cellulite. Plast Reconstr Surg. 2010;125(6):1788-96.

FURTHER READING

1. Avram MM. Cellulite: a review of its physiology and treatment. Journal of Cosmetic Laser Therapy. 2004;6:181-5.
2. Dover J, Burns J, Coleman S, et al. A prospective clinical study of noninvasive cryolypolysis for subcutaneous fat layer reduction—Interim report of available subject data. Presented at the Annual Meeting of the American Society for Laser Medicine and Surgery, April 2009, National Harbor, Maryland.
3. Hamilton EC, Greenway FL, Bray GA. Regional fat loss from the thigh in women using 2% aminophylline. Obesity Research. 1993;1:95S.
4. Hexsel DM, Mazzuco R. Subcision: a treatment for cellulite. International Journal of Dermatology. 2000;39:539-44.
5. Klein KB, Zelickson B, Riopelle JG, et al. Non-invasive cryolipolysis for subcutaneous fat reduction does not affect serum lipid levels or liver function tests. Lasers Surg Med. 2009;41(10):785-90.
6. Kligman AM, Pagnoni A, Stoudemayer T. Topical retinol improves cellulite. Journal of Dermatologic Treatment. 1999;10:119-25.
7. Manstein D, Laubach H, Watanabe K, et al. Selective cryolysis: a novel method of non-invasive fat removal. Lasers Surg Med. 2008;40(9):595-604.
8. Mirrashed F, Sharp JC, Krause V, et al. Pilot study of dermal and subcutaneous fat structures by MRI in individuals who differ in gender, BMI, and cellulite grading. Skin Research and Technology. 2004;10:161-8.
9. Nurnberger F, Muller G. So-called cellulite: an invented disease. The Journal of Dermatologic Surgery and Oncology. 1978;4:221-9.
10. Pierard-Franchiemont C, Pierand GE, Henry F, et al. A randomized, placebo controlled trial of topical retinal in the treatment of cellulite. American Journal of Clinical Dermatology; 2000.pp.1369-74.
11. Querleux B, Cornillon C, Jolivet O, et al. Anatomy and physiology of subcutaneous adipose tissue by in vivo magnetic resonance imaging and spectroscopy: relationships with sex and presence of cellulite. Skin Research and Technology. 2002;8:118-24.
12. Rosales-Berber IA, Diliz-Perez E. Controlled cooling of subcutaneous fat for body reshaping. Presented at the 15th World Congress of the International Confederation for Plastic, Reconstructive and Aesthetic Surgery, 2009, New Delhi, India.
13. Rossi ABR, Vergnanini AL. Cellulite: a review. Journal of the European Academy of Dermatology and Venereology. 2000;14:251-62.
14. Rotunda AM, Avram MM, Avram AS. Cellulite: Is there a role for injectables? Journal of Cosmetic Laser Therapy. 2005;7:147-54.

CHAPTER

13

Laser Treatment in Asians

Henry Hin Lee Chan

INTRODUCTION

Laser surgery in Asians differs from Caucasians in several aspects. First of all, the skin of Asian people with a higher epidermal melanin content is more prone to adverse effects including postinflammatory hyperpigmentation (PIH). The higher epidermal content acts as competing chromophobes for deeper laser-targeted lesions such as port-wine stain or laser-assisted hair removal and therefore, effective skin cooling is essential to reduce the risk of complication. Photoaging in Asians also presented with more pigmentary conditions including lentigines, seborrheic keratosis with wrinkling presenting later on in life as compared with Caucasians. In a Korean study, Chung et al.[1] found both pigmentary changes and wrinkling to be the major features of photoaging in Asians. However, moderate to severe wrinkling becomes apparent only at about 50 years, which is a decade or two later than age-matched Caucasians.[2]

Another important factor is the relatively low risk of skin cancer among Asians. Taking geographical factor into consideration(data within the same state), the prevalence of nonmelanoma skin cancer among American born Asians is about 10 times less than that seen in Caucasians. For melanoma, the risk among Asians is also much lower with the incidence among Japanese women being 2.04 per million population as compared with 130.9 per million among the Italian data. The implication is that laser is frequently used to treat lesions including congenital melanocytic nevi.

This chapter will review the use of laser for cosmetic indication in Asians with more emphasis on the mean to avoid complication such as post-inflammatory hyperpigmentation.

Cosmetic laser surgery in Asians can be categorized into the following types:

- Treatment of pigmentary conditions
- Treatment of vascular conditions
- Skin rejuvenation.

LASER FOR THE TREATMENT OF CONGENITAL PIGMENTARY CONDITIONS

While lasers can be most effective for the treatment of nevus of Ota, the outcome is much less impressive among patients with café au lait patch and Becker's nevi. The use of fractional resurfacing together with pigment laser has improved the outcome of these resistant lesions.

Café au lait Patch (Figs 13.1A and B)

The uses of lasers for the treatment of café au lait patch have led to variable results. An earlier study that examined the use of continuous-mode 511-nm copper vapor laser demonstrated good to excellent results in 15 out of 16 patients after two treatment sessions,[3] such findings have not been found to be consistent. 510-nm pulsed-dye laser and erbium: YAG laser have also been shown to be effective in some cases.[4-6]

Among all the lasers, quality-switched (QS) lasers yielded the most inconsistent results with high recurrence rates and increased darkening as the main complication. In a study using QS 694-nm ruby laser

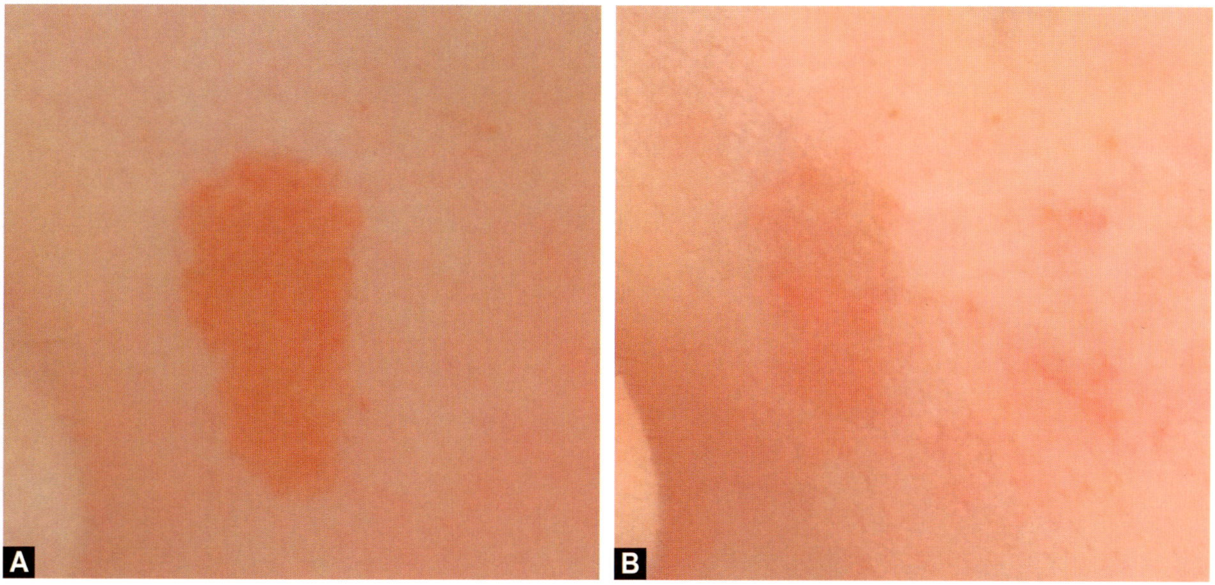

Figs 13.1A and B: (A) Café au lait at baseline; (B) After treatment with long-pulsed Alexandrite (Alex) laser

and QS 532-nm Nd:YAG laser, it was found that the degree of improvement varied across the lesions.[7] One hypothesis was that QS lasers failed to remove the follicular melanocytic component of the café au lait macules (CALM).

The author's current approach is to use a long-pulsed pigment laser, such as normal mode ruby laser (NMRL) or long-pulsed Alexandrite (LP Alex) laser without cooling, to target not only the epidermal melanocytes but also the follicular melanocytes and in doing so, improve to clinical outcome. Typical laser parameters are LP Alex 755 nm; 10-mm spot size; 3-ms pulse duration; 25–40 J/cm^2 with ashen gray appearance as the main clinical endpoint. In one study of 33 patients with CALM, NMRL was shown to have a lower risk of recurrence (42.4%) compared to QS ruby laser (81.8%) three months after a single treatment.

More recently, for lesions that failed to improve after three treatment sessions, 1927-nm thulium fiber laser has been used to further enhance the treatment outcome. Patients are treated with LP Alex laser in one session to be followed in 4 weeks time by non-ablative resurfacing with 1927-nm thulium fiber laser (treatment level 11, 20 mJ) (Figs 13.1A and B) Some patients with more resistant lesions appear to benefit from such a combined approach.

Becker's Nevus (Figs 13.2A and B)

Previous literature looking at the use of argon and CO_2 lasers indicated high risk of scarring or permanent hypopigmentation. Similar disappointing result was observed with the use of QS ruby laser that led to postoperative increase in pigmentation after 4 weeks.[8]

A study comparing the use of erbium: YAG laser to QS 1064-nm Nd:YAG laser in 22 patients with a follow-up of 2 years showed that erbium: YAG laser was significantly better even after one treatment.[9]

In the author's practice, they treat Becker's nevi similar to café au lait patches and use a long-pulsed pigmented laser to remove hair and pigmentation, however textural change is a possible complication. More recently, they combined 1927-nm thulium fiber laser with long-pulsed Alexandrite laser using similar parameters as that they used for café au lait patch. The advantage is that beside greater degree of improvement, the texture changes that previously seen among patients treated with long pulsed pigment laser alone can also improve with the nonablative fractional resurfacing (Figs 13.2A and B).

Melanocytic Nevi (Figs 13.3A and B)

The use of laser for the treatment of melanocytic nevi is controversial especially among Caucasians as the main issue is the potential delay in the diagnosis of neoplastic changes. Indeed, previous studies indicated reports of histological atypia in patients with melanocytic nevi that were treated by carbon dioxide laser and laser for hair removal.[11,12] Due to genetic variation, the risk of melanoma is much lower among Asians and the incidences of

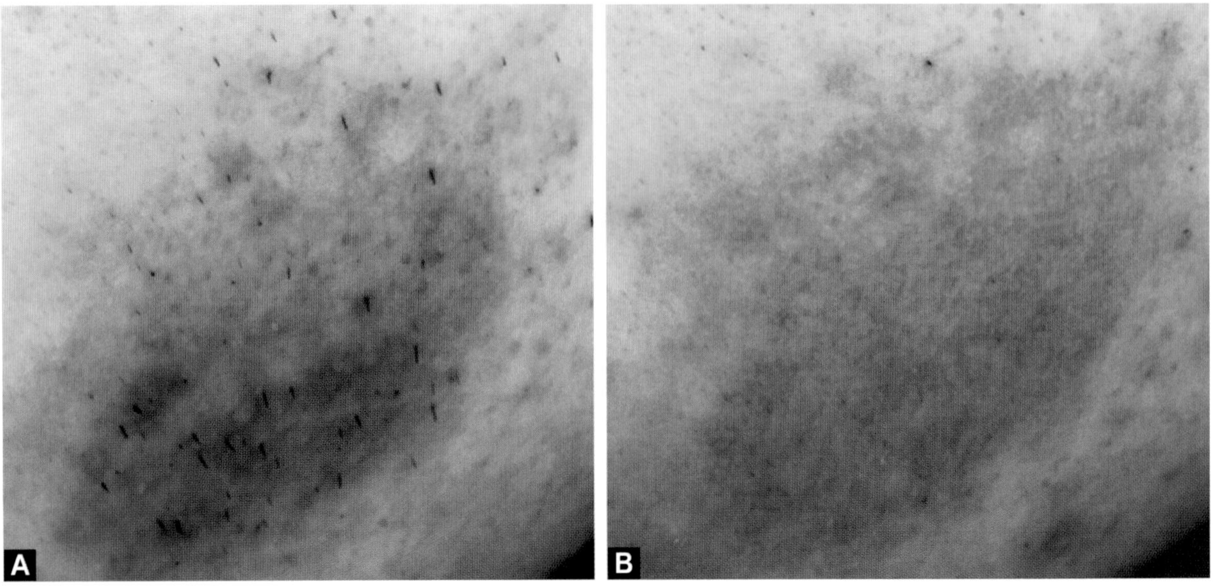

Figs 13.2A and B: (A) Becker's nevus at baseline; (B) After four treatment sessions with long-pulsed Alexandrite and 1927-nonablative fractional resurfacing (NAFR) at alternate treatment sessions

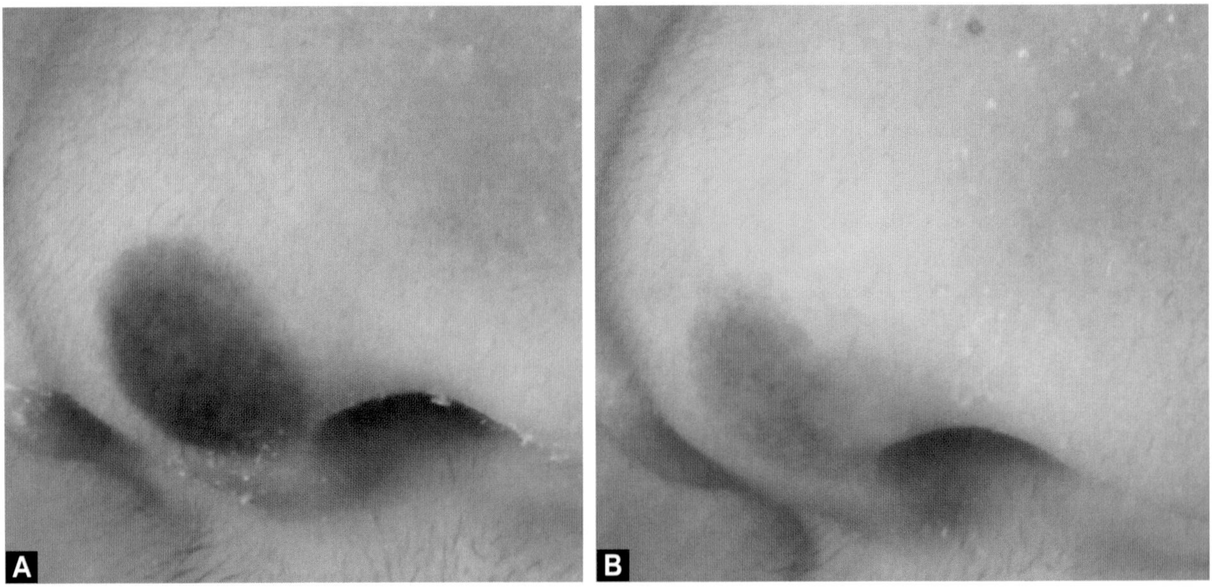

Figs 13.3A and B: (A) Congenital melanocytic nevi at baseline; (B) After eight treatment sessions with long-pulsed Alexandrite and quality-switched (QS) ruby and three sessions with NAFR 1927 nm

melanoma has been reported to be between 0.2 and 2.2 per 1,00,000 among Asians, much lower than in Caucasians.[13] Furthermore, the most common sites for the development of melanoma among skin of color are non sun-exposed areas, such as palmar, plantar, subungual and mucosal surfaces. As a result, the use of laser for the treatment of melanocytic nevi is a popular practice in Asian countries.

Different pigment lasers have been used in the removal of melanocytic nevi. Treatment of congenital melanocytic nevi using a QS ruby laser was found to achieve an average clearance of 76% after eight treatment sessions.[14] The use of a QS ruby followed immediately, or 2 weeks later, with the normal mode ruby laser (NMRL) can lead to 52% of visible decrease in pigment without complete histological clearance.[15]

The short and long-term histological findings of congenital nevi that have been treated with the NMRL indicate that subtle microscopic scars that reach 1 mm in diameter are frequent. It was proposed that such scars cover the underlying nevus cells, that leads to cosmetic improvement.[16] Better cosmetic result has been reported by first using a NMRL to remove the epidermis, followed immediately by multiple passes of a QS ruby laser.[17] This approach allows the effective removal of the epidermis and in doing so enables a greater degree of penetration by the QS ruby laser, of which multiple passes further enhance the clinical efficacy. The typical laser parameters in the author's practice are LP Alex 755 nm, 10-mm spot size; 3-ms pulse duration and 15–25 J/cm^2. Immediately after treatment, wet gauze is used to remove the epidermis. This is then to be followed by QS ruby laser, 5-mm spot size, 3–4 J/cm^2 with repeated passes until mild bleeding occurs. The author now also treats the lesion with 1927-nm thulium fiber laser in alternative sessions to improve treatment outcome and also reduce the risk of texture changes. Treatment interval should be spaced at 4–6 weekly (Figs 13.3A and B).

Nevus of Ota (Figs 13.4A and B)

Nevus of Ota is a dermal melanocytic hematoma characterized clinically by mottled, dusky blue and brown hyperpigmentation. The pigmentation carries significant psychosocial impact and often affects the skin and mucous membranes innervated by the first and second branches of the trigeminal nerve. Histologically, ectopic melanocytes can be seen in the dermis. This condition is more common among Asians and affects about 0.6% of the population. QS ruby, QS Alexandrite and QS 1064 nm Nd:YAG lasers have all been used to achieve good clinical outcome[18-20] (Figs 13.4A and B). Previous studies indicated that three or more treatment sessions are necessary before any clinical improvement can be observed. Clinical endpoint is defined as immediate whitening for QS ruby and Alex lasers, and immediate whitening with punctuate bleeding for QS 1064-nm Nd:YAG laser. The treatment interval should initially be 6 to 8 weeks and towards the end of the treatment, when the lesion has lightened significantly requiring higher fluence to achieve the clinical endpoint, treatment interval should be lengthened to several months.

QS ruby is shown to be associated with the lowest number of treatment sessions but greater risk of hypopigmentation. Besides hypopigmentation, other potential complications include erythema after laser procedure, transient postinflammatory hyperpigmentation, texture changes and repigmentation which can occur among 0.6 to 1.2% of patients.[21]

The number of treatment sessions has been shown to be related with several factors, including

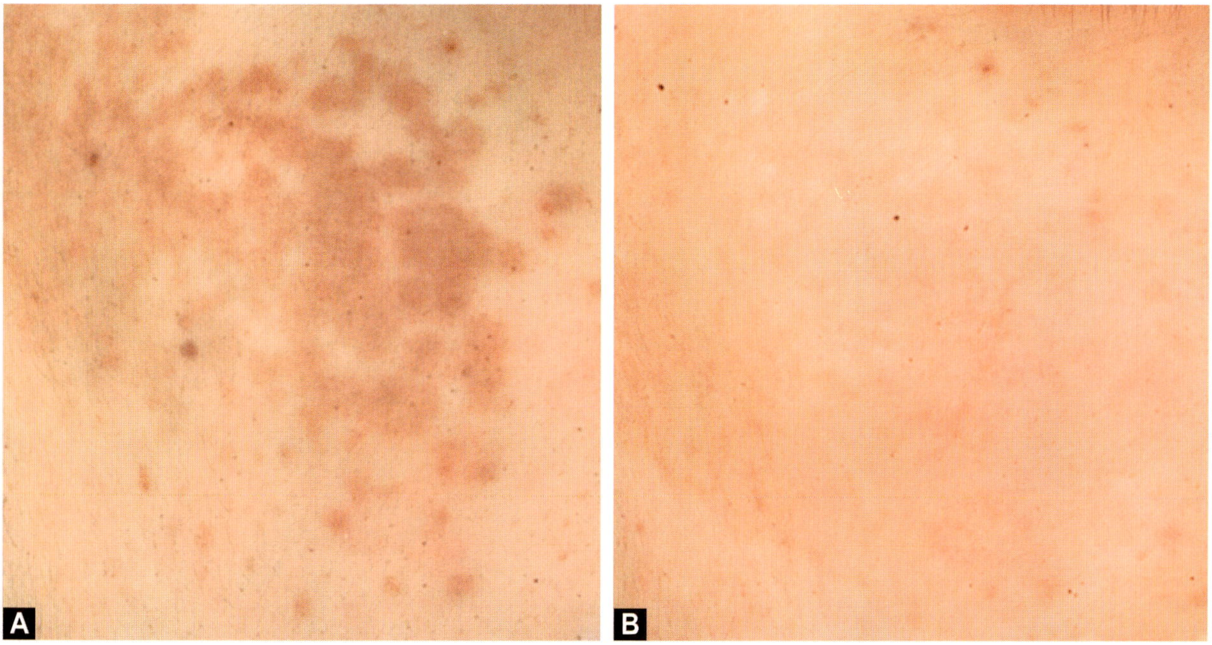

Figs 13.4A and B: (A) Nevus of Ota at baseline; (B) After four treatment sessions with QS ruby laser

the age when treatment is initiated with younger age group patients requiring lesser treatment sessions and also lowest risk of complication.[22] Indeed to avoid the potential psychosocial impact, early treatment is recommended so that complete clearing can be obtained before schooling. Periorbital involvement was also found to be associated with more treatment sessions.[23] Recently, a study of 10 Asian patients with dermal pigmented lesions (three of which were nevus of Ota) showed that the use of QS Alex laser delivered with compression was associated with a lower risk of purpura and dyspigmentation when compared with laser treatment without compression.[24] The efficacy was not compromised with compression. Diascopy caused emptying of the cutaneous blood vessels and hence reduced the risk of laser injury to blood vessels.

Fractional resurfacing was recently found to be effective in the removal of nevus of Ota in a patient that failed to respond after QS 1064-nm Nd:YAG laser.[25] More recently, picoseconds laser has been introduced and was found to be effective for the treatment of resistant tattoo and whether such type of laser offered additional benefit for patient with nevus of Ota remains to be seen.[26]

LASER AND LIGHT SOURCES FOR THE TREATMENT OF ACQUIRED PIGMENTARY CONDITIONS

Lasers and intense pulsed light sources are commonly used for the treatment of acquired pigmentary conditions in Asians and the degree of response varies depending upon the skin type, the type of lesion and other factors including recent sun exposure. Although Asians are often classified as Fitzpatrick skin type III and IV, such classification is not accurate. Detail history regarding response to sun exposure can assist in determining high risk individuals with those more prone to sun tan carry a higher risk of complication. Any sun exposure in the few weeks prior to laser treatment can predispose patients with ethnic skin to a higher risk of postinflammatory hyper- or hypopigmentation. Hence, the use of sunscreens and topical depigmenting agents for at least 2 weeks prior to any such treatment can help reduce the risk of PIH.

There are now many lasers and intense pulse light sources that can be effective in the treatment of acquired pigmentary conditions and appropriate selection of the device used can optimize the treatment outcome and reduce the risk of complication.

LASER AND INTENSE PULSED LIGHT TREATMENT FOR FRECKLES AND LENTIGO (FIGS 13.5 AND 13.6)

Freckles and lentigines are benign pigmented lesions commonly seen in Asians. Freckles occur in younger age groups and are relatively uniform in distribution, size and color. Histologically, they are characterized by epidermal hypermelanosis without

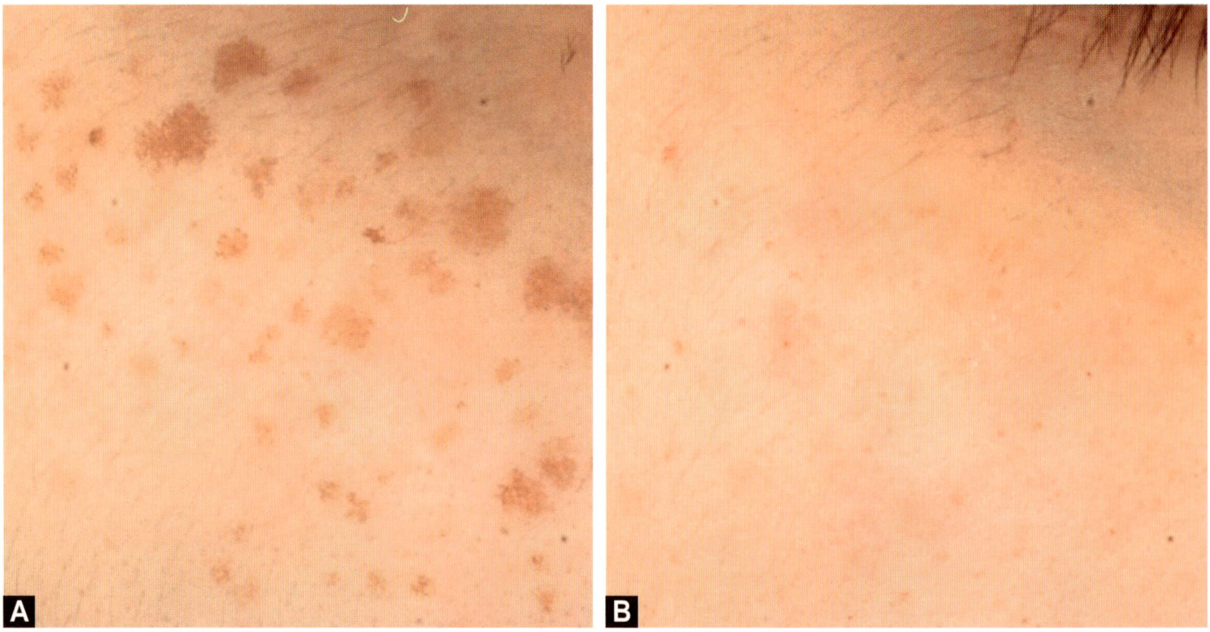

Figs 13.5A and B: (A) Freckles and lentigo at baseline; (B) After one treatment session with QS 532-nm Nd:YAG laser

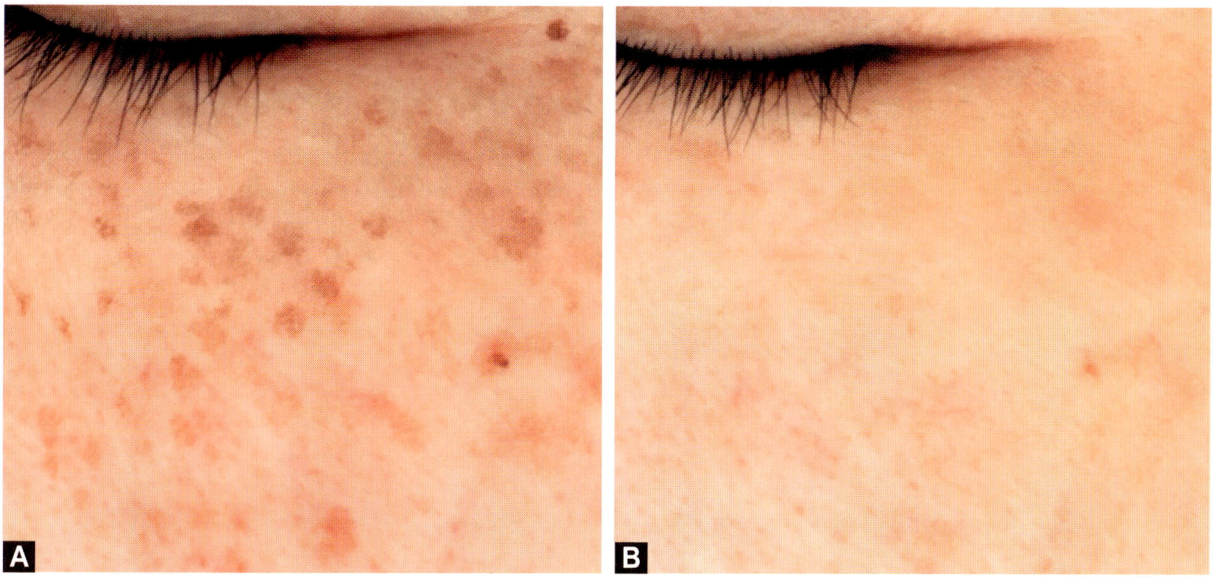

Figs 13.6A and B: (A) Freckles at baseline; (B) After two treatment sessions with long-pulsed (LP) 532-nm KTP laser

an increase in melanocyte numbers. Lentigines tend to appear later and vary in size, color and distribution. Histologically, both epidermal hypermelanosis and increase in melanocyte numbers are seen. Anderson et al. were the first to demonstrate the efficacy of Q-switched (QS) lasers in the removal of cutaneous pigmentation.[27] Previous studies have indicated that while Q-switched (QS) lasers can be most effective for the treatment of freckles and lentigo in Caucasians, they can be associated with a higher risk of complication among Asians with PIH risk estimated to be 10 to 25%.[28,29] QS lasers generate not only photothermal effect but also photomechanical, resulting in excessive degree of inflammatory reaction and therefore, higher degree of PIH. On the other hand, long-pulsed pigmented lasers or IPL can be most effective as they only generated photothermal injury and in doing so, reduce the risk of PIH. By matching the pulse width of the long-pulsed pigmented lasers or IPL (millisecond domain) to the thermal relaxation time of the epidermis (10 milliseconds), the risk of thermal injury to the dermis is minimized. Several studies in the last decades have demonstrated the efficacy and lower risk of complication when comparing the use of long-pulsed pigmented lasers to QS laser in the removal of freckles and lentigo in Asians.[29,30] In a recent retrospective study that examined four different pigmented lasers (QS 532 Nd:YAG; LP 532 KTP laser with contact cooling; long-pulsed 595-nm pulsed-dye laser with compression; long-pulsed Alexandrite 755-nm laser).[31] Long-pulsed 532 KTP laser was found to be the most effective with the least complication (Figs 13.5 and 13.6).

In the author's practice, treatment options are offered to patients in order to obtain the appropriate informed consent. Patients are informed that if they choose QS lasers, the advantage of such treatment is that the number of sessions required to obtain significant degree of improvement (defined as more than 75% of clearing) is about one to two but there is a week of downtime with redness and swelling lasting a couple of days and crust that usually takes a week to fall off. The risk of PIH for freckles is lower and is estimated to be about 5–10% but with solar lentigo such risk can increase to 10–20%. To reduce the risk of unnecessary laser to the surrounding normal skin, the smallest spot size is used and the lowest possible fluence that would induce immediate whitening should be chosen. Typical laser parameter for QS 532 Nd:YAG laser used is 2-mm spot size and 0.6 to 0.8 J/cm^2.

For long-pulsed pigment laser, the author's recent publication indicated the smallest spot size together with cooling device can be particularly effective with a lowest risk of complication especially postinflammatory hyperpigmentation.[31] The appropriate clinical endpoint for long-pulsed pigment laser is slight dark-gray appearance. Typical treatment parameters for a long-pulsed 532 KTP laser with cooling is 2–3 mm spot size, pulsed duration 2 ms and fluence between 8 J/cm^2 and 14 J/cm^2. For LP 595-nm pulsed-dye laser with compression, typical parameters are 1.5-ms pulse width, 7-mm spot size with compression and fluence at the range of 10–13 J/cm^2. For LP Alexandrite (Alex) laser, typical parameter is 10-mm spot size and 25–35 J/cm^2 with a pulsed duration of 3 ms.

Intense pulsed light source has also been used for the treatment of freckles and lentigo and can be most effective if there is significant contrast between lesional and nonlesional skin. However, if the contrast is low either the operator used below threshold fluence to avoid complication in which cases, clinical outcome diminished or above threshold fluence was used and complications including foot-printing hypopigmentation can develop. Clinical endpoint varies depending upon the type of IPL used. For IPL with a shorter pulsed duration (2–3 ms), slight gray darkening is the appropriate clinical endpoint. For longer-pulsed width IPL, there is often an absence of immediate endpoint. Patient's subjective feedback is therefore important to determine the appropriate parameters used.

Nonablative fractional resurfacing can be used to improve freckles and lentigines to some degree but is not as specific as pigment laser and therefore is often used if the patient requested improvement of other skin components such as acne scar, skin texture as well as lentigines.

● MELASMA (FIGS 13.7 AND 13.8)

Melasma is a common acquired pigmentary condition among female Asian patients that can be most challenging for the clinician to treat. Several factors are known to be associated with the development of melasma such as sun exposure, genetic, hormonal factors including pregnancy and oral contraceptive. A recent transcriptomic gene study indicated increased epidermal hyperpigmentation as the main abnormality in melasma.[32] The numbers of melanocytes were not significantly increased. Angiogenesis has also been shown to play a role in the pathogenesis of melasma.

As melasma is chronic in nature, sun protection and topical bleaching agents remain to be the first line treatment with second line therapeutic options being minor office-based procedures such as chemical peel, microdermabrasion and vitamin C iontophoresis. Laser and light source should only be used among resistant cases.

Previous studies indicated that high fluence QS laser and 510-nm pulsed-dye laser can be associated with darkening of melasma with unpredictable outcome.[33,34] For IPL, the results were also inconsistent. In one study that examined the

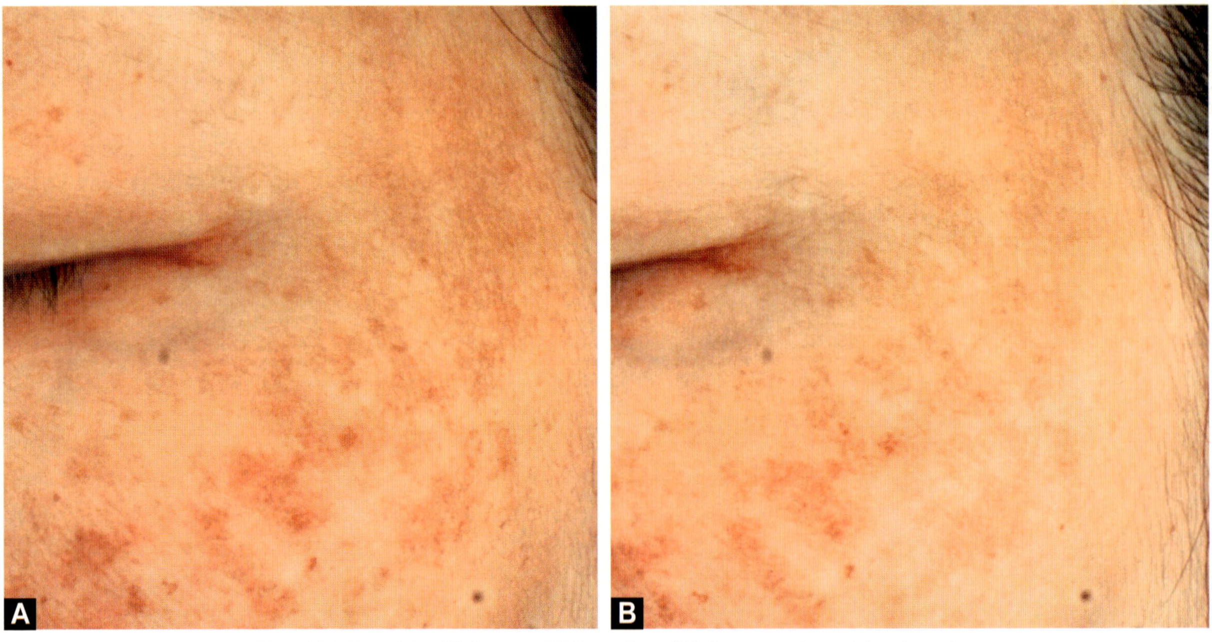

Figs 13.7A and B: Melasma. (A) Baseline; (B) One month post treatment 1927 thulium laser energy 10mJ, treatment level 6, 4 passes

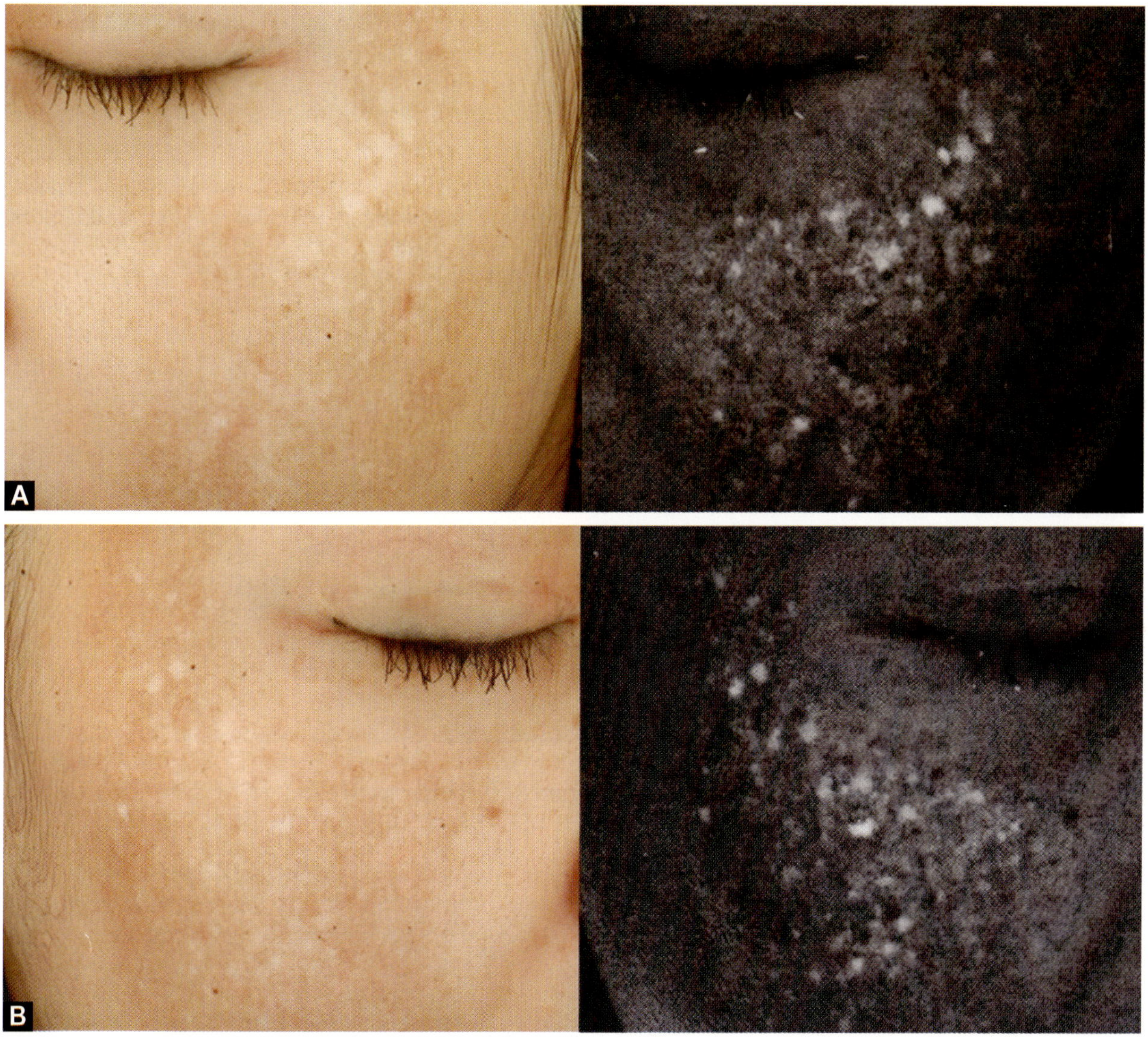

Figs 13.8A and B: Hypopigmentation after nine QS 1064 laser treatments for melasma

use of IPL (570-nm and 590 to 615-nm filters in 4-week intervals for a total of four treatments) for the treatment of melasma indicated that melasma improved by 39.8% compared to only 11.6% in the control group.[35] Two patients in the intense pulsed light group experienced transient postinflammatory hyperpigmentation, and partial repigmentation was noted 24 weeks after the last treatment session. In a more recent study, 89 patients with melasma were treated with an intense pulse light source device with a uniform pulse profile. They were able to achieve excellent results (77.5% of treated subjects had over 50% improvement 3 months after treatment) with low risk of increase in pigmentation (3%).[36] This was despite the lack of topical bleaching agents during the study period. Their findings differ significantly from previous data. Although the uniform profile of this IPL device may be one of the reasons for such observation as suggested by the investigators, other factors are more likely to contribute to the differences in clinical outcome including geographical location of the tested site and recruitment criteria.

Ablative lasers are probably the only devices that can lead to a potential cure. The objective was to ablate the abnormal clonal melanocytic expansion and in doing so, lead to a long-term cure.[37,38] However, given the known associated adverse effects of ablative lasers including prolonged erythema, pigmentary disturbance, risk of infection as well as scarring, their use has become much less popular in recent years. Fractional resurfacing has replaced ablative procedure in the last several years as the main resurfacing procedure and early study indicated good success rate using nonablative fractional resurfacing for the treatment of melasma with 90% of patients have some degree of improvement after treatment with nonablative fractional resurfacing with 1550-nm laser.[39] However more recent studies indicated such treatment to be less impressive. In a Korean study that treated 24 melasma patients with four treatments of the same device, investigators observed clinical improvements in 60% of the patients and in 44% at 4 weeks after treatment, but the figures decreased to 52% and 35%, respectively, at 24 weeks after treatment.[40] Two European studies also indicated less impressive findings with one single blinded control study indicating no significant difference between the group with the laser and sunblock as compared with sunblock alone.[41,42]

More recently, 1927-nm thulium fiber laser has been introduced as a new nonablative fractional resurfacing laser for the treatment of melasma.[43] The author's group examined the use of such laser for the treatment of melasma among Chinese patients and while there was temporary improvement, most patients experience recurrence 3 months after treatment[44] (Figs 13.7A and B).

Laser toning involves the use of large spot size, low fluence, QS 1064-nm Nd:YAG laser (6–8 mm spot size, 1.6–2.3 J/cm^2) in the treatment of melasma and has gained much popularity in Asian countries in recent years.[45] Mild erythema is used as the clinical endpoint and treatment is often performed in 1–2 weekly intervals. While melasma can certainly be lightened with such treatment, prolonged treatment can lead to mottled depigmentation which is utmost difficult to manage[46] (Figs 13.8A and B). Furthermore, relapse of melasma, and in some cases, rebound can occur. More recently, it has been proposed to combine bleaching agents, microdermabrasion with laser toning and by reducing the frequency of treatment sessions (monthly instead of weekly) and reduces the numbers of passes (three rather than 10's); it has been suggested to be an effective treatment with a lower risk of complication.[47] Further prospective clinical trial is necessary to verify the efficacy and adverse effect rate of such approach.

Vascular endothelial growth factor (VEGF) has been implicated to play a role in the pathogenesis of melasma and indeed, telangiectasia is not uncommon within melasma.[48] As a result, vascular lasers can also be used to treat the vascular aspects either on its own or in combination with laser toning.[49]

ACQUIRED BILATERAL NEVUS OF OTA-LIKE MACULES (ABNOM OR HORI'S MACULES)

Hori's macules (Figs 13.9A and B) are dermal hyperpigmentation commonly seen in Asian patients that affects approximately 0.8% of the population.

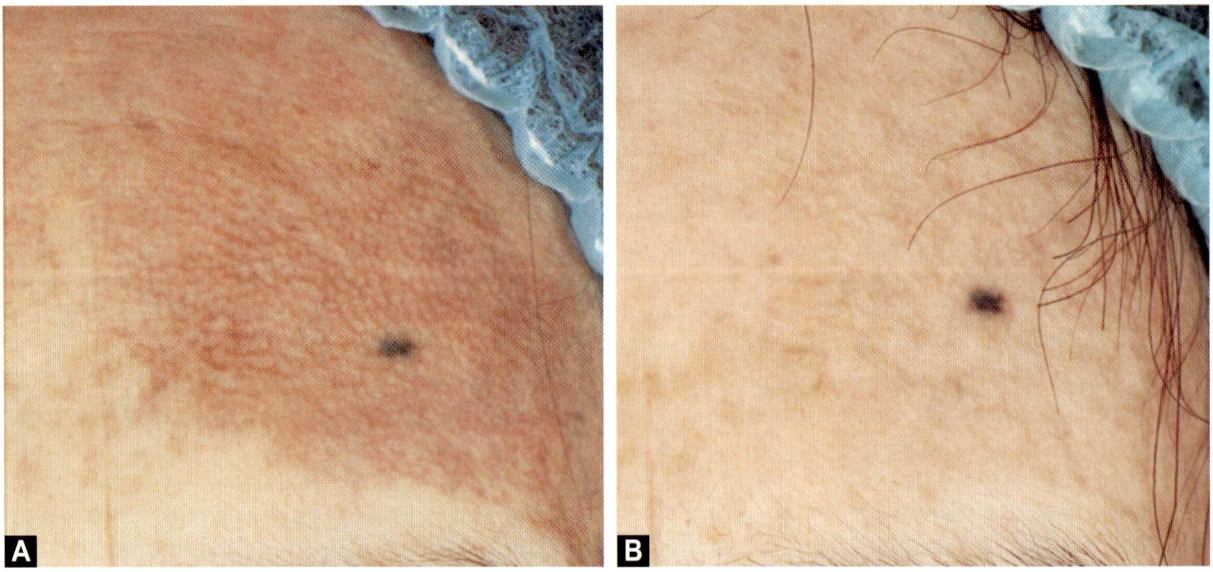

Figs 13.9A and B: (A) Hori's macules at baseline; (B) After three treatment sessions with QS ruby laser

Hori's macules present as bilateral blue-gray macules typically located over the malar region in a symmetrical pattern. Other areas can also be affected including lateral temples, alae nasi, eyelids and foreheads. Histologically, dermal melanocytes are dispersed in the papillary and middle part of the dermis.[50]

Unlike nevus of Ota, the pigmentation of Hori's macules is acquired, has a late onset in adulthood, and does not affect the mucosa. Melasma and Hori's macules can coexist in some patients. Like nevus of Ota, QS lasers have been shown to be effective for the treatment of Hori's macules. QS ruby, QS Alex and QS 1064-nm Nd:YAG have all been found to achieve complete clearance with postinflammatory hyperpigmentation (PIH) that ranged from 7% to 73% with QS ruby associated with the greatest degree of improvement and lowest risk of PIH.[51-53] Combined laser therapy has also been found to be effective. One study indicated that QS 532-nm Nd:YAG used in conjunction with QS 1064-nm Nd:YAG can achieve better result than either laser on its own.[54] Another study indicated that ablative laser, used first to remove the epidermis, allows better penetration of the QS ruby and obtained superior result as compared with QS-ruby laser on its own.[55] More recently, to avoid the downtime associated with high fluence QS lasers, low fluence laser toning with QS laser has also been advocated but the number of treatment sessions increased significantly requiring a mean treatment sessions of 11 for 46.7% of the treated patients to have over 75% degree of improvement.[56]

LASER TREATMENT OF VASCULAR LESIONS IN ASIANS (FIGS 13.10A TO D)

Vascular-specific lasers induce vessel injury, and have been used to target vascular lesions such as port-wine stains (PWS), telangiectasia, scars as well as for nonablative skin rejuvenation. One of the principal absorption peaks of oxyhemoglobin is at 577 nm, with a smaller peak around 700–1100 nm.

Asians, with greater epidermal melanin content, are at a higher risk of adverse effects such as vesiculation and pigmentary changes after laser treatments of vascular lesions. Furthermore, with the epidermal melanin acting as a competing chromophore for hemoglobin, higher fluence or more treatment sessions are necessary to produce the desirable clinical endpoint. Before the development of epidermal cooling, studies indicated that the treatment of port-wine stains in Asians was associated with a greater risk of complication including transient postinflammatory hyperpigmentation and texture changes.[57,58] Adequate skin cooling allows epidermal protection, and in doing so improves safety and efficacy. Several cooling methods, including cold gel, air cooling, cryogen spray cooling (CSC), and contact cooling with a sapphire window, can be used in conjunction with vascular laser. Among all cooling techniques, cryogen spray cooling with pulsed-dye laser (PDL-CSC) has been well looked into and its role in the treatment of vascular lesions among Asians is now well established. In a retrospective study, Chang and Nelson found that PDL-CSC could enhance clinical efficacy, and a higher fluence could be used without any increase in complication rate for the treatment of port-wine stains in Asians.[59] Several others studies had since confirmed their findings.[60] Typical treatment parameters for port-wine stains among Asians are PDL 11–13 J/cm^2, 7-mm spot size, 1.5-ms pulse width with dynamic cooling device (DCD) set at 40 ms/20 ms delay. The clinical endpoint is purpura without epidermal whitening.

Although PDL can often lead to significant degree of clearing, complete blanching of PWS is rarely seen. It has been suggested that regeneration and revascularization of photocoagulated blood vessels due to angiogenesis occurs as part of the skin's normal healing process.[61] The heterogeneity of vessels characteristic of PWS require the use of different spot sizes, fluencies, pulse widths and dynamic cooling, depending on vessel size and anatomic location. As for oxyhemoglobin, besides the principal absorption peaks at 577 nm, there is a smaller peak around 700–1100 nm. With the development of epidermal cooling, longer wavelengths laser that were previously used for the treatment of pigmentation can now be also used for the treatment of vascular lesions.[62,63] The advantages of these lasers include greater depth of penetration and also bulk tissue heating which can be effective for the treatment of hypertrophic lesions. Combination of PDL with LP 755-nm Alex lasers has been used. Previous studies indicated resistant PWS especially those that were hypertrophic can be particularly responsive to the treatment of LP Alex either alone or in combination with PDL[62] (Figs 13.10A to D). Serious side-effects were infrequent that included pain, edema, bullae,

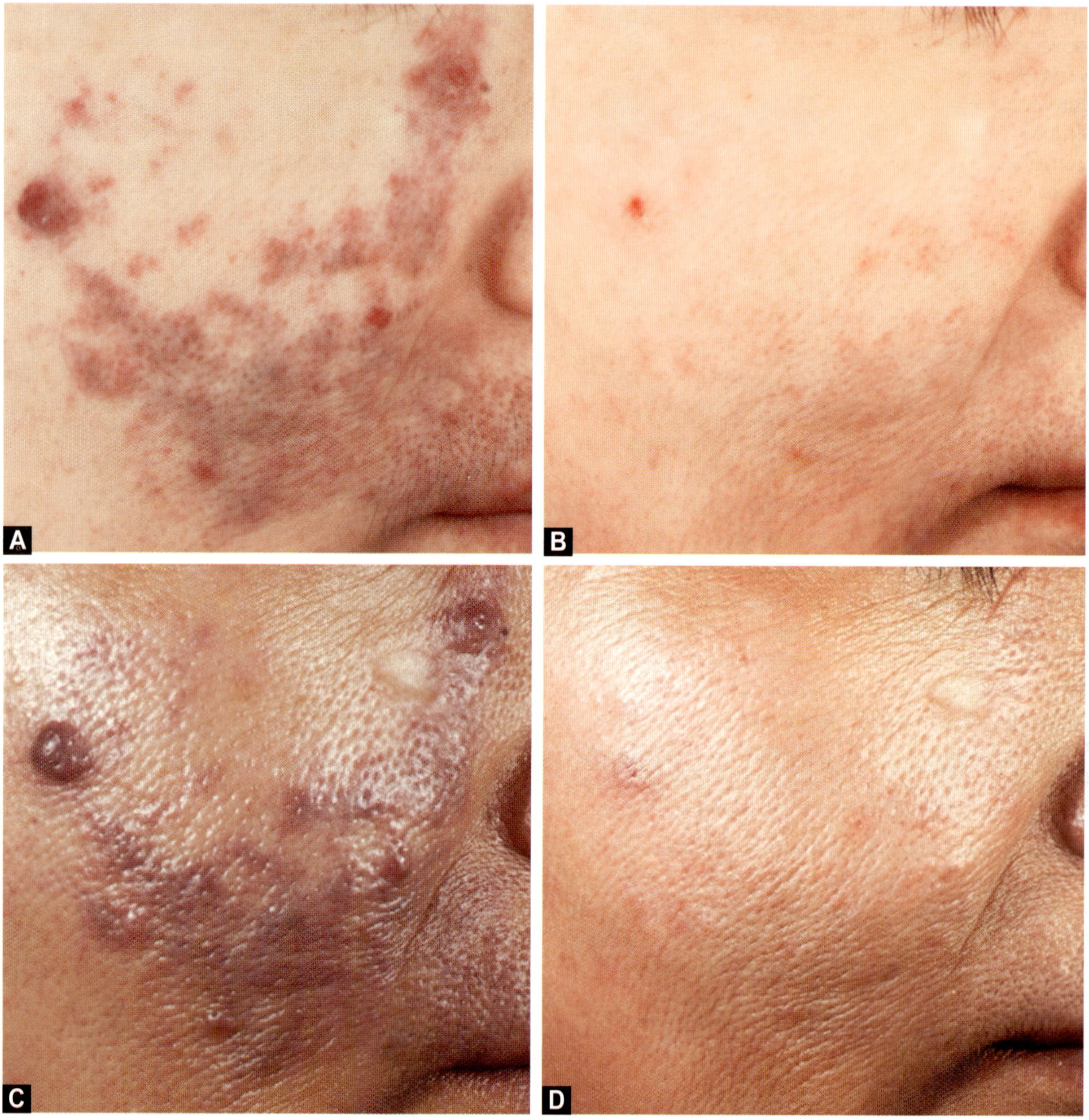

Figs 13.10A to D: (A) Hypertrophic port-wine stain at baseline (cross polarized image); (B) After eight treatment sessions with combined LP Alex and PDL 595 nm; (C) Hypertrophic port-wine stain at baseline (parallel polarized image); (D) After eight treatment sessions with combined LP Alex and PDL 595 nm

crusting and rare scarring. Beside LP Alex, the study did also indicate the role of LP 1064-nm Nd:YAG laser for the treatment of lip PWS. Combined 595-nm and 1064-nm laser irradiation has also been recommended for recalcitrant and hypertrophic PWS.[63]

Facial telangiectasia is a common dermatological complaint and may be associated with rosacea, photodamage, prolonged topical corticosteroid use, liver disease, radiodermatitis and connective tissue disease. Pulsed-dye laser is presently regarded as the treatment of choice, due to its excellent efficacy and safety profile. However, purpura and/or PIH can occur at the treated site and is generally unacceptable to most patients, and hence studies were performed to compare the efficacy of purpuric and subpurpuric PDL treatment for facial telangiectasia. In a split-face study, purpuric settings achieved a greater reduction in telangiectasia density in 82% of patients (7-mm spot size, 10-ms pulse duration, fluence 8.5–10 J/cm^2, DCD 30-ms spray and 20-ms delay interval).[64] Another study showed subpurpuric treatment with PDL (7-mm spot size, pulse duration 6 ms, fluence 7–9 J/cm^2) resulted in 75% of patients achieving greater than 25% improvement after a single treatment.[65] This is generally preferred due to minimal downtime but there is the need for more treatments to achieve the desired outcome. Further studies have suggested the use of dual wavelength laser treatments with sequential subpurpuric delivery of 595 nm and 1064-nm radiation demonstrating better results when compared with single wavelength treatment after a single treatment session.[66]

For facial telangiectasia among Asians the typical treatment parameters are 595-nm PDL; 10-mm spot size; 10-ms pulse width; 13 J/cm^2; DCD 40/20 ms with immediate vessel disappearance as the clinical endpoint.

The use of PDL has additionally been proven to be effective in the treatment of hypertrophic scars and keloids, which are more common in darker skinned patients. Previous studies comparing the use of purpuric and subpurpuric PDL in the improvement of hypertrophic scar indicated subpurpuric dose to be associated with a greater degree of efficacy as purpuric dose can lead to excessive injury that can result in worsening of the scar. With the appropriate parameters, improvements in skin texture, bulk and scar texture have been reported.[67] Typical treatment parameters are 595-nm PDL, 12-mm spot size, 0.45 ms, 4.5–5.0 J/cm^2 with DCD set at 40/20 ms at monthly intervals.

ABLATIVE, NONABLATIVE AND FRACTIONAL SKIN RESURFACING (FIGS 13.11 AND 13.12)

Ablative resurfacing with carbon dioxide (CO_2) and Er:YAG lasers have long been the gold standard. They target water as a chromophore, leading to epidermal and dermal vaporization and ablation of 100 to 200 μm in depth. Although clinically effective in improving rhytides, atrophic scarring and dyschromia, there is significant associated downtime and potential side-effects, including persistent erythema, hyper- and hypopigmentation, infection, and even scarring, especially in dark skin.[68]

Photoaging in Asians tends to present with more pigmentary conditions including lentigines, seborrheic keratosis with wrinkling presenting later on in life as compared with Caucasians. Nonablative skin rejuvenation involves the use of cooling to protect the epidermis and then delivery of laser or IPL to the dermis, leading to dermal injury and subsequent collagen regeneration was popular among Asians.[69-71] Often multiple devices are used at the same time to achieve the desirable effect with reduction of lentigines, facial telangiectasia and mild

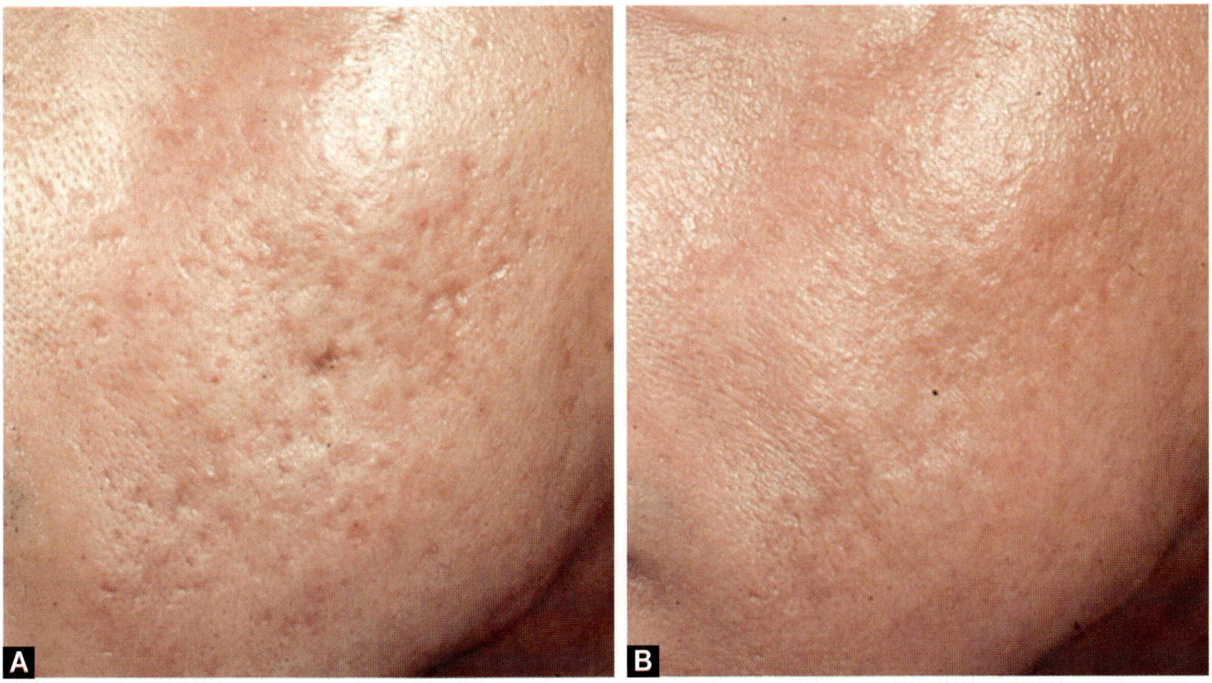

Figs 13.11A and B: (A) Acne scars at baseline; (B) After eight treatment sessions with NAFR with 1550 nm

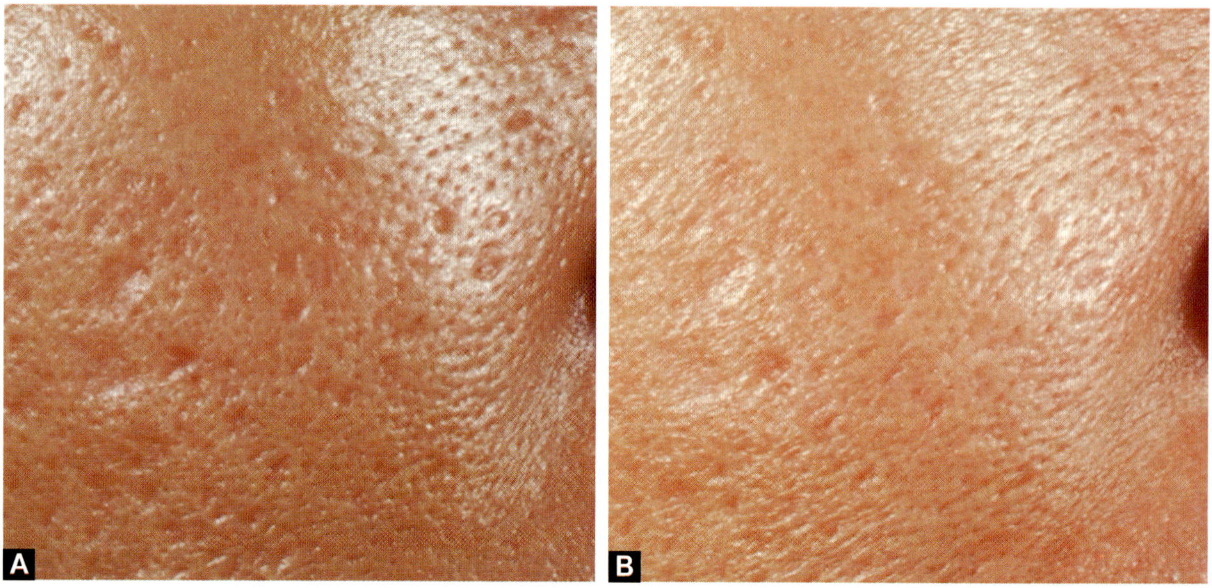

Figs 13.12A and B: (A) Acne scars at baseline; (B) Eight months after a single treatment with ablative CO_2 fractional resurfacing

degree improvement of skin texture and rhytides typically after a series of monthly treatments. There is little downtime associated and low adverse effects.

The development of fractional photothermolysis has revolutionized skin rejuvenation and resurfacing, attempting to achieve comparable clinical results to ablative lasers, but with a safety profile more similar to nonablative technologies.[72] The 1550-nm erbium-doped fiber nonablative laser was the first fractional laser approved for clinical use. By creating an array of microscopic treatment zones (MTZs) with controlled width, depth and density, a fixed percentage of the skin is thermally coagulated in each treatment session, leaving an intact stratum corneum. Healthy tissue surrounding these MTZs allow for rapid healing and re-epithelialization within one day. This technology has proven to be effective in improving photoaging, dyschromia, rhytides, atrophic scarring and poikiloderma.[73,74] Nonablative fractional resurfacing (NAFR) used for acne scarring in Asian skin carries a high risk of PIH. Studies have indicated that treatment density, rather than energy, is a stronger determining factor in the development of PIH.[75] Further studies have confirmed that by reducing the number of passes and the total treatment density, but increasing the treatment sessions from three to six to compensate for the reduced passes, clinical efficacy remains statistically improved whilst reducing the PIH risk in Asians from 18.2% to 6%.[76] (Figs 13.11A and B). Besides 1550 nm, other wavelengths have also been used for nonablative fractional resurfacing including 1440 and 1927 nm. 1927-nm thulium fiber laser can be particularly effective for the treatment of pigmentary condition and is often used in combination with 1550 nm for skin rejuvenation in Asians.

Ablative fractional resurfacing (AFR) has been investigated for photorejuvenation and acne scarring in Asian skin. A recent study has demonstrated the efficacy of the 10,600-nm fractional CO_2 laser in the treatment of wrinkles in Asian patients.[77](Figs 13.12A and B). However, the rate of PIH was high with 55.5% and 11.1% at 1 and 6 months post treatment, respectively. Erythema was a common side-effect which was found in all patients though most of them resolved in 1 week. Another group Trelles et al. has used fractional Er:YAG laser for skin rejuvenation.[78] Erythema was again a common side-effect seen in all skin types. However, only patients with type IV skin suffered from PIH beyond 2 months. There is another recent study by a Korean Group comparing the clinical efficacies of 1550- and 1565-nm Er:glass lasers in the treatment of periorbital wrinkles.[79] It showed that both 1550- and 1565-nm Er:glass lasers were safe and effective modalities in the treatment of periorbital wrinkles. There was no significant difference between the two devices in terms of efficacy and side-effects. Post-treatment erythema and localized edema were observed in all patients and generally resolved within 2–3 days after the treatment. Three of 20 patients (15%) noted a darkening of their pre-existing pigmentary lesions. One patient developed PIH caused by contact dermatitis induced by the topical anesthetic cream. These pigmentary alterations resolved in all patients within 2 months.

CONCLUSION

With the appropriate selection of device and parameters, laser surgery can be used effectively for the treatment of pigmentary and vascular lesions in Asians. Fractional resurfacing can be used for skin rejuvenation and the risk of PIH can be lowered with lower density and increased number of treatment sessions.

REFERENCES

1. Chung JH. Photoaging in Asians. Photodermatol Photoimmunol Photomed. 2003;19:109-21.
2. Chan HH, Jackson B. Laser treatment on ethnic skin. In: Photodermatology. Lim HW, Honigsmann H, Hawk JLM (Eds). Informa Healthcare. New York; 2007. pp. 417-32.
3. Somyos K, Boonchu K, Somsak K, et al. Copper vapour laser treatment of cafe-au-lait macules. Br J Dermatol. 1996;135:964-8.
4. Alora MB, Arndt KA. Treatment of a cafe-au-lait macule with the erbium:YAG laser. J Am Acad Dermatol. 2001;45:566-8.
5. Alster TS. Complete elimination of large cafe-au-lait birthmarks by the 510-nm pulsed dye laser. Plast Reconstr Surg. 1995;96:1660-4.
6. Alster TS, Williams CM. Cafe-au-lait macule in type V skin: successful treatment with a 510 nm pulsed dye laser. J Am Acad Dermatol. 1995;33:1042-3.
7. Grossman MC, Anderson RR, Farinelli W, et al. Treatment of cafe au lait macules with lasers. A clinicopathologic correlation. Arch Dermatol. 1995;131:1416-20.
8. Kopera D, Hohenleutner U, Landthaler M. Quality-switched ruby laser treatment of solar lentigines and Becker's nevus: a histopathological and immunohistochemical study. Dermatology. 1997;194: 338-43.
9. Trelles MA, Allones I, Moreno-Arias GA, et al. Becker's naevus: a comparative study between erbium: YAG and Q-switched neodymium:YAG; clinical and histopathological findings. Br J Dermatol. 2005; 152:308-13.
10. Nanni CA, Alster TS. Treatment of a Becker's nevus using a 694-nm long-pulsed ruby laser. Dermatol Surg. 1998;24:1032-4.
11. Drummer R, Kempf W, Burg TG. Pseudo-melanoma after laser therapy. Dermatology. 1998;197:71-3.
12. Soden CE, Smith K, Skelton H. Histological features seen in changing nevi after therapy with an 810 nm pulsed diode laser for hair removal in patients with dysplastic nevi. Int J Dermatol. 2001;40:500-4.
13. Chan HH. Laser treatment of nevomelanocytic nevi – Can results from an Asian study be applicable to the white population? Arch Dermatol. 2002;138:535.
14. Waldorf HA, Kauvar AN, Geronemus RG. Treatment of small and medium congenital nevi with the Q-switched ruby laser. Arch Dermatol. 1996;132:301-4.
15. Duke D, Byers HR, Sober AJ, et al. Treatment of benign and atypical nevi with the normal-mode ruby laser and the Q-switched ruby laser: clinical improvement but failure to completely eliminate nevomelanocytes. Arch Dermatol. 1999;135:290-6.
16. Imayama S, Ueda S. Long- and short-term histological observations of congenital nevi treated with the normal-mode ruby laser. Arch Dermatol. 1999;135:1211-8.
17. Kono T, Nozaki M, Chan HH, et al. Combined use of normal mode and Q-switched ruby lasers in the treatment of congenital melanocytic naevi. Br J Plast Surg. 2001;54:640-3.
18. Geronemus RG. Q-switched ruby laser therapy of nevus of Ota. Arch Dermatol. 1992;128:1618-22.
19. Watanabe S, Takahashi H. Treatment of nevus of Ota with the Q-switched ruby laser. N Engl J Med. 1994;331:1745-50.
20. Chan HH, King WW, Chan ES, et al. In vivo trial comparing patients' tolerance of Q-switched Alexandrite (QS Alex) and Q-switched neodymium: yttrium-aluminum-garnet (QS Nd:YAG) lasers in the treatment of nevus of Ota. Lasers Surg Med. 1999;24:24-8.
21. Kono T, Nozaki M, Chan HH, et al. A retrospective study looking at the long-term complications of Q-switched ruby laser in the treatment of nevus of Ota. Lasers Surg Med. 2001;29:156-9.
22. Kono T, Chan HH, Ercocen AR, et al. Use of Q-switched ruby laser in the treatment of nevus of Ota in different age groups. Lasers Surg Med. 2003;32:391-5.
23. Chan HH, Lam LK, Wong DS, et al. Nevus of Ota: a new classification based on the response to laser treatment. Lasers Surg Med. 2001;28:267-72.
24. Kono T, Groff WF, Chan HH, et al. Comparison study of a Q-switched alexandrite laser delivered with versus without compression in the treatment of dermal pigmented lesions. J Cosmet Laser Ther. 2007;9:206-9.
25. Kouba DJ, Fincher EF, Moy RL. Nevus of Ota successfully treated by fractional photothermolysis using a fractionated 1440-nm Nd:YAG laser. Arch Dermatol. 2008;144:156-8.

26. Saedi N, Metelitsa A, Petrell K, et al. Treatment of tattoos with a picosecond alexandrite laser: a prospective trial. Arch Dermatol. 2012 Sep 17:1-4. [Epub ahead of print]
27. Anderson RR, Margolis RJ, Watenabe S. Selective photothermolysis of cutaneous pigmentation by Q-switched Nd:YAG laser pulses at 1064, 532 and 355 nm. J Invest Dermatol. 1989;93:28-32.
28. Murphy MJ, Huang MY. Q-switched ruby laser treatment of benign pigmented lesions in Chinese skin. Am Acad Med, Singapore. 1994;23:60-6.
29. Chan HH, Fung WK, Ying SY, et al. An in vivo trial comparing the use of different types of 532 nm Nd:YAG lasers in the treatment of facial lentigines in Oriental patients. Dermatol Surg. 2000;26:743-9.
30. Wang CC, Sue YM, Yang CH, et al. A comparison of Q-switched alexandrite laser and intense pulsed light for the treatment of freckles and lentigines in Asian persons: a randomized, physician-blinded, split-face comparative trial. J Am Acad Dermatol. 2006;54:804-10.
31. Ho SG, Chan NP, Yeung CK, et al. A retrospective analysis of the management of freckles and lentigines using four different pigment lasers on Asian skin. J Cosmet Laser Ther. 2012;14:74-80.
32. Kang HY, Suzuki I, Lee DJ, et al. Transcriptional profiling shows altered expression of wnt pathway- and lipid metabolism-related genes as well as melanogenesis-related genes in melasma. J Invest Dermatol. 2011;131:1692-700.
33. Grekin RC, Shelton RM, Geisse JK, et al. 510-nm pigmented lesion dye laser: its characteristics and clinical uses. J Dermatol Surg Oncol. 1993;19:380-7.
34. Taylor CR, Anderson RR. Ineffective treatment of refractory melasma and postinflammatory hyperpigmentation by Q-switched ruby laser. J Dermatol Surg Oncol. 1994;20:592-7.
35. Wang CC, Hui CY, Sue YM, et al. Intense pulsed light for the treatment of refractory melasma in Asian patients. Dermatol Surg. 2004;30:1196-200.
36. Li YH, Chen JZ, Wei HC, et al. Efficacy and safety of intense pulsed light in treatment of melasma in Chinese patients. Dermatol Surg. 2008;34:693-700.
37. Manaloto RM, Alster T. Erbium:YAG laser resurfacing for refractory melasma. Dermatol Surg. 1999; 25:121-3.
38. Angsuwarangsee S, Polnikorn N. Combined ultrapulse CO_2 laser and Q-switched alexandrite laser compared with Q-switched alexandrite laser alone for refractory melasma: split-face design. Dermatol Surg. 2003;29:59-64.
39. Rokhsar C, Fitzpatrick RE. The treatment of melasma with fractional photothermolysis: a pilot study. Dermatol Surg. 2005;31:1645-50.
40. Lee HS, Won CH, Lee DH, et al. Treatment of melasma in Asian skin using a fractional 1550nm laser: an open study. Dermatol Surg. 2009;35: 1499-504.
41. Karsai S, Fischer T, Pohl L, et al. Is non-ablative 1550-nm fractional photothermolysis an effective modality to treat melasma? Results from a prospective controlled single-blinded trial in 51 patients. J Eur Acad Dermatol Venereol. 2012;26:470-6.
42. Barysch MJ, Rümmelein B, Kolm I, et al. Split-face study of melasma patients treated with non-ablative fractionated photothermolysis (1540 nm). J Eur Acad Dermatol Venereol. 2012;26:423-30.
43. Niwa Massaki AB, Eimpunth S, Fabi SG, et al. Treatment of melasma with the 1,927-nm fractional thulium fiber laser: a retrospective analysis of 20 cases with long-term follow up. Lasers Surg Med. 2012 Dec 19.[Epub ahead of print]
44. Ho SG, Yeung CK, Chan NP, et al. A retrospective study of the management of Chinese melasma patients using a 1927 nm fractional thulium fiber laser. J Cosmet Laser Ther. 2013 Feb 5. [Epub ahead of print]
45. Polnikorn N. Treatment of refractory dermal melasma with the MedLite C6 Q-switched Nd:YAG laser: two case reports. J Cosmet Laser Ther. 2008; 10:167-73.
46. Chan NPY, Ho SGY, Shek SYN, et al. A case series of facial depigmentation associated with low fluence Q-switched 1064 nm Nd:YAG laser for skin rejuvenation and melasma. Lasers Surg Med. 2010;42:712-9.
47. Kauvar AN. Successful treatment of melasma using a combination of microdermabrasion and Q-switched Nd:YAG lasers. Lasers Surg Med. 2012;44:117-24.
48. Kim EH, Kim YC, Lee ES, et al. The vascular characteristics of melasma. J Dermatol Sci. 2007;46:111-6.
49. Passeron T, Fontas E, Kang HY, et al. Melasma treatment with pulsed-dye laser and triple combination cream: a prospective, randomized, single-blind, split-face study. Arch Dermatol. 2011;147:1106-8.
50. Hori Y, Kawashima M, Oohara K, et al. Acquired, bilateral nevus of Ota-like macules. J Am Acad Dermatol. 1984;10:961-4.
51. Kunachak S, Leelaudomlipi P, Sirikulchayanonta V. Q-switched ruby laser therapy of acquired bilateral nevus of Ota-like macules. Dermatol Surg. 1999; 25:938-41.
52. Lam AY, Wong DS, Lam LK, et al. A retrospective study on the efficacy and complications of Q-switched alexandrite laser in the treatment of acquired bilateral nevus of Ota-like macules. Dermatol Surg. 2001;27:937-41.
53. Polnikorn N, Tanrattanakorn S, Goldberg DJ. Treatment of Hori's nevus with the Q-switched Nd:YAG laser. Dermatol Surg. 2000;26:477-80.
54. Ee HL, Goh CL, Khoo LS, et al. Treatment of acquired bilateral nevus of Ota-like macules (Hori's nevus) with a combination of the 532 nm Q-switched Nd:YAG laser followed by the 1064 nm Q-switched Nd:YAG is more effective: prospective study. Dermatol Surg. 2006;32:34-40.

55. Manuskiatti W, Sivayathorn A, Leelaudomlipi P, et al. Treatment of acquired bilateral nevus of Ota-like macules (Hori's nevus) using a combination of scanned carbon dioxide laser followed by Q-switched ruby laser. J Am Acad Dermatol. 2003;48:584-91.
56. Cho SB, Park SJ, Kim MJ, et al. Treatment of acquired bilateral nevus of Ota-like macules (Hori's nevus) using 1064 nm Q-switched Nd:YAG with low fluence. Int J Dermatol. 2009;48:1308-12.
57. Asahina A, Watanabe T, Kishi A, et al. Evaluation of the treatment of port-wine stains with the 595 nm long pulsed dye laser: a large prospective study in adult Japanese patients. J Am Acad Dermatol. 2006;54:487-93.
58. Ho WS, Chan HH, Ying SY, et al. Laser treatment of congenital facial port-wine stains: long-term efficacy and complications in Chinese patients. Lasers Surg Med. 2002;30:44-7.
59. Chang CJ, Nelson JS. Cryogen spray cooling and higher fluence pulsed dye laser treatment improve port wine stain clearance while minimizing epidermal damage. Dermatol Surg. 1999;25:767-72.
60. Chiu CH, Chan HH, Ho WS, et al. Prospective study of pulsed dye laser in conjunction with cryogen spray cooling for treatment of port wine stains in Chinese patients. Dermatol Surg. 2003;29:909-15.
61. Nelson JS, Geronemus RG, Huikeshoven M, et al. Redarkening of port wine stains 10 years after laser treatment. The New England Journal of Medicine. 2007; 356:2745.
62. Izikson L, Nelson JS, Anderson RR. Treatment of hypertrophic and resistant port wine stains with a 755 nm laser: a case series of 20 patients. Lasers Surg Med. 2009;41:427-32.
63. Kono T, Frederick Groff W, Chan HH, et al. Long-pulsed neodymium:yttrium-aluminium-garnet laser treatment for hypertrophic port-wine stains on the lips. J Cosmet Laser Ther. 2009;11:11-3.
64. Alam M, Dover JS, Arndt KA. Treatment of facial telangiectasia with variable-pulse high-fluence pulsed-dye laser: comparison of efficacy with fluences immediately above and below the purpura threshold. Dermatol Surg. 2003;29: 681-5.
65. Jasim ZF, Woo WK, Handley JM. Long-pulsed (6-ms) pulsed dye laser treatment of rosacea-associated telangiectasia using subpurpuric clinical threshold. Dermatol Surg. 2004;30:37-40.
66. Karsai S, Roos S, Raulin C. Treatment of facial telangiectasia using a dual-wavelength laser system (595 and 1,064 nm): a randomized controlled trial with blinded response evaluation. Dermatol Surg. 2008;34:702-8.
67. Nouri K, Elsaie ML, Vejjabhinanta V, et al. Comparison of the effects of short- and long-pulse durations when using a 585-nm pulsed dye laser in the treatment of new surgical scars. Lasers Med Sci. 2010;25:121-6.
68. Nanni CA, Alster TS. Complications of carbon dioxide laser resurfacing: an evaluation of 500 patients. Dermatol Surg. 1998;24:315-20.
69. Alam M, Hsu T, Dover JS, et al. Nonablative laser and light treatments: histology and tissue effects: a review. Lasers Surg Med. 2003;33:30.
70. Chan HH, Lam LK, Wong DS, et al. Use of 1320nm Nd:YAG laser for wrinkle reduction and the treatment of atrophic acne scarring. Lasers Surg Med. 2004; 34:98-103.
71. Chua SH, Ang P, Khoo LS, et al. Nonablative 1450-nm diode laser in the treatment of facial atrophic acne scars in type IV to V Asian skin: a prospective clinical study. Dermatol Surg. 2004;30:1287-91.
72. Manstein D, Herron GS, Sink RK, et al. Fractional photothermolysis: a new concept for cutaneous remodeling using microscopic patterns of thermal injury. Lasers Surg Med. 2004;34:426-38.
73. Review of fractional photothermolysis: treatment indications and efficacy. Dermatol Surg. 2009; 35:1445-61.
74. Alexiades-Armenakas MR, Dover JS, Arndt KA. The spectrum of laser skin resurfacing: nonablative, fractional, and ablative laser resurfacing. J Am Acad Dermatol. 2008;58:719-37.
75. Kono T, Chan HH, Groff WF, et al. Prospective direct comparison study of fractional resurfacing using different fluences and densities for skin rejuvenation in Asians. Lasers Surg Med. 2007;39:311-4.
76. Chan NP, Ho SG, Yeung CK, et al. The use of non-ablative fractional resurfacing in Asian acne scar patients. Lasers Surg Med. 2010;42:710-5.
77. Chan NP, Ho SG, Yeung CK, et al. Fractional ablative carbon dioxide laser resurfacing for skin rejuvenation and acne scars in Asians. Lasers Surg Med. 2010;42:615-23.
78. Trelles MA, Mordon S, Velez M, et al. Results of fractional ablative facial skin resurfacing with the erbium:yttrium-aluminium-garnet laser 1 week and 2 months after one single treatment in 30 patients. Lasers Med Sci. 2009;24:186-94.
79. Jung JY, Cho SB, Chung HJ, et al. Treatment of periorbital wrinkles with 1550- and 1565-nm Er:glass fractional photothermolysis lasers: a simultaneous split-face trial. J Eur Acad Dermatol Venereol. 2011; 25:811-8.

CHAPTER 14

Lasers and Energy-Based Devices for the Consumer: The Future of Esthetic Energy-Based Devices

Eric F Bernstein, Tobin C Island

INTRODUCTION

In the last ten years, over-the-counter energy-based medical devices for dermatological applications have transitioned from nascent to the most rapidly growing category in the $40B global annual consumer beauty market.[1-3] For the purposes of this chapter, we define energy-based medical devices as medical devices that employ light (laser or otherwise), radiofrequency radiation, ultrasound, or other similar types of radiated, nonchemical energy that is transmitted into the skin with enough energy and/or power to affect the structure or function of the skin. This definition distinguishes products that work by transmitting energy into the skin (such as laser hair removal) from those that work on the surface (such as epilators or razors) or by chemical means, and this definition is consistent with the United States Food and Drug Administration (US FDA) definition of a medical device. We exclude nonmedical devices in this chapter, even though they may employ at least some transmitted energy (such as acoustic toothbrushes or acoustic skin brushes) for brevity, consistency, and because a regulatory clearance provides at least some assurance of safety and effectiveness of the claimed dermatological effect.

The growth in home-based energy devices is being driven by improving technology, better understanding of the dermatological applications themselves and how to adapt them for home use, regulatory environments that are now well experienced with predicate prescription therapies, and huge global market forces for beauty products, especially those that offer better efficacy than cosmetic products but at a lower cost than professionally-administered and/or prescription therapies. Home devices (that can be used indefinitely and on multiple body locations) often cost less than a single visit to a dermatologist (for what is usually a multi-visit therapy for each of multiple body areas). Such devices are an example of the so-called "disruptive innovation" that can emerge if a new product category delivers similar performance —it need not be equivalent—to existing solutions that are much more expensive.[2,4]

In this chapter, we discuss some of the key enabling technologies for home devices, briefly survey the currently available devices, provide example case studies comparing specifications and performance to prescription devices used in the clinic, and predict future directions. We aim to provide the reader a scientifically-based perspective that can be used to help appropriately inform his/her patients about these devices and help guide this burgeoning field. Like many emerging fields, there is a wide variation in the effectiveness, safety, and quality among the existing products, and while the medical professional does not employ these devices directly, medical personnel can play an important role developing, testing, regulating, educating, and advising consumers—both now and, increasingly, in the future as these products continue to advance and popularize.

OVERVIEW OF OFFICE-BASED ESTHETIC LASERS AND ENERGY-BASED DEVICES

Since the birth of modern pulsed or scanned lasers for dermatologic use in the mid-1980s, there has been an explosive growth in the number and type of devices entering the market. This has dramatically expanded the number of conditions that can be successfully treated with lasers, and now also other energy-based devices. There are a number of broad categories of devices for treating a myriad of dermatologic conditions. These include devices for: removal of unwanted blood vessels and associate conditions, hair removal, skin resurfacing including photoaging and acne scarring, tattoo removal and removal of pigmented lesions, treatment of acne, skin tightening, body contouring, cellulite and fat reduction, and treatment of hyperhidrosis. Some devices for treating the above conditions are ideally suited to home use, while others are not and may never be.

Modern dermatologic lasers use pulses of laser energy, or scanned beams that to the target tissues behave as pulses, to selectively target chromophores within the skin, while relatively ignoring non-target surrounding tissue. This "selective photothermolysis" is based on a seminal work by Anderson and Parrish demonstrating that target tissue can be removed without damaging surrounding non-target structures.[5-7] Because we are treating living human skin, the effect of lasers and energy-based devices is often more than simply removing target tissue. Laser or energy-based device treatment stimulates an inflammatory cascade that can induce skin remodeling, wound healing, and other inflammatory-induced effects, dramatically increasing the range of conditions that respond to laser and energy-based device treatments. Additionally, lasers or energy-based devices can also interact with the tissue through photochemical processes (such as employed in certain acne phototherapy), nondestructive tissue heating (such as that used in nonablative, nonfractionated remodeling), and photobiological processes (such as the presumed mitochondrial mechanisms for certain low-level-light-therapy).

Lasers and light sources such as intense pulsed light sources (IPLs) that target vascular lesions can be used to treat a variety of vascular lesions and conditions where hypervascularity is central to the condition to be treated. For example, vascular lasers emitting yellow-orange (585–595 nm) or green (532 nm) light can selectively target unwanted blood vessels and remove facial telangiectasias, lower extremity spider veins, vascular birth marks such as port-wine stains, as well as diffuse redness caused by much smaller facial vessels.[8-19] These devices can also improve striae[14] by improving redness and inducing minimal to moderate skin remodeling, as well as improving rosacea,[18] including both the diffuse redness and the papular component, treat psoriasis,[15] and verrucae,[13] and improve erythematous scars,[19] by not only removing the redness but also by remodeling disordered collagen and other extracellular matrix components in the dermis. Generally, it is thought that a critical minimum fluence is necessary for the destruction of unwanted blood vessels, and that low-level laser or broad-spectrum light is relatively ineffective for removing unwanted blood vessels. In-office professional lasers for removing unwanted blood vessels and treating conditions where vascularity plays a major role are generally relatively high-energy, expensive devices. Developing safe and effective devices that target unwanted blood vessels has not yet made it to the home-use market. Low-energy devices can affect inflammation and temporarily reduce redness or inflammation, and some home devices in this category (particularly for treating acne) are on the market.

Although lasers for treating unwanted blood vessels are among the first widely-used devices exploiting selective photothermolysis, laser hair removal[20-27] is currently the most popular laser procedure worldwide. Laser hair removal works by selectively targeting melanin pigment in hair shafts to cause damage, which then fortunately induces a selective inflammatory response that stimulates a prolonged resting phase in affected hair follicles. A number of hair follicles may also be thermally destroyed during laser hair removal, but inflammation appears to play the major role in laser hair removal. This can be illustrated by the fact that paradoxical unwanted hair growth can be induced by these same lasers, particularly in rare circumstances often involving hormonal abnormalities, indicating that opposite effects on the hair follicle can occur based on the type and fluence of laser light delivered and the induced thermal destruction and inflammation.[28] Professional in-office hair removal lasers often employ cooling devices to reduce the temperature of the epidermis, limiting unwanted damage to the epidermis, and thus side-effects. Sufficient heating still occurs at the deeper level of the hair bulge and bulb, despite cooling of the more superficial epidermis. Since these lasers target melanin pigment, the epidermis is an unwanted target, since it too contains melanin, although in significantly less amounts than darkly-pigmented hair shafts. Lasers that penetrate deeply into the skin and that are beyond the wavelengths that target vascular chromophores are used for laser hair removal. These include the retired 694-nm ruby laser,[23,24] the 755-nm alexandrite laser,[25-27] the 810-nm diode laser,[20-22,26,27] and the 1,064-nm neodymium-doped, yttrium, aluminum, garnet (Nd:YAG) laser.[26] In addition, because melanin pigment absorbs a broad band of wavelengths with absorption decreasing with increasing wavelength, IPLs can also be used for hair removal, especially if filtered to remove most of the noneffective longer wavelengths. The longer wavelength lasers such as the Nd:YAG laser provide some selective advantage in sparing epidermal melanin pigment in more darkly pigmented individuals while still maintaining the ability to sufficiently damage hair, resulting in very effective laser hair removal in people with Fitzpatrick skin types IV–VI.[26] This is somewhat surprising given that the Nd:YAG wavelength is absorbed both by epidermal and hair shaft melanin pigment. Home devices for light-based hair removal utilize both inexpensive laser light sources and IPLs, but have not as yet been able to incorporate active skin cooling due to cost and device size limitations, nor may skin cooling ultimately be found necessary in home devices, perhaps especially if home devices are limited to a smaller subset of subjects (such as Fitzpatrick skin types I–IV, or only those with darker hair colors) than professional devices. Still, laser- and IPL-based home hair removal devices are a major class of home light-based esthetic devices. Darker skin types must be screened out at this time to reduce the risk of injuring the skin with consumer units, so home hair removal devices generally have integrated pigment measuring capabilities to avoid treatment of darkly pigmented individuals. It is also worth noting that effective home devices may intentionally offer different levels of benefit than each other and/or professional systems. For example, some home devices may provide permanent hair removal whereas others may provide only temporary hair removal, depending on technical output specifications, treatment regimens, and user characteristics. While temporary hair removal may not be practical in the clinic, consumers may find it worthwhile if it competes effectively on cost, time and convenience versus traditional shaving and waxing. Likewise, home devices offer the opportunity for frequent or even daily treatment regimens, which are impractical in the clinic but could provide new benefits to consumers in the home.

Laser tattoo removal is accomplished in-office by the use of powerful quality-switched (Q-switched) lasers capable of emitting nanosecond-domain laser pulses with extremely high peak powers.[29-38] The need for such short pulse-duration lasers is centered on the fact that the target particles, consisting of tattoo granules aggregated in cutaneous macrophages, are relatively small compared to blood vessels or hair shafts targeted by other laser modalities. Prolonged heating of these small granules allows heat to spread from the target particles to surrounding skin, increasing the risk of scarring. This is dramatically illustrated when viewing tattoos treated by IPLs, which often demonstrate significant scarring and keloid formation, from their millisecond-domain pulses. Q-switched lasers used to treat tattoos include the 694-nm ruby laser[29-32,38], the 755-nm alexandrite laser[35-38], and the 1,064-nm Nd:YAG laser[32-34,37,38] which by incorporating the potassium titanyl phosphate (KTP) crystal also emits 532-nm laser light. Technology to inexpensively and safely deliver Q-switched laser energy in the home setting has not been developed and may be out of reach even for the distant future. Q-switched lasers are also used for treating epidermal melanin pigment such as freckles, lentigos, and café au lait macules. Because the pigment in these lesions is located in the epidermis and not the dermis as with tattoos, IPLs are also used to remove freckles and lentigos.[39] Effective treatment of melasma by lasers is controversial and minimally effective in select cases at best, which may be due to the significant inflammatory component at work in areas affected by melasma. Freckles and lentigos may be amenable to home treatment with IPLs, however, the low margin between therapy and side-effects and the need for evaluation of pigmented lesions by professionals for cancer screening will likely limit such devices from broad-scale use in the consumer market.

Resurfacing lasers that target water are used to treat photoaging and acne scarring, and exert most effect on the textural changes associated with these conditions. Thus, fine lines and wrinkles, enlarged pores and the depressions of acne scarring improve following treatment with these lasers. Generally, wavelengths that are absorbed by water are used, and skin is either ablated or removed, in the case of carbon dioxide (CO_2)[40-45] and Erbium:YAG (Er:YAG)[46-48] lasers. Carbon dioxide lasers emit at 10,600 nm and ablate skin and leave a zone of denatured dermal collagen behind, which stimulates a wound healing response following treatment.[40-45] Less tissue can be removed with other wavelengths such as that delivered by the Er:YAG laser emitting at 2,940 nm, which leave less damaged dermal collagen behind than the CO_2 laser.[40-49] This can often result in less hemostasis and less immediate tissue tightening from treatment with the Er:YAG, as opposed to the CO_2 laser. These fully-ablative resurfacing lasers can yield significant photoaging benefits but generally come with substantial downtime and comparatively high levels of side-effects. There have been no home devices developed with this modality nor does it appear likely any time soon.

There are also water-absorbed, resurfacing lasers that provide no tissue ablation, simply tissue heating and the induction of inflammation, as with diode lasers that emit at 1,320 nm, 1,450 nm, or a host of other wavelengths available from the telecommunications industry.[50-53] These lasers incorporate various strategies to cool the skin such as forced air or cryogen spray cooling, thus eliminating tissue ablation.[50-53] Home devices in this category are likely limited by the expense of high optical power requirements and critical cooling and safety systems, as well as the low margin between effective therapy and side-effects. No home devices in this category have come to market to-date.

The biggest advance seen with lasers that target water has come with the proliferation of fractionated lasers.[54-59] The concept is to reduce the side-effects that occur following large-area confluent treatment by treating only a smaller percentage of the skin surface with each treatment, and administering a series of treatments. Although five treatments targeting 20% of a treatment area might indeed equate to a single 100% treatment when ablating inanimate objects, skin is a living organ and thus an open wound where the entire skin surface has been treated heals in a very different way than a fractionated treatment where islands of normal tissue are left untreated. Nonetheless, fractionated lasers have revolutionized the use of water-targeting lasers for the treatment of photoaging, acne scarring and a host of other conditions. Both ablative CO_2 and nonablative 1,550-nm fiber or other 1,320-nm or 1,450-nm diode lasers, as well as partially ablative 1,927-nm thulium-doped fiber lasers have been produced as fractionated lasers.[54-59] Fractionated laser treatment resulting in zones of thermal damage separated by nontreated or partially-treated skin can be accomplished in many ways; (e.g. macrolenses, microlenses, optical scanners, mechanical scanners, grids, screens and fiber rasterization) to make tiny zones of injury in treated areas. Although CO_2 lasers cannot be produced for the home market in a cost-effective or safe manner, diode lasers emitting in the wavelengths absorbed by water can, and have, been developed for consumer use. Fractionated lasers that leave zones of untreated skin between small treatment zones are available for skin rejuvenation and can be incorporated into a general skin care regimen.

Other energy-based technologies not utilizing light such as radiofrequency (RF)-emitting devices, microwave-emitting devices, focused high-frequency ultrasound, and even controlled tissue cooling have been used in multiple esthetic applications in the clinic.[60-65] RF-emitting devices have been used to treat skin sagging associated with photoaging.[60,61] RF devices that deliver RF energy deeply in the dermis have been used to stimulate tissue tightening,[61] while more superficially administered RF energy is being used to treat photoaging and acne scarring.[60] The proposed mechanism of action is the treatment of deep layers of dermal connective tissue to stimulate tissue tightening or tissue remodeling. Microwave devices are being used to destroy the fat layer between the dermis and subdermal fat, and in doing so can eliminate sweat glands thus treating hyperhidrosis.[62,63] A device that delivers controlled cooling to subdermal fat has been developed for fat layer reduction.[65] This device causes selective damage to fat that then induces apoptosis in fat cells, thus reducing the fat layer in treated areas. Devices emitting superficial RF energy may be adapted for home use in the future, if the cost and size of these devices can be sufficiently limited. Likewise, controlled cooling would appear to be adaptable to home use, maybe requiring sensors to ensure proper temperature profiles.

An entire class of devices that are ideally suited to the home market are mid-level and low-level light sources, such as light-emitting diodes (LEDs), that administer continuous or modulated light with relatively narrow band widths at relatively low fluences that generally act via a photochemical or photobiological mechanism, not a thermal one.[66,67,70] An example of mid-level light sources are the blue light devices (arc lamps and more recently LED sources) that have been used in physician offices for treating acne.[66,67,70] The blue wavelengths target porphyrins present in acne bacteria resulting in free-radical production, thus destroying the acne bacteria. Numerous home devices based on these principles, predominately for acne, are already on the market utilizing LEDs. An example of low-level light sources acting on purported biological pathways are various other light sources emitting a whole range of visible wavelengths that have been used in physician offices to improve photodamaged skin, reduce or prevent the inflammation associated with various laser treatments, and to stimulate hair growth or to destroy fat. Devices that emit low-level, narrow-band light are ideally suited to home use because they are extremely safe, and sources such as LEDs can be very inexpensive to produce. Furthermore, as mentioned earlier, the home domain where regular treatments (daily or multi-daily) are required, and a lower threshold for efficacy than expected for physician treatments (e.g. mildly superior to cosmetic topical agents), provides an opportunity for low-level light devices that does not necessarily exist in the clinic. Because the energy is of a relatively low fluence, the effectiveness of these devices for treating photodamage, acne, acne scarring, unwanted fat, or to induce hair growth may be quite variable between various applications and devices. The ultimate success of this category will likely depend on achieving improved efficacy from the current stable of devices, as well as further advances in technology, which in turn will depend upon developing a better understanding of the underlying mechanisms of actions of these devices so that they can be optimized for different applications. The authors expect a steady increase of home devices that will utilize LEDs with photobiological and photochemical mechanisms—some of which will provide efficacy and some of which will provide little or none—as the underlying science is advanced.

DEVICES DEVELOPED FOR HOME USE

Tables 14.1 to 14.3 list the home energy-based devices known to the authors to be currently cleared by the

Table 14.1: Cleared over-the-counter (OTC) hair removal devices

Mfgr	*Name of Device*	*510k Number*	*Cleared Name*	*FDA Cleared Indications*	*Type*
Hair Removal					
Home Skinovations	Silk'n SensEpil (US: Flash & Go)	K103184, K082298, K072906	Silk'n Flash N' Go	Flash N Go is an over-the-counter device intended for the removal of unwanted hair. Flash N Go is also intended for permanent reduction in hair regrowth defined as a long-term, stable reduction in hair counts following a treatment regimen	OTC
Remington	i-Light Intense Pro	K103560, K120080	Shaser IPL Hair Removal System	The Shaser IPL is an over-the-counter device intended for hair removal	OTC
TRIA Beauty	TRIA Hair Removal Laser	K120737, K053527, K090820	TRIA HRL	TRIA is an over-the-counter device intended for adjunctive use with shaving for hair removal sustained with periodic treatments. TRIA is also intended for permanent reduction in hair regrowth defined as a long-term, stable reduction in hair counts following a treatment regime. Permanent hair reduction is defined as long-term, stable reduction in the number of hairs regrowing when measured out to 6,9 and 12 months after the completion of the treatment regimen	OTC

Table 14.2: Cleared OTC acne treatment devices

Mfgr	*Name of Device*	*510k Number*	*Cleared Name*	*FDA Cleared Indications*	*Type*
Acne Devices					
Syneron Beauty	Tanda Skincare System: Tanda Clear	K080591	Tanda Skincare System	The Tanda Skincare System is generally indicated to treat dermatological conditions. Specifically, blue light modules are indicated to treat mild-to-moderate inflammatory acne	OTC
PhotoMedex	Omnilux Clear-U	K081307	Omnilux Clear-U	The Omnilux Clear-U is intended to emit energy in the red and blue region of the spectrum, specifically indicated to treat mild-to-moderate acne on the face	OTC
Therative	Thermaclear	K060653	ThermaClear	ThermaClear is indicated for the treatment of individual acne pimples in persons with mild-to-moderate inflammatory acne	OTC
Silver Bay	Baby Blue	K093963	Quasar Blue Light Therapy System	The Quasar Blue Light Therapy System is intended to provide photo therapeutic light to the body. The Quasar Blue Light Therapy System is generally indicated to treat dermatological conditions. The Quasar Blue Light Therapy System is specifically indicated to emit visible blue/violet light to treat mild-to-moderate inflammatory acne vulgaris	OTC
Radiancy	No! No! Skin	K102477	no!no! Skin	The no!no! Skin is intended to provide phototherapeutic light and heat to the body and is generally indicated to treat dermatological conditions. It is specifically indicated for the treatment of individual acne pimples in persons with mild-to-moderate inflammatory acne	OTC
LumaTherm	Zeno	K043377	Zeno	Zeno is indicated for the treatment of individual acne pimples in persons with mild-to-moderate inflammatory acne	OTC
Solta Medical	CLARO SX	K090744	CLARO	The CLARO is indicated for the treatment of individual acne pimples in persons with mild-to-moderate inflammatory acne	OTC
TRIA Beauty	TRIA Skin Perfecting Blue Light	K090312	Tria Skin Perfecting Blue Light	The device is generally indicated to treat dermatological conditions and specifically indicated to treat mild-to-moderate inflammatory acne vulgaris. It is intended for over-the-counter use	OTC

Table 14.3: Cleared OTC skin rejuvenation devices

Mfgr	*Name of Device*	*510k Number*	*Cleared Name*	*FDA Cleared Indications*	*Type*
Anti-aging					
Home Skinovations	Silk'n Reju or Face FX (Silk'n FaceFX in US by HomeSkinovations)	K110301	Silk'n FX	Silk'n FX is an over-the-counter device indicated to emit energy in the red and IR region of the spectrum for use in dermatology for the treatment of periorbital wrinkles	OTC
PhotoMedex	Omnilux New U	K072459	Onmilux New-U	The Omnilux New-U is intended to emit energy in the red and IR region of the spectrum for use in dermatology for the treatment of periorbital wrinkles	OTC
LED Intellectual Properties LLC	LightStim by LightStim International, Inc.	K101190	Light for Wrinkles	The Light for Wrinkles is an over-the-counter handheld device intended for use in the treatment of periorbital wrinkles	OTC
Palomar Medical Technologies	Palovia Skin Renewing Laser	K090525	LOI System	The LOI System is an over-the-counter device intended for treatment of periorbital wrinkles	OTC
Syneron Beauty	Tanda Regenerate	K103415	Tanda Max System	The Tanda Max System is intended for the treatment of wrinkles, rhytides and fine lines in the periorbital region	OTC
Ageless Beauty Corp.	EVIS MD Platinum Red Light Therapy	K082247	Evis MD Platinum Red Light Therapy	The Evis MD Platinum Red Light Therapy device is intended to provide light to the body. Generally indicated to dermatology use for the treatment of superficial, benign vascular and pigmented lesions "such as but not limited to solar lentigines, sun spots, liver spots and age spots".	OTC

US FDA and available on the US market at the time of this writing in the areas of hair removal (3 devices), acne treatment (8 devices), and skin rejuvenation (6 devices). This chapter will describe selective examples of these devices based on high market share and/or representative technology, as well as selected devices that are not currently FDA cleared and/or available in international markets but are noteworthy in understanding the home device market.[66-85]

Hair Removal

Some examples of consumer hair-removal devices are shown in Figures 14.1A and B.

Tria

The Tria Hair Removal Laser ($395; Tria Beauty, Inc., Pleasanton, CA) is notable as the only laser hair-removal over-the-counter (OTC) device available on the US market and the first with a permanent hair reduction indication. It is indicated for temporary and permanent hair reduction for Fitzpatrick skin types I–IV and individuals with brown and black hair color. The device is a diode laser with a wavelength of 808 nm, a spot size of 1 cm diameter, a maximum pulse repetition rate of 1 Hz, and an energy output ranging from 7–22 J/cm^2 selectable by the user. These parameters can be compared to a professional, in-office diode laser such as the Lumenis LightSheer ST (Lumenis Inc., Santa Clara, CA) which has wavelength of 808 nm, spot size of 1 cm diameter, maximum pulse repetition rate of 2 Hz, and an energy output of 10–40 J/cm^2, a pulse-duration from 10 ms to 400 ms typically averaging 30 ms, and contact cooling. The Tria home-based device has similar characteristics except for a lower maximum repetition rate and fluence, a pulse-duration averaging between 100 ms and 500 ms, and a lack

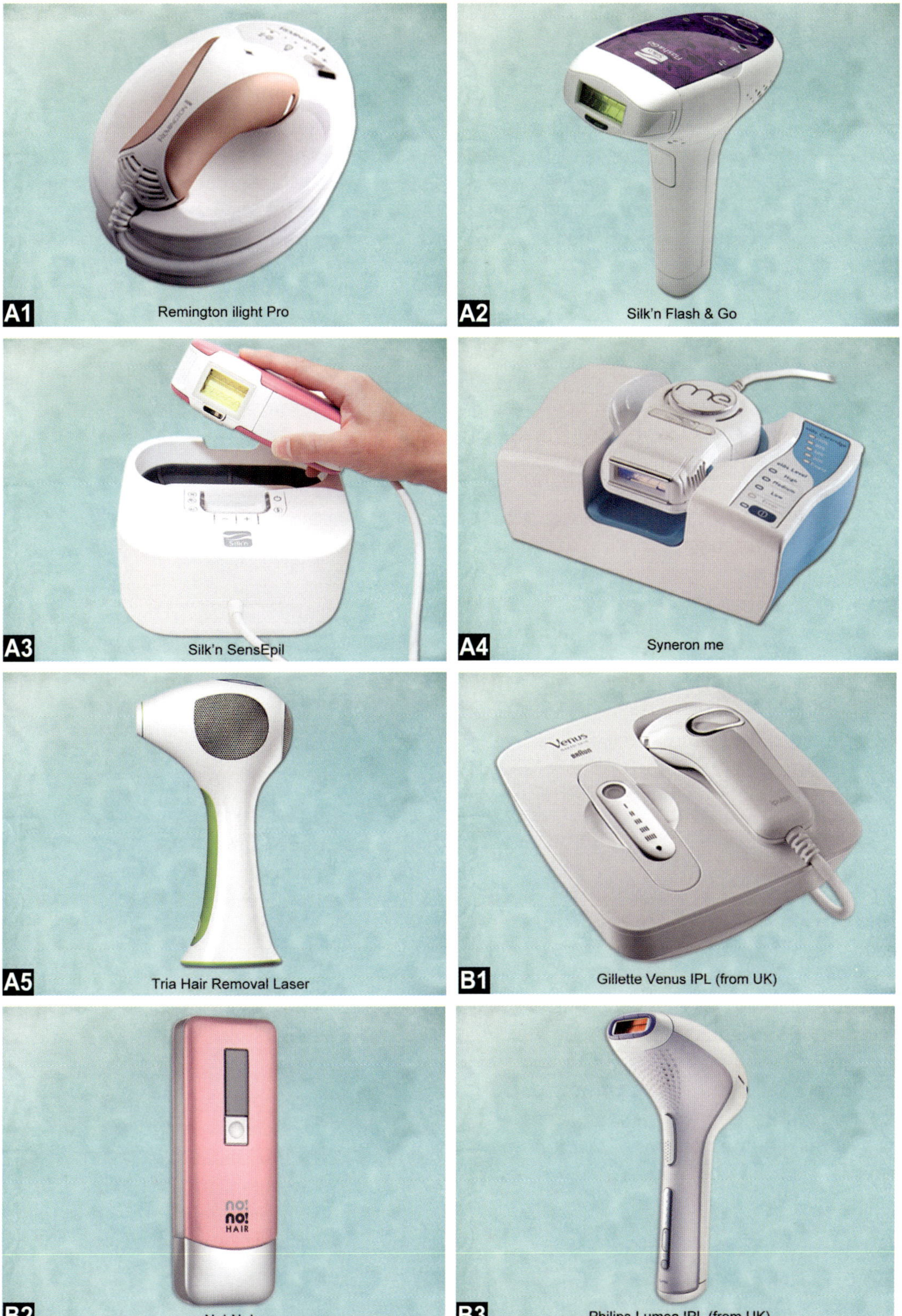

Figs 14.1A and B: (A) Consumer hair removal devices cleared by the United States Food and Drug Administration (US FDA) (at the time of the writing of this chapter); (B) Notable consumer hair removal devices not cleared by the US FDA (at the time of the writing of this chapter)

of contact cooling. Therefore, the home device will be slower to use and may be less effective or require more treatments to achieve similar outcomes, as compared to in-office hair-removal lasers. There are two peer-reviewed clinical studies with the Tria laser, both with blinded hair counts and one with a shaving control, that indicate that the device provides both a temporary and permanent hair-removal effect that lasts at least one year after a series of treatments for indicated users.[68-70]

The Tria device is also notable for two new pieces of safety technology—skin color sensing and eye safety optics—that go beyond typical contact sensing. The Tria skin color sensor is an optical sensor that measures the color of the skin and disables the laser output if the epidermis has too much melanin for safe use, thereby preventing use by nonindicated skin types. All home hair-removal devices subsequently cleared by the US FDA now have a similar technology. The Tria eye safety technology makes the laser output safe for the retina even if it were accidentally pulsed into the eye while in direct contact with the cornea, according to the manufacturer. To accomplish this, the device includes optics that diffuse the light so that the retinal fluence is below the class 1 eye safety limits established by international standards (e.g. IEC 60825). These safety features are good examples of technological advancement by home device manufacturers that will further enable the home device market.

Home Skinovations

Home Skinovations, Ltd.(Yokneam, Israel) has two IPL devices on the US market: Silk'n SensEpil ($499) and Silk'n Flash&Go ($299).[68-72] The devices are indicated for temporary and permanent hair reduction and are notable as the first cleared IPL devices on the market and the first OTC clearance allowing facial use. The devices are cleared for treating Fitzpatrick skin types I–IV and brown and black hair colors. The devices are flashlamp-based with a filtered spectrum from about 475 to 1100 mm, a spot size of about 3 cm^2, a pulse-width of 5 ms, a pulse repetition frequency of 4.1 seconds, and a fluence range of 3–7 J/cm^2. Comparing to an in-office IPL such as the IPL-containing Lumenis One (Lumenis Inc., Santa Clara, CA) which has a similar broadband wavelength range from 515–1,200 nm with interchangeable filters (although in-office devices generally have greater filtering), spot sizes of 5.2 and 1.2 cm^2, a pulse repetition rate of up to 1 Hz, and an energy output of 10–40 J/cm^2, one can see that the home IPL has a moderately lower maximum repetition rate and substantially lower fluence. Therefore, the home device will be slower to use and is likely less effective than its professional, office-based, IPL counterparts.[72-79] It is also notable that the home IPL device delivers about one-third the fluence of the Tria laser, presumably because the broadband light may be more strongly absorbed by melanin, and has a shorter pulse duration and higher peak powers, with about twice the coverage rate. Lasers have a better safety and efficacy profile for professional in-office hair-removal devices, however, they are more expensive to build. Future innovations in technology for home-based devices will determine which technology, if any, wins out in the home device market.

Remington/Shaser

Remington (DeForest, WI) has the only other FDA-cleared OTC hair-removal device on the US market in the form of its Light Pro IPL device ($249). It is cleared for temporary hair removal for Fitzpatrick skin types I–IV and brown or black hair. It is not currently cleared for facial use or permanent hair reduction. The iLight Pro has a 2.2-cm^2 spot size, a delay of 6 seconds between pulses and a maximum fluence of 10 J/cm^2. Compared to the Silk'n devices, the iPulse offers a somewhat higher maximum fluence (10 J/cm^2 vs 7 J/cm^2) which might be achieved by Remington's pulse stretching circuitry which provides mildly better skin safety by allowing greater heat diffusion during the pulse. Like the other devices, it employs a skin color sensor to prevent use on dark skin types and a skin contact sensor that requires the output window to be placed against the skin in order to fire. Since eye safety standards do not exist for IPLs (unlike lasers), it is not possible to independently certify eye safety although one research group published results concluding that the iPulse and the Silk'n devices are safe regarding the retina.[73-76] The device is most notable for longer IPL pulse-durations and its relatively low price ($245 vs $499 Home Skinovations and $395 Tria).

Syneron/Candela (Irvine, CA)

The Syneron Beauty division of the medical laser company sells the mē (£399; also marketed by

HoMedics), a combined IPL and radiofrequency (RF) device, in some non-US markets, and has received FDA 510k clearance from the US FDA. The device is notable for the combination of energy sources including IPL and RF as well as the mechanical epilator and mechanical shaver accessories. In typical use, the consumer moves the device across the skin and the leading epilator first pulls the hair out of the follicle and then IPL and RF pulses follow. This gives an immediate hair removal effect (the same as other epilators) and the potential for longer-term hair removal provided by the IPL/RF energy, although removal of the pigmented hair shaft may reduce the efficacy of the subsequent light energy.

Other Notable Hair Removal Devices

While not FDA-cleared nor available in the US, several other devices are of particular mention:

- *CyDen/Proctor and Gamble (P&G) (Swansea, UK)*: CyDen is a United Kingdom (UK)-based manufacturer of IPL hair removal systems sold under the Cyden, Boots, and now Gillette brand in some ex-US markets. The devices are advertised in the UK for temporary and permanent hair removal on Fitzpatrick skin types I– IV. CyDen was recently acquired by P&G, which presumably indicates the large consumer multinational company was sufficiently convinced of at least minimum levels of safety and efficacy and of a compatible business model. The CyDen technology is characterized by its pulse control which reportedly delivers the flashlamp pulse in longer and more controlled pulses compared to traditional IPLs, which could provide somewhat better skin safety and thereby more energy into the hair follicle.
- *Palomar/Gillette (Burlington, MA and Cincinnati, OH)*: In the OTC hair removal category, Palomar is most notable for its multi-year joint development and royalty agreement with Gillette for a home hair-removal product, although that agreement is now apparently somewhat dissolved. Palomar received the industry's first OTC clearance for a home hair-removal device—a diode laser—in 2006 but as of this writing no product has been commercialized. Gillette, now a P&G company, markets an IPL device based on the CyDen IPL called the Gillette Venus Naked Skin in the UK.
- *Philips Electronics (Amsterdam, The Netherlands)*: The multinational consumer giant markets an IPL device named the Lumea outside the US. This is a well-designed filtered flashlamp device that is battery powered with a modern industrial design. It has a maximum fluence range of 2.0–6.5 J/cm^2 a pulse duration of 2.5–7.0 ms, a spot size of 3 cm^2, a repetition rate of 4.5 seconds, and is marketed as providing temporary hair removal that lasts for months. Especially noteworthy is a well-done study by the Philips researchers that showed that the IPL device was effective at causing confined localized heating in the hair follicle and matrix that induced temporary, but not permanent, hair removal.[77]
- *Radiancy/PhotoMedex (Radnor, PA)*: Radiancy, recently merged with PhotoMedex, and manufactures and markets the No!No! Hair for hair removal. This device is a hot-wire razor in which an electrically heated wire about 1 cm in length that is held just above the skin (about 0.5 mm) by mechanical roller/standoffs and severs the surface hair by burning it as the user glides over the skin. One peer-reviewed publication (independent hair counts but no controls) claims a hair removal effect lasting multiple weeks,[78] but another publication (with independent hair counts and a control) found no differences compared to razor blade shaving.[79]
- *Epila Laser Hair Remover (BNB Medical Company, Ltd, Seoul, Korea)*: This is a low-power diode laser available in some ex-US markets. It has a small spot size (about 1 mm) that with focusing optics can produce high fluence at the skin surface but the zone of high fluence beneath the skin would be small, so efficacy is likely limited.
- *Rio Laser Hair Removal (The Dezac Group, Ltd, Cheltenham, UK)*: This is another low-power diode laser available in some global markets. Similar to the Epila in spot size and total power, some models of the Rio have a scanner to automatically move the laser across the skin, although the low power and small spot size is nevertheless expected to result in limited efficacy.

Acne Treatment

Some examples of consumer acne treatment devices are shown in Figure 14.2.

As shown in Table 14.2, acne is currently the largest category of home devices in terms of number of devices with eight legally available devices in the United States. The devices can be categorized

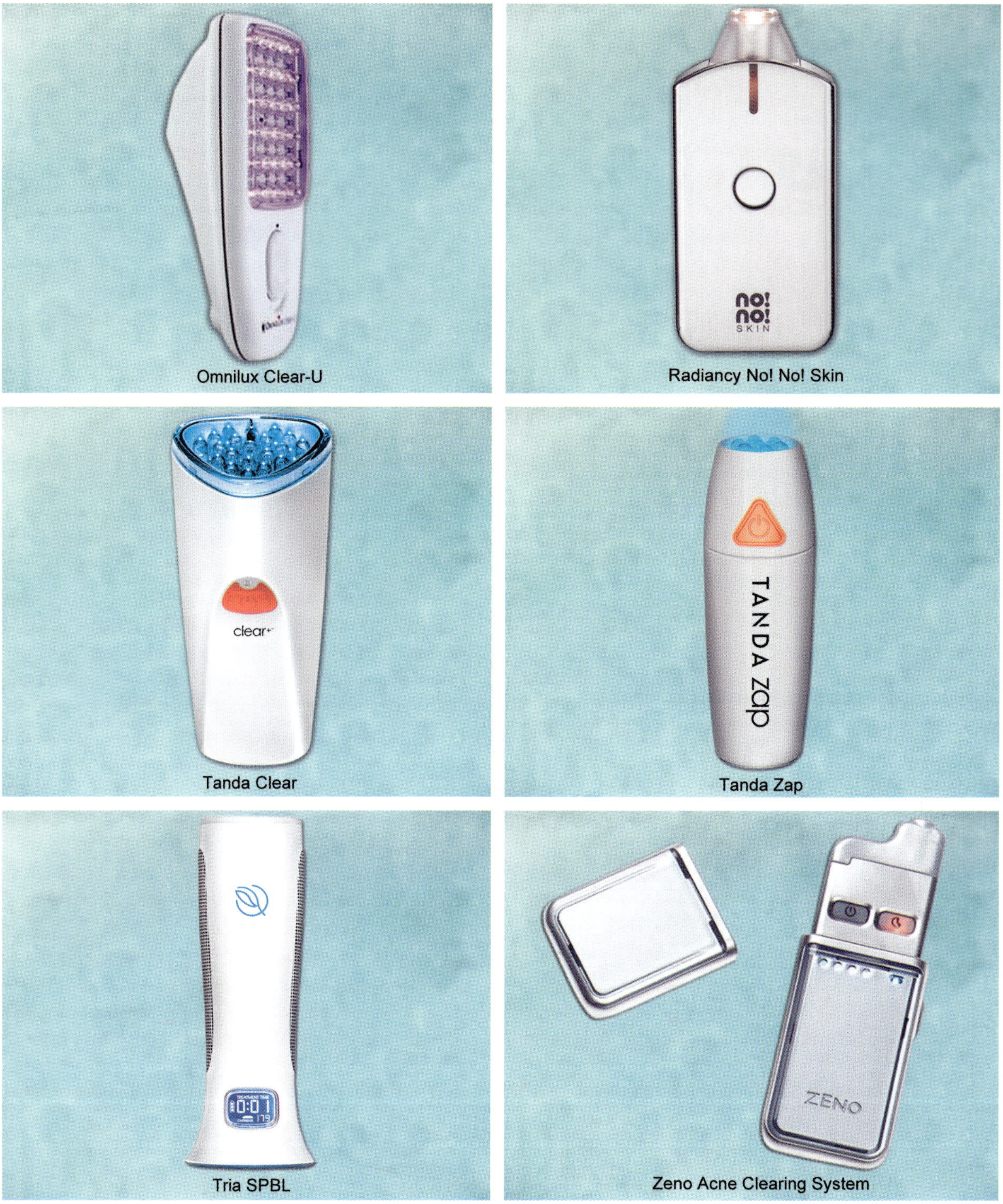

Fig. 14.2: Consumer acne treatment devices cleared by the US FDA (at the time of the writing of this chapter)

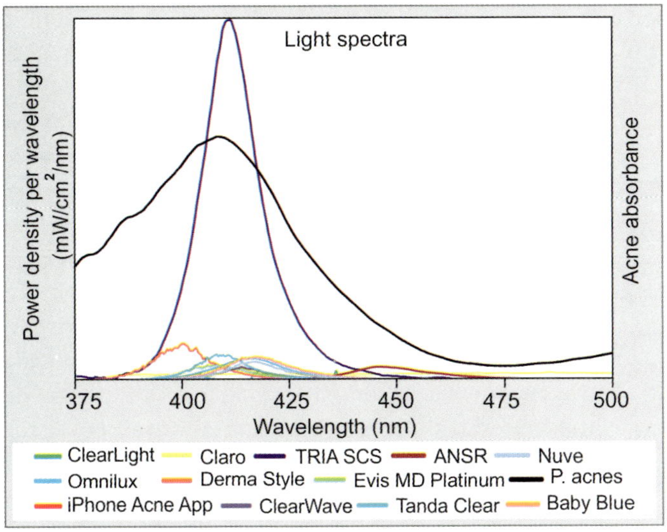

Fig. 14.3: Light intensity as a function of wavelength for consumer acne treatment devices

into two types based on the use mode: those that treat individual lesions (colloquially known as "zit zappers") and those that are area-based (like the full-face panel devices more typical of the office setting). The devices can also be broadly categorized based upon mechanism of action: heat-based devices and light-based devices. Even more so than with hair removal, there are substantial differences in technology, efficacy, and price between these acne devices, with some likely offering minimal efficacy to others that have energy outputs similar (or even surpassing if used daily in a concentrated fashion) in-office devices. As an example, see Figure 14.3 that plots the relative light intensity as a function of wavelength for many of the most common light-based devices on the market along with the action spectrum for *P. acnes*, where the wide-range of outputs can be readily seen.

Individual Lesion Devices

Zeno

The Zeno Acne Clearing Device ($249 at introduction, now with multiple related models ranging from about $20–$200), manufactured by Tyrell/Zeno (Houston, TX), was the pioneer in this type of device, receiving the first FDA clearance in 2005 for a heat-based, single pimple treatment device, indicated for mild-to-moderate inflammatory acne. While there are multiple models now available, they all generally have a small tip (about 3 mm diameter) that is heated electrically by a battery pack. The user is instructed to hold the tip on an inflammatory lesion, press a button to initiate the heating, wait for 1–2 minutes, and repeat 2–4 times per day. It is claimed that the temperature rise inhibits the *P. acnes* bacteria.

Therma Clear

Similar to the Zeno, the ThermaClear Acne Clearing Device (Therative, Inc., San Francisco, CA; $149, not readily available at the time of this writing) has an electrically heated tip that is used to help speed clearance of individual pimples but with a shorter treatment time of several seconds per pulse.

No!No! Skin (PhotoMedex, Radnor, PA)

This device obtained FDA clearance in 2008 with the indication for treating mild-to-moderate inflammatory pimples. It consists of a small tip that is held over the individual lesion from which white light and heat is delivered from a small grain of wheat light bulb. A published clinical study that compares treated and untreated lesions (although the type of lesion differed significantly between the control and active arms) suggests that the time of clearance of the pimples can be mildly improved by using the device as instructed.[80]

Claro

The Claro device (Solta Medical, about $200) is notable in that it is the only IPL device cleared for OTC acne therapy, and, furthermore, for treating individual lesions. Like all IPLs, it produces a short flash of white light (producing heat and light in the tissue) that in this case is directed into an inflamed lesion by holding the light output window at the tip of the device against the lesion.

Large-Area Devices

Most of the home OTC devices are in the category of area-based devices, designed not to treat individual lesions but to treat an area of skin with multiple lesions. These devices are almost exclusively panels of LEDs producing fairly distinct bands of light radiation. Most are in the blue wavelengths targeting Soret-band porphyrin absorption but some include infrared and/or visible wavelengths targeting the Q-band or simple heating that may be beneficial for treating acne.

Clear-U

This LED panel-based device (PhotoMedex, $349) employs infrared (IR) and visible LEDs and is indicated for mild-to-moderate inflammatory acne. The output is about 0.8 W at 40 mW/cm^2 with a 30 cm^2 window that user holds this against their skin in the same location for a 20 min treatment session once per week, giving a light dose of about 30 J/cm^2 per week. Sadick et al. published a study comparing lesions counts to baseline (no untreated control) that showed a reduction in inflammatory lesions by 20%, 38%, 63% and 69% after 2, 4, 8 and 12 weeks of treatment, respectively.[80]

Tanda Clear

The US FDA-cleared Tanda Clear (Syneron, Irvine, CA) employs blue LEDs combined with sonic vibration and gentle warming and has an output of about 0.6 W at 50 mW/cm^2 over a 12-cm^2 window, currently selling for $195. The user is instructed to hold the device in a fixed location for 3 minutes daily twice per day, which results in a light dose of about 125 J/cm^2 per week. Gold et al. found a reduction in lesions compared to baseline (no untreated control) of 22%, 41% and 36% after 1, 4 and 8 weeks of the phototherapy, respectively.[83] Syneron also introduced the US FDA-cleared Tanda Zap—an acne spot treatment device utilizing LEDs, with both a Pink Zap and Blue Zap, at a very low price point of $49.

Tria

Also utilizing blue LEDs, the Tria Skin Perfecting Blue Light (TRIA Beauty, $250) differs in that it uses much higher intensity (400 mW/cm^2) light, and that the user glides the device over the treatment area rather than holding it in a fixed spot. Used according to the instruction manual with 5 minutes daily for each approximately 12 cm^2 area, it delivers a weekly dose of about 200 J/cm^2. Wheeland et al. found a reduction in inflammatory lesions compared to baseline (no untreated control) of 31%, 45% and 60% at 1, 3 and 6 weeks, respectively.[70] The same study also reported benefit when the device is used for the same treatment time across the whole face, although the lesions count reduction was less (about half of the benefit from the concentrated dose) as would be expected since the average delivered fluence was reduced.[70] Wheeland and Dhawan performed a similar study with the Tria blue light device whereby they also employed a complementary daily topical regimen and found that the topicals provided some incremental benefit (about 20%).[71]

Other Panel-Based Devices

Other panel-based devices on the market include Baby Blue (Silver Bay, $250), DPL Nuvi (LED Technologies, $130), Evis MD Platinum (Evis Beauty, $115), ClearWave (Verilux, $130) and Silk'n Blue (Home Skinovations, Ltd) which can all be generally characterized as fixed panel, low output power devices producing about 0.3 W or less of output light.

Skin Rejuvenation

Some examples of consumer skin rejuvenation devices are shown in Figures 14.4A and B.

The most rapidly emerging new group of home devices is for skin rejuvenation, and this category is expected to ultimately dominate the home device field since the majority of existing consumer skin care spending is related to anti-aging treatments. Table 14.3 lists the devices currently cleared. The current market is characterized by two types of devices: fractionated lasers and low level light therapy (LLLT) devices. The fractionated lasers mimic their in-clinic cousins by delivering coagulated micro-thermal zones (MTZs) but do so with more frequent sessions (daily or 2 times per week versus monthly for an in-office device), with lower pulse energy (up to 15 mJ versus up to 70 mJ for in-office devices), and with lower density of laser treatment zones (a few

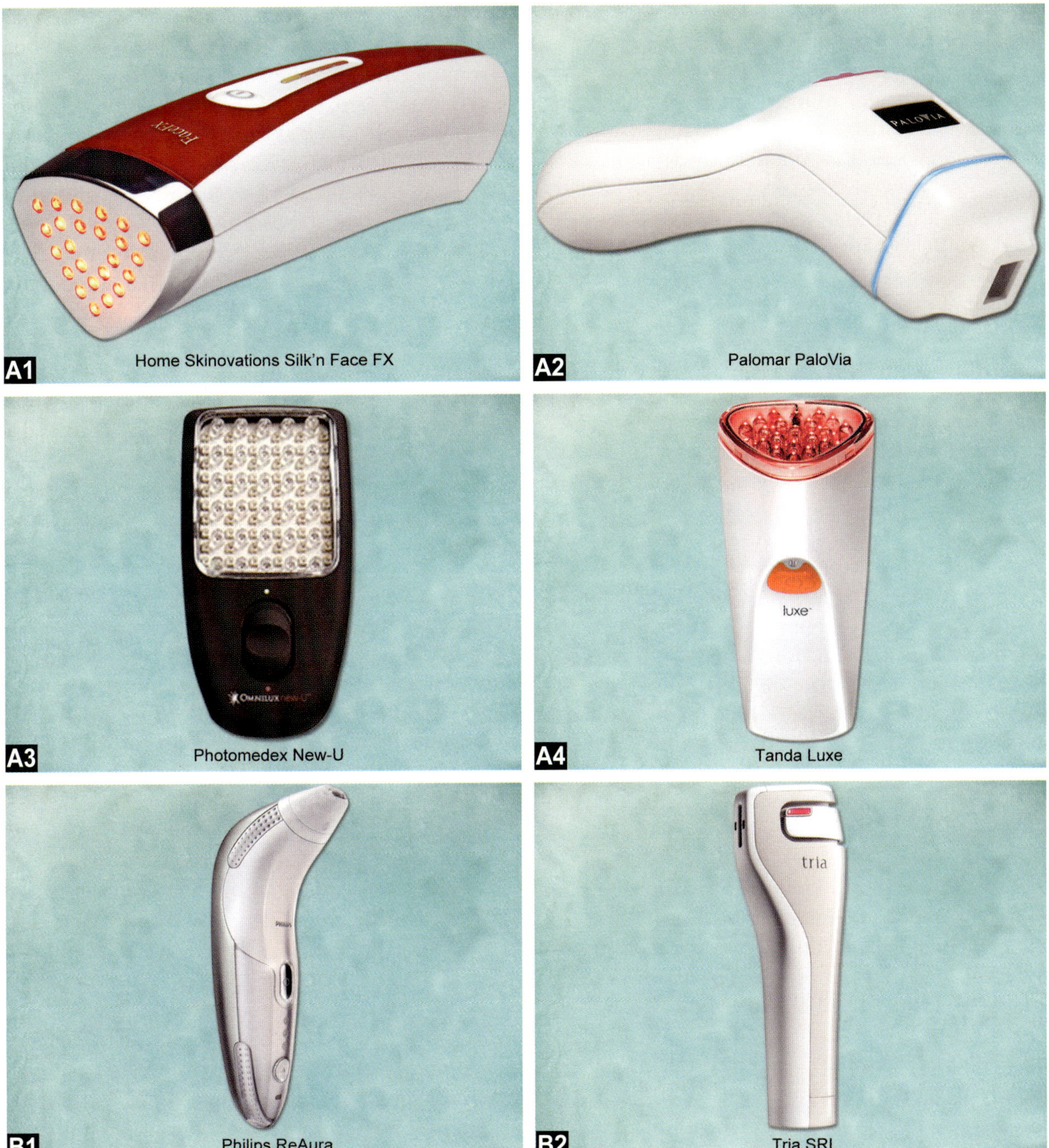

Figs 14.4A and B: (A) Consumer skin rejuvenation devices cleared by the US FDA (at the time of the writing of this chapter); (B) Notable consumer skin rejuvenation devices not cleared by the US FDA (at the time of the writing of this chapter)

percent of the skin area for at-home devices versus 30–50% typically for in-office devices). The LLLT anti-aging devices generally do not have an in-office analog and tend to offer a much lower level of benefit albeit at typically lower cost and low or no side-effects.

Fractionated Lasers

PaloVia

At present, the PaloVia (Palomar Medical Technologies, $500) is currently the only FDA-cleared home fractionated laser on the US market. This device is a 1410-nm diode laser cleared for periorbital wrinkle reduction in 2009 and is currently sold in retail stores, by television retail, e-commerce, and through physicians' offices. It is a stamping type of device where the user holds the output window (about 1 cm^2) against the skin and internally a fiber optic is rasterized in an x-y fashion to deliver a pattern of microscopic thermal injury zones to the skin. The user moves the device to the adjacent skin and repeats the process 10–15 times for each periorbital region. The wavelength is 1410 nm for water absorption with a maximum pulse energy of 15 mJ that nonablatively coagulates tissue in a zone about 200–250 microns deep by 300–350 microns wide with a treatment zone density of about 36–72 treatment zones/cm^2. Leyden et al. performed a user study of about 136 subjects, 36 of whom were enrolled in a pilot study and 100 were enrolled in the pivotal study.[83] For subjects enrolled in the pilot study, 80% demonstrated improvement following 4 weeks of daily treatments, while 60% demonstrated improvement after the maintenance treatment period and this benefit persisted for 3 months following the end of the maintenance period, decreasing to 40% of subjects after 4 months of no treatment.[83] Subjects in the pivotal study used the device daily for 4 weeks and then twice a week in maintenance mode for 12 weeks. Blinded observations compared to baseline (no untreated control was used) were made by a panel of graders who found 90% of subjects had at least a one point improvement in Fitzpatrick Wrinkle Scale and 76% had similar improvement after the maintenance phase.[83] Side-effects were essentially mild versions of in-office fractionated treatments, including erythema and mild discomfort.

Other Notable Fractionated Lasers

Philips, in a development program with Solta Medical (Hayward, CA) which manufactures the pioneering Fraxel line of in-office fractionated lasers, is offering the ReAura ($1300) home fractional device in Europe. The ReAura device uses a gliding mode of operation, similar to the in-office Fraxel Dual (Solta Medical, Hayward, CA), and thus has the ability to treat large areas (whole face, hands, décolletage) in a single session. In use, the consumer moves the device slowly across the skin and pulses are automatically scanned across a 1 cm aperture to deliver the two-dimensional array of microthermal zones. As per the instruction manual, users should treat themselves two times per week for 8–12 weeks. Full-face treatments take about 25 minutes with the ReAura.

Tria Beauty also has developed a fractionated laser for home use, known as the Tria Skin Rejuvenating Laser (SRL), available for sale outside the US (available in Canada and the European Union; $499). Like the Philips device, the Tria SRL is a gliding large-area device that the users move across their skin to deliver the fractionated treatment but with a treatment speed about twice as fast as ReAura, resulting in treatment times of about 4 minutes per day for facial treatments. Its instruction manual suggests daily use for 8 weeks followed by a rest period of 4 weeks. The device has generally similar output parameters as the ReAura and PaloVia (e.g. 1425 nm, 12 mJ/ pulse) so one would expect generally similar results.

Nonfractionated Lasers

The anti-aging field is more crowded when it comes to nonfractionated home skin care devices with no fewer than five cleared devices (see Table 14.3). These devices offer comparatively low output levels distributed (essentially) uniformly on the skin (i.e. not in a fractionated manner) and generally employ LEDs as the light source. Representative devices are:

- *Tanda Luxe (Syneron, $195)*: The US FDA-cleared Luxe is similar to the Tanda acne device except with a red light LED panel rather than blue light, and is now combined with a light sonic vibration and gentle warming features. The device is cleared for periorbital wrinkle treatment. The red light is claimed to boost cellular energy to increase collagen, elastin and microcirculation.
- *OmniLux New-U (PhotoMedex, $300)*: It uses infrared LEDs in a home-use panel version similar in some output parameters to the company's prescription panel LED system. In a published study, Sadick reported that subjects noted improvement of fine lines and wrinkles.[82]
- *LightStim for Wrinkles (LightStim, $249)*: The LightStim uses a panel of infrared and red LEDs and is FDA-cleared for facial wrinkles.
- *Silk'n Face FX (Home Skinovations, $300)*: Another small panel of red LEDs emitting at 645 nm, this device is FDA-cleared for treating periorbital wrinkles. Consumers are instructed to use it for 20 minutes three times per week.

OTHER APPLICATIONS (FIG. 14.5)

While hair removal, acne, and anti-aging currently dominate the home energy-based device market, there are important other applications with cleared and shipping products, and the potential for strong growth, particularly: hair growth stimulation, fat treatment, and psoriasis phototherapy, among others.

A standout in the hair growth field is the Hair Max Laser Comb (Lexington International, $300) which received FDA clearance in 2007. A randomized, double blinded, controlled clinical study showed the low-level laser device can moderately increase hair growth.[85] More devices in this category are expected (based on increasing office-based clearances for hair growth devices) and, like the other LLLT devices, more expansion is expected as the fundamental mechanisms of action are better understood and can be optimized.

Although there are currently no FDA-cleared OTC devices for fat removal, the FDA has cleared for prescription use a low-level light phototherapy system (Zerona, Erchonia, Inc.) and a noninvasive cold therapy technique (CoolSculpting, Zeltiq) that are indicative of the kinds of technologies that can reasonably be envisioned to be adapted to home use. Therefore, the authors expect fat removal home devices in the not too distant future, although they caution that skepticism remains high for the LLLT systems based on limited quality research and experience.

Levia (Lerner Medical Devices, cost unknown) is an at-home psoriasis treatment that employs UVB phototherapy and is now available through physician-directed use (i.e. users must obtain a prescription but can use the device at home). It consists of a console and a handpiece about the size of a hair dryer that has a 3 cm^2 output window from which UVB is emitted. The use mode is stamping. A fiber-optic comb can be attached for treating the scalp. This home device is intended for individuals with chronic, small area psoriasis and can provide a convenient, cost-effective solution compared to the multiple office visits typically required for UVB

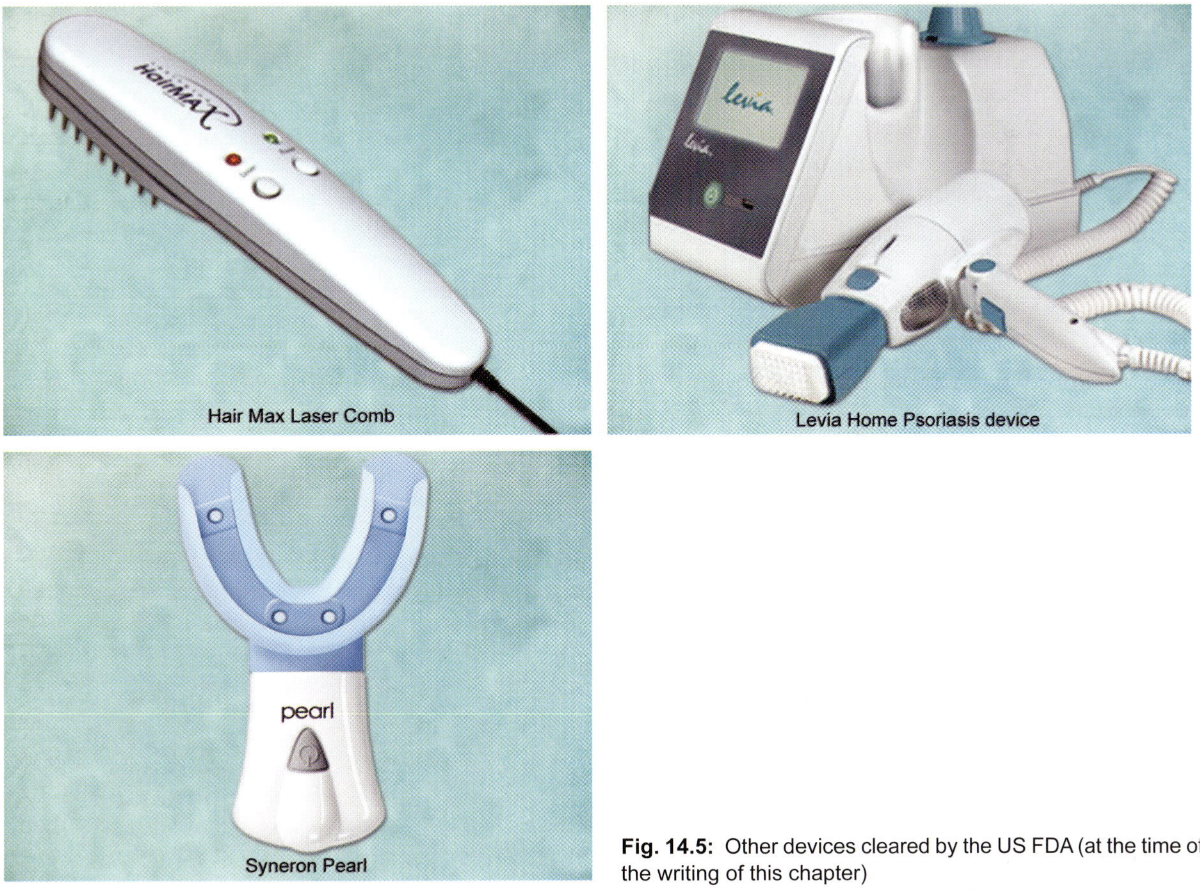

Fig. 14.5: Other devices cleared by the US FDA (at the time of the writing of this chapter)

phototherapy. It is an example of where a home device has the potential to significantly grow a medical therapy like UVB administration because of greater convenience and lower cost.

Syneron has introduced a consumer teeth whitening system that uses ionic technology to activate a topical whitening gel. The electric current activates a hydrogen peroxide whitening gel to whiten teeth in the home setting. The device is used five times a day for 5 days and currently retails for $195.

THE FUTURE

The market for home-use energy-based devices has been growing steadily over the last decade and the authors expect that trend to continue, and indeed, to likely accelerate. This is being driven by: (a) improved technology—particularly lower cost energy sources such as high-power LEDs and laser diodes and "smart" sensors which allow safer use in the home environment, (b) greater sophistication and understanding by manufacturers in adapting physician devices to home use—successful OTC devices are not just watered-down office-based devices, (c) a wider range of indications, applications and techniques emerging from the professional space, and (d) unabated strong global market forces. Perhaps the best evidence of the likelihood of growth is the emergence of large, multinational consumer companies (in addition to the start-ups and medical laser companies from the last decade) developing, partnering, and marketing these devices, including Philips in hair removal and fractionated anti-aging home devices, Proctor & Gamble in hair removal, as well as programs for development of home devices by L'Oreal, Unilever, and Johnson & Johnson. As with any developing market (and many developed markets, for that matter), the authors expect that there will continue to be a wide range of quality among these devices—from those that offer minimal (or no) benefit to those that offer levels of benefits that are comparable to, or even in some applications superior to, physician-administered treatments. In this chapter, the aim was to provide the reader a scientifically-based perspective based on output specifications and clinical data of a range of devices that can be used to help appropriately inform his/her patients about these devices and help appropriately understand this burgeoning field.

REFERENCES

1. Skin Deep: Taking Home the Lasers, Pulsers and Sonic Care; October 5, 2011. Available from: http://www.nytimes.com/2011/10/06/fashion/assessing-those-laser-pulsing-light-and-sonic-skin-care-products-for-home-use.html?_r=0
2. Metelitsa AL, Green JB. Home-use laser and light devices for the skin: an update. Semin Cutan Med Surg. 2011;30:144-7.
3. Cosmetics market research summary. Available from: http://www.aginskyconsulting.com/downloads/ACG%20Industry%20Summary%20Reports%20-%20Q4-07/ACG%20Russian%20Cosmetics%20Market%20Overview.pdf
4. Gan SD, Graber EM, Laser Hair Removal. A Review Dermatol Surg. 2013;39:823-38.
5. Anderson RR, Parrish JA. Microvasculature can be selectively damaged using dye lasers: a basic theory and experimental evidence in human skin. Lasers Surg Med. 1981;1(3):263-76.
6. Parrish JA, Anderson RR, Harrist T, et al. Selective thermal effects with pulsed irradiation from lasers: from organ to organelle. J Invest Dermatol. 1983;80 Suppl:75s-80s.
7. Anderson RR, Jaenicke KF, Parrish JA. Mechanisms of selective vascular changes caused by dye lasers. Lasers Surg Med. 1983;3(3):211-5.
8. Bernstein EF, Kornbluth S, Brown DB, et al. Treatment of spider veins using a 10 millisecond pulse-duration frequency-doubled neodymium YAG laser. Dermatol Surg. 1999;25(4):316-20.
9. Adrian RM. Treatment of leg telangiectasias using a long-pulse frequency-doubled neodymium:YAG laser at 532 nm. Dermatol Surg. 1998;24(1):19-23.
10. Tan OT, Kerschmann R, Parrish JA. The effect of epidermal pigmentation on selective vascular effects of pulsed laser. Lasers Surg Med. 1984;4(4):365-74.
11. Garden JM, Tan OT, Parrish JA. The pulsed dye laser: its use at 577 nm wavelength. J Dermatol Surg Oncol. 1987;13(2):134-8.
12. Alster TS, Wilson F. Treatment of port-wine stains with the flashlamp-pumped pulsed dye laser: extended clinical experience in children and adults. Ann Plast Surg. 1994;32(5):478-84.
13. Tan OT, Hurwitz RM, Stafford TJ. Pulsed dye laser treatment of recalcitrant verrucae: a preliminary report. Lasers Surg Med. 1993;13(1):127-37.
14. McDaniel DH, Ash K, Zukowski M. Treatment of stretch marks with the 585-nm flashlamp-pumped pulsed dye laser. Dermatol Surg. 1996;22(4):332-7.
15. Zelickson BD, Mehregan DA, Wendelschfer-Crabb G, et al. Clinical and histologic evaluation of psoriatic plaques treated with a flashlamp pulsed dye laser [see comments]. J Am Acad Dermatol. 1996;35(1):64-8.

16. Zelickson BD, Kilmer SL, Bernstein E, et al. Pulsed dye laser therapy for sun damaged skin. Lasers Surg Med. 1999;25(3):229-36.
17. Bernstein EF, Lee J, Lowery J, et al. Treatment of spider veins with the 595 nm pulsed-dye laser [see comments]. J Am Acad Dermatol. 1998;39(5 Pt 1):746-50.
18. Bernstein EF, Kligman A. Rosacea treatment using the new-generation, high-energy, 595 nm, long pulse-duration pulsed-dye laser. Lasers Surg Med. 2008;40:233-9.
19. Alster TS. Improvement of erythematous and hypertrophic scars by the 585-nm flashlamp-pumped pulsed dye laser. Ann Plast Surg. 1994;32(2):186-90.
20. Grossman MC. What's new in cutaneous laser research. Dermatol Clin. 1997;15:1-8.
21. Campos VB, Dierickx CC, Farinelli WA, et al. Hair removal with an 800-nm pulsed diode laser. J Am Acad Dermatol. 2000;43:442-7.
22. Lou WW, Quintana AT, Geronemus RG, et al. Prospective study of hair reduction by diode laser (800 nm) with long-term follow-up. Dermatol Surg. 2000;26:428-32.
23. Grossman MC, Dierickx CC, Farinelli W, et al. Damage to hair follicles by normal mode Ruby lasers. J Am Acad Dermatol. 1996;35:889-94.
24. Dierickx CC, Grossman MC, Farinelli WA, et al. Permanent hair removal by normal-mode ruby laser. Arch Dermatol. 1998;134:837-42.
25. Görgü M, Aslan G, Aköz T, et al. Comparison of Alexandrite laser and electrolysis for hair removal. Dermatol Surg. 2000;26:37-41.
26. Bouzari N, Tabatabai H, Abbasi Z, et al. Laser hair removal: comparison of long-pulsed Nd:YAG, long-pulsed Alexandrite, and long-pulsed diode lasers. Dermatol Surg. 2004;30(4 Pt 1):498-502.
27. Handrick C, Alster TS. Comparison of long-pulsed diode and long-pulsed Alexandrite lasers for hair removal: a long-term clinical and histologic study. Dermatol Surg. 2001;27:622-6.
28. Bernstein EF. Hair growth induced by diode laser treatment. Dermatol Surg. 2005;31:584-6.
29. Taylor CR, Gange RW, Dover JS, et al. Treatment of tattoos by Q-switched ruby laser: a dose-response study. Arch Dermatol. 1990;126:893-9.
30. Scheibner A, Kenny G, White W, et al. A superior method of tattoo removal using the Q-switched ruby laser. J Dermatol Surg Oncol. 1990;16:1091-8.
31. Ashinoff R, Geronemus RG. Rapid response of traumatic and medical tattoos to treatment with the Q-switched ruby laser. Plast Reconstr Surg. 1993;91:841-5.
32. Kilmer SL, Anderson RR. Clinical use of the Q-switched ruby and the Q-switched Nd:YAG (1064 nm and 532 nm) lasers for treatment of tattoos. J Dermatol Surg Oncol. 1993;19:330-8.
33. Kilmer SL, Lee MS, Grevelink JM, et al. The Q-switched Nd:YAG laser effectively treats tattoos: a controlled, dose-response study. Arch Dermatol. 1993;129:971-8.
34. Jones A, Roddey P, Orengo I, et al. The Q-switched Nd:YAG laser effectively treats tattoos in darkly pigmented skin. Dermatol Surg. 1996;22:999-1001.
35. Fitzpatrick RE, Goldman MP. Tattoo removal using the alexandrite laser. Arch Dermatol. 1994;130:1508-14.
36. Alster TS. Q-switched alexandrite laser treatment (755 nm) of professional and amateur tattoos. J Am Acad Dermatol. 1995;33:69-73.
37. Leuenberger ML, Mulas MW, Hata TR, et al. Comparison of the Q-switched alexandrite, Nd:YAG, and ruby lasers in treating blue-black tattoos. Dermatol Surg. 1999;25:10-4.
38. Zelickson BD, Mehregan DA, Zarrin AA, et al. Clinical, histologic, and ultrastructural evaluation of tattoos treated with three laser systems. Lasers Surg Med. 1994;15:364-72.
39. Hellwig S, Schönermark M, Raulin C. Treatment of vascular malformations and pigment disorders of the face and neck by pulsed dye laser, Photoderm VL and Q-switched ruby laser. Laryngorhinootologie. 1995;74(10):635-41.
40. Fitzpatrick RE, Goldman MP. Advances in carbon dioxide laser surgery. Clin Dermatol. 1995;13:87-95.
41. Ross EV, Grossman MC, Duke D, et al. Long-term results after CO2 laser skin resurfacing: a comparison of scanned and pulsed systems. J Am Acad Dermatol. 1997;37:709-18.
42. Thomsen S. Pathologic analysis of photothermal and photomechanical effects of laser-tissue interactions. Photochem Photobiol. 1991;53:825-35.
43. Kirsch KM, Zelickson BD, Zachary CB, et al. Ultrastructure of collagen thermally denatured by microsecond domain pulsed carbon dioxide laser. Arch Dermatol. 1998;134:1255-9.
44. Ellis DL, Weisberg NK, Chen JS, et al. Free electron laser infrared wavelength specificity for cutaneous contraction. Lasers Surg Med. 1999;25:1-7.
45. Kauvar A, Waldorf H, Geronemus R. A histopathological comparison of "Char-free" carbon dioxide lasers. Dermatol Surg. 1996;22:343-8.
46. Bass LS. Erbium: YAG laser skin resurfacing: preliminary clinical evaluation. Ann Plast Surg. 1998;40:328-34.
47. Adrian RM. The erbium: YAG laser: facts and fiction. Dermatol Surg. 1998;24:296.
48. Goldman MP, Manuskiatti W. Combined laser resurfacing with the 950-microsec pulsed CO_2 + Er: YAG lasers. Dermatol Surg. 1999;25:160-3.
49. Collawn SS. Combination therapy: utilization of CO_2 and Erbium: YAG lasers for skin resurfacing. Ann Plast Surg. 1999;42:21-6.

50. Leclère FM, Magalon G, Philandrianos C, et al. Prospective ex-vivo study on thermal effects in human skin phototypes II, IV and VI: a comparison between the 808, 1064, 1210 and 1320-nm diode laser. J Cosmet Laser Ther. 2012;14:7-13.
51. Bernstein EF. A multiplexed 1,440 and 1,320 nm laser for treatment of chronic photodamage. J Drugs Dermatol. 2011;10:1266-70.
52. Bernstein EF. Double-pass, low-fluence laser treatment using a large spot-size 1,450 nm laser improves acne. Lasers Surg Med. 2009;41:116-21.
53. Bernstein EF. A pilot investigation comparing low-energy, double pass 1,450 nm laser treatment of acne to conventional single-pass, high-energy treatment. Lasers Surg Med. 2007;39:193-8.
54. Latowsky BC, Abbasi N, Dover JS, et al. A randomized, controlled trial of four ablative fractionated lasers for photoaging: a quadrant study. Dermatol Surg. 2012;38:1477-89.
55. Uebelhoer NS, Ross EV, Shumaker PR. Ablative fractional resurfacing for the treatment of traumatic scars and contractures. Semin Cutan Med Surg. 2012;31:110-20.
56. Hunzeker CM, Weiss ET, Geronemus RG. Fractionated CO_2 laser resurfacing: our experience with more than 2000 treatments. Aesthet Surg J. 2009;29: 317-22.
57. Weiss ET, Brauer JA, Anolik R, et al. 1927-nm fractional resurfacing of facial actinic keratoses: a promising new therapeutic option. J Am Acad Dermatol. 2013;68:98-102.
58. Moody MN, Landau JM, Goldberg LH, et al. 450-nm diode laser in combination with the 1550-nm fractionated erbium-doped fiber laser for the treatment of steatocystoma multiplex: a case report. Dermatol Surg. 2012;38:1104-6.
59. Chiu RJ, Kridel RW. Fractionated photothermolysis: the Fraxel 1550-nm glass fiber laser treatment. Facial Plast Surg Clin North Am. 2007;15:229-37.
60. Yeung CK, Chan NP, Shek SY, et al. Evaluation of combined fractional radiofrequency and fractional laser treatment for acne scars in Asians. Lasers Surg Med. 2012;44(8):622-30.
61. Taub AF, Garretson CB. Treatment of acne scars of skin types II to V by sublative fractional bipolar radiofrequency and bipolar radiofrequency combined with diode laser. J Clin Aesthet Dermatol. 2011;4(10):18-27.
62. Hong HC, Lupin M, O'Shaughnessy KF. Clinical evaluation of a microwave device for treating axillary hyperhidrosis. Dermatol Surg. 2012;38(5):728-35.
63. Johnson JE, O'Shaughnessy KF, Kim S. Microwave thermolysis of sweat glands. Lasers Surg Med. 2012;44(1):20-5.
64. Jewell ML, Solish NJ, Desilets CS. Noninvasive body sculpting technologies with an emphasis on high-intensity focused ultrasound. Aesthetic Plast Surg. 2011;35(5):901-12.
65. Avram MM, Harry RS. Cryolipolysis for subcutaneous fat layer reduction. Lasers Surg Med. 2009; 41(10):703-8.
66. Ammad S, Gonzales M, Edwards C, et al. An assessment of the efficacy of blue light phototherapy in the treatment of acne vulgaris. J Cosmet Dermatol. 2008;7(3):180-8.
67. Tremblay JF, Sire DJ, Lowe NJ, et al. Light-emitting diode 415 nm in the treatment of inflammatory acne: an open-label, multicentric, pilot investigation. J Cosmet Laser Ther. 2006 ;8(1):31-3.
68. Wheeland RG. Permanent hair reduction with a home-use diode laser: safety and effectiveness 1 year after eight treatments. Lasers Surg Med. 2012;44(7):550-7.
69. Wheeland RG. Simulated consumer use of a battery-powered, hand-held, portable diode laser (810 nm) for hair removal: a safety, efficacy and ease-of-use study. Lasers Surg Med. 2007;39(6):476-93.
70. Wheeland RG, Koreck A. Safety and effectiveness of a new blue light device for the self-treatment of mild-to-moderate acne. J Clin Aesthet Dermatol. 2012;5(5):25-31.
71. Wheeland RG, Dhawan S. Evaluation of self-treatment of mild-to-moderate facial acne with a blue light treatment system. J Drugs Dermatol. 2011;10(6):596-602.
72. Mulholland RS. Silk'n—a novel device using Home Pulsed Light for hair removal at home. J Cosmet Laser Ther. 2009;11(2):106-9.
73. Haedersdal M, Beerwerth F, Nash JF. Laser and intense pulsed light hair removal technologies: from professional to home use.Br J Dermatol. 2011;165 (Suppl 3):31-6.
74. Emerson R, Town G. Hair removal with a novel, low fluence, home-use intense pulsed light device. J Cosmet Laser Ther. 2009;11(2):98-105.
75. Town GA, Ash C, Eadie E, et al. Measuring key parameters of intense pulsed light (IPL) devices. J Cosmet Laser Ther. 2007;9(3):148-60.
76. Ash C, Town G, Bjerring P. Relevance of the structure of time-resolved spectral output to light-tissue interaction using intense pulsed light (IPL). Lasers Surg Med. 2008;40:83-92.
77. Roosen GF, Westgate GE, Philpott M, et al. Temporary hair removal by low fluence photoepilation: histological study on biopsies and cultured human hair follicles. Lasers Surg Med. 2008;40(8):520-8. doi: 10.1002/lsm.20679.
78. Spencer JM. Clinical evaluation of a handheld self-treatment device for hair removal. J Drugs Dermatol. 2007;6(8):788-92.
79. Biesman BS. Evaluation of a hot wise hair removal device compared to razor shaving. Lasers Surg Med. 2013;45:283-95.

80. Sadick NS. Handheld LED array device in the treatment of acne vulgaris. J Drugs Dermatol. 2008;7(4):347-50.
81. Gold MH, Sensing W, Biron JA. Clinical efficacy of home-use blue-light therapy for mild-to-moderate acne. J Cosmet Laser Ther. 2011;13(6):308-14.
82. Sadick NS, Laver Z, Laver L. Treatment of mild-to-moderate acne vulgaris using a combined light and heat energy device: home-use clinical study. J Cosmet Laser Ther. 2010 ;12(6):276-83.
83. Leyden J, Stephens TJ, Herndon JH. Multicenter clinical trial of a home-use nonablative fractional laser device for wrinkle reduction. J Am Acad Dermatol. 2012;67(5):975-84.
84. Sadick NS. A study to determine the efficacy of a novel handheld light-emitting diode device in the treatment of photoaged skin. J Cosmet Dermatol. 2008;7(4):263-7.
85. Leavitt M, Charles G, Heyman E, et al. HairMax LaserComb laser phototherapy device in the treatment of male androgenetic alopecia: a randomized, double-blind, sham device-controlled, multicenter trial. Clin Drug Investig. 2009;29(5):283-92.

Index

Page number followed by *f* and *t* indicates figure and table respectively.

O

P

Q

R